THE SULTAN'S SEX POTIONS

The Sultan's Sex Potions

Arab Aphrodisiacs in the Middle Ages

Naṣīr al-Dīn al-Ṭūsī

A Critical Edition, Translated and Introduced by

Daniel L. Newman

SAQI

Published 2014 by Saqi Books

ISBN 9780863567476
eISBN 9780863567520

First published 2014 in Great Britain by

SAQI
26 Westbourne Grove
London W2 5RH
www.saqibooks.co.uk

A full CIP record for this book is available from the British Library.

Printed and bound by TJ International

Contents

Preface 7
Note on Transliteration 10
Symbols and Abbreviations 12

INTRODUCTION

Chapter 1: Arabic Erotic Literature 15
- The Genre: History and Typology 20
- Sources 27
- Features 36
- When East Meets West 49

Chapter 2: The Author 57

Chapter 3: The Sultan's Potions 63
- Contents and Structure 63
- The Manuscripts 68

TRANSLATION

The Book of Sexual Stimulants and the Sultan's Potions 85

Appendix: List of Erotological Works 163
Bibliography 183
Index of Proper Names 199
Index of Arabic Terms 202
Index of English Terms 205

Arabic Text [Arabic pagination 3]
Arabic Index of Proper Names [Arabic pagination 69]
Arabic Index of Terms [Arabic pagination 70]

Preface

When the Emirati-born family guidance counsellor Widād Lūtā published her book, *Sirrī li 'l-ghāya, muᶜāshara al-zawjiyya: uṣūl wa ādāb* (usually translated as 'Top Secret: Sexual Guidance for Married Couples'), in 2009, it caused quite a furore in the traditional Gulf state. In the same period, there was a similar vehement reaction to the publication of other works deemed contrary to present-day mores, whether it be those offering an unorthodox interpretation of sexuality within Islam, such as *Ḥayra Muslima* ('A Muslim Woman's Confusion', 2009) by the Tunisian feminist Ulfa Yūsuf, or Muṣṭafā Fatḥī's novel *Balad al-Wilād* ('The Boys' Country', 2009), which chronicles homosexuality in contemporary Egyptian society.

In today's globally wired age, of course, it is not just the printed word that must be considered, with satellite television and the Internet being much more pervasive, prominent and powerful media. In addition to the proliferation of private (usually foreign) sex channels, the past decade has also seen the appearance of programmes dealing with sexual health and relationships on mainstream Arab media, as well as on web forums and, of course, blogs. The response by Arab society in general to all of these has been one of severe censure, often including accusations of unreligiousness and transgression against local culture.

While, to the casual observer, this response may not be surprising within a modern context, it is less so when seen in its broader historical context. Arabic literature has a long and extremely rich tradition in sexology, with the first examples emerging as early as the ninth century. On the whole, contemporary Arabic-speaking readers are as unfamiliar with this aspect of their heritage as Western audiences are.

This book presents a critical edition, translation and study of one such text from the past – the thirteenth century, to be precise – which deals with a core subject within the genre, aphrodisiacs, and provides a unique insight into the role of sexuality in the Islamic world in the Middle Ages. Its author, a famous Persian scholar, wrote not in his native Persian (Farsi), but in the scholarly lingua franca of his age, Arabic.

The Introduction will provide a brief overview of Arabic erotological literature and attempt to highlight some of its salient topics and authors, as well as the context of its creation.

It is something of a contradiction that a preface usually represents not the start of the book, but rather its end, as it is usually written when the creative work has been completed. This preface is no exception to this rule. At the same time, it is also an opportunity to acknowledge assistance that has been provided by others that has facilitated the task – which always proves to be more arduous than was initially imagined, or indeed bargained for.

First and foremost, I should like to thank Ms Whitney Stanton for the unstinting support – both editorial and otherwise – that she has given me in the course of the making of the book.

Secondly, a particular word of thanks is due to the staff of the libraries in Paris (Bibliothèque nationale), Tunis (Dār al-Kutub al-Waṭaniyya), Berlin (Staatsbibliothek), Glasgow (University of Glasgow), Cairo (Dār al-Kutub wa 'l-Wathā'iq al-Qawmiyya) and Alexandria (Bibliotheca Alexandrina). In Alexandria, my gratitude goes especially to Dr Ahmed Mansour, who generously provided me with some key resources.

The book constitutes the start of a project that will result in the translation of a number of other medieval Arabic erotic works, and so the manuscripts that have been my companions for such a long time will remain so for the foreseeable future.

Note on Transliteration

The style of transcription of Arabic words in this book is that of the *Encyclopaedia of Islam* (2nd edn), with the following deviations: kh = kh; dj = j; sh = sh; ḳ = q. The transcription does not reflect the regressive assimilation (*idghām*) of the lateral in the definite article 'al' with the so-called 'sun letters' (t, th, d, r, z, s, sh, ṭ, ẓ, ṣ, ḍ, n): for example *al-Shām* (and not *ash-Shām*). In line with common usage, *hamza* is not transcribed in word-initial positions, whereas the so-called 'nunation' (*tanwīn*) – regular indefinite inflectional noun endings – is dropped throughout (except in some cases for the accusative singular *-an*), as are the anaptyctic vowels of catenated speech. Place names appear in their common historical English forms – for example Cairo (instead of al-Qāhira) – or in transliteration, usually followed by an English equivalent in brackets, when it involves little-known towns or areas for which no established English form is available, such as 'Alamūt'. Arabic technical terms are transliterated and italicized, except for words that have gained currency in English, such as 'Islam', 'Muslim', 'hadith' or 'imam'. The plurals of isolated Arabic words appear in the singular with the English regular plural *-s* marker – *dirhams* instead of *darāhim*.

As regards dates, only the Gregorian ones are given, with the dates of the Muslim (lunar) Hijra calendar (which starts in 622

AD, the year in which the Prophet Muḥammad emigrated from Mekka to Medina) added in the event of overlaps or ambiguity, in which case the Hijra calendar year comes first – for example 1236/1820–21.

Symbols and Abbreviations

[A]	Berlin manuscript
[B]	Glasgow manuscript
BN	Bibliothèque nationale (Paris)
[C]	Cairo manuscript
CA	Classical Arabic
EI^{1}	*Encyclopaedia of Islam* (1st edn)
EI^{2}	*Encyclopaedia of Islam* (2nd edn)
GAL	C. Brockelmann 1937–46
GALS	C. Brockelmann 1937–46, Supplement
GAS	F. Sezgin 1967–84
Gr.	Greek
Lat.	Latin
pl.	plural
sg.	singular

(ب)	Berlin Mss
(ق)	Cairo Mss
(غ)	Glasgow Mss

<	derived from
{ }	text in margin of Mss
+	addition
-	omission
?	doubtful reading

INTRODUCTION

CHAPTER ONE

Arabic Erotic Literature

In spite of the recently increased attention attracted by gender and sexuality in modern Islamic societies, the history of the discourse of sexuality and eroticism in the Arab-Muslim tradition remains to be written. This is all the more surprising in view of the unparalleled richness of erotological and erotic literature.

Until the 1960s, interest in the subject was driven by the prurient appetites of a segment of the Victorian readership for whom the reputedly sexually permissive East proved an irresistible attraction. The leading exponent in this movement was, of course, Richard Burton, who was only too willing not only to pander to, but also to invigorate this myth – particularly through his translations of *The Arabian Nights* (1885–88) and *The Perfumed Garden* (1886). The latter was a rather free rendition of a sixteenth-century erotic manual written by the Tunisian scholar al-Nafzāwī, entitled *al-Rawḍ al-ʿāṭir fī nuzhat al-khāṭir* ('The Perfumed Garden of Sensual Delight').

Burton's translation is weighed down by Oriental(ist) views – or, rather, prejudices – about Arab-Muslim sexuality, couched in a pseudo-scholarly purple prose, complete with mock critical apparatus offering the author's salacious comments on the arcana and idiosyncrasies of 'Muhammedan' sexual practices (particularly homosexuality), often invoking divine endorsement by proxy.

This resulted in a translation that inflates the thin source text to several hundred pages. For instance, Chapter 5 ('On Intercourse') is one of the shortest – a mere seven lines in the Arabic printed edition – but takes up three pages in Burton's text. The following is a brief example of the translation strategy. The chapter ends as follows in Arabic:

> *fa idhā qaḍayta ḥājataka fa-lā taqūmu ᶜanhā qiyāman tatarāmā fīhi al-ᶜajala wa la-yakun dhālika ᶜalā yamīnika yarfaq*[1]

This is rendered by the most recent translator as: 'When you have satisfied your desire, do not be in a hurry to rise from her but do so gently, on your right hand side.'[2]

Burton's rendition is, to put it mildly, somewhat 'expansive':

> And after the enjoyment is over, and your amorous struggle has come to an end, be careful not to get up at once, but withdraw your member cautiously. Remain close to the woman, and lie down on the right side of the bed that witnessed your enjoyment. You will find this pleasant, and you will not be like a fellow who mounts the woman after the fashion of a mule, without any regard to refinement, and who, after the emission, hastens to get his member out and to rise. Avoid such manners, for they rob the woman of all her lasting delight.

> In short, the true lover of coition will not fail to observe all that I have recommended; for, from the observance of my recommendations will result the pleasure of the woman, and these rules comprise everything essential in that respect.
>
> God has made everything for the best![3]

Burton's translation was based on the earliest French published version (1886), authored by the mysterious 'Baron R***', rather than on the Arabic text.[4] It was, however, entirely in keeping with Burton's own modus operandi in his rendition of *Alf Layla wa Layla* (revealingly titled *The Arabian Nights' Entertainments*) – this time from the Arabic original – in which the translator is highly 'visible', to use a popular term in contemporary translation studies,[5] on almost every page, whether through textual embellishment or notes replete with foreign phrases, especially for the more 'delicate' issues. Though clearly aimed at conveying the scholarly credentials of the author, the commentary only increases the already considerable exoticness – or 'foreignization', if you will – of the convoluted Victorian prose, which often collapses under the weight of its own pretentiousness. Secondly, and more importantly, it also conveyed much of Burton's views on sexuality, in general, and that of the 'Orientals', in particular.

One might say that the *text* clearly chose its mediator, who became an *actor*, rather than a 'trans-actor', as the translation became a rewriting of 'the Other' within a preconceived framework, which is dealt with in great detail in the 'Terminal Essay'[6] to his translation of the Arabian Nights. The fourth part of the essay deals with the 'Social Condition' and it is here that Burton expounds on the '*turpiloquium*' in Eastern societies. It includes sections on 'Woman', 'Pornography' and, most controversially, 'Pederasty', which he proceeds 'to discuss … sérieusement, honnêtement, historiquement; to show it in decent nudity not in suggestive fig-leaf or feuille de vigne'![7]

One of the more famous sections is that on the so-called 'Sotadic Zone', which in the Burtonian *Weltanschauung* encompasses areas whose populations are inclined towards pederasty. It includes parts of Europe (southern France, Spain, Italy and Greece), Northern Africa and most of Asia, but its epicentre is 'Asia Minor and Mesopotamia now occupied by the "unspeakable Turk," a race of born pederasts.'[8]

In the world of Victorian pornography, Burton's *Perfumed Garden* was an instant hit, and inspired others to produce their own 'translations' of Eastern sexual culture. In the first half of the twentieth century the 'genre' subsided, but it is clear from A. Edwardes's *Jewel in the Lotus* (1963) that the Burtonian view and attitude towards Oriental(ist) sexuality endured for much longer.

Arabic erotic literature is a wide-ranging subject, cutting across many centuries and genres. While the output is primarily associated with belles-lettres (*adab*), particularly the *mujūn* (dissolute) poetry by the likes of Abū Nuwās (756–814) and Bashshār Ibn Burd (714–784), the present discussion will centre on works that fall under the heading of erotological literature written in Arabic, irrespective of author origins.

A comprehensive study of medieval Arabic erotological and sexual literature has yet to be written, not least because of the large number of primary sources that remain in manuscript form, while others have scarcely been studied. That is not to say that the field is still a blank canvas, as a number of scholars have produced ground breaking work dealing with Islamicate[9] sexuality in history.[10] Recent decades have also seen a growing interest in specific themes, such as homosexuality, both in history[11] and the present,[12] transvestism,[13] hermaphroditism,[14] transsexualism,[15] Islamic jurisprudence (especially with regard to homosexuality),[16] and the role of sexuality in contacts between Muslim and Western cultures.[17]

The spectre of Orientalism is never far away, albeit in a more modern, and far more surreptitious, guise; for instance, in a number of cases the discourse regarding homosexuality in the Muslim (Arab) world has borrowed – and re-gendered – tropes from historical Orientalism concerning Eastern women. Within this discourse, the submissive Eastern temptress is replaced by her masculine counterpart, the lascivious virile Eastern male.[18]

The first observation is that the overwhelming majority of scholarship on sexual and erotological literature has been conducted by Western scholars. Secondly, the interest in the subject as an academic field has hitherto resulted in only a handful of scholarly editions of the primary sources. Many re-editions of books are emendated, with the editors' barely veiled distaste causing them to omit words that run counter to prevailing morals. In the most extreme cases, this involves the omission of entire chapters that are deemed inconsistent with the shariah.[19]

This distinctly modern, Victorian-inspired morality extends to high literature as well, with modern editions of Abū Nuwās's work excluding his *mujūn* verse, to the extent that the poems in question were the object of a separate edition, enticingly titled *al-Nuṣūṣ al-muḥarrama* ('The Forbidden Texts').[20]

Translations of the primary texts are few and far between, and those that exist are problematic, as many are based on non-authoritative sources (often unidentified by the translator), in the above-mentioned Victorian style, or are 'secondary' renditions, i.e. relayed through a third language.[21]

The Genre: History and Typology

Chief among the erotological and sexological literature are sex manuals and guides, (semi-)fictional works, and medical treatises – and often a combination of all three – which generally contain details on sexual health, hygiene, regimens and disorders, as well as various treatments, remedies and medicines.

The genre first emerged at the turn of the ninth century, with a large number of works being produced especially in the period up to the thirteenth century. The overlap between the sexual and erotic, on the one hand, and the technical–medical and 'spiritual', on the other, is a salient aspect of this type of literature, as religious injunctions are often juxtaposed with medical prescription and erotic titillation.

Several are known only by their titles, while a large number remain in manuscript form. In principle, this category excludes works that deal with profane, chaste love, such as *Kitāb al-Zahra* by Muḥammad Ibn Dāwūd al-Ẓāhirī (d. 910) and *Rawḍat al-qulūb wa nuzhat al-muḥibb wa 'l-maḥbūb* by al-Shayzarī (twelfth century).[22] But things are never straightforward, and even these contain some stories and anecdotes associated with the erotic/erotological genre.

One of the mainstays in the majority of the erotological corpus is the inclusion of aphrodisiacs, with some authors devoting an entire treatise to them – for example *Adwiyat al-Bāh* ('Medicines for Sexual Intercourse') by al-Qusṭanṭīnī (d. 1568), the anonymous *Risāla fī dhikr adwiyat al-bāh* ('Treatise on Medicines for Sexual Intercourse'), and al-Ṭūsī's *Kitāb albāb al-bāhiyya wa 'l-tarākīb al-sulṭāniyya*, which forms the object of this study.[23]

Sexual health and erotology were often discussed in the medical literature, which may conveniently be subdivided into a number of categories.[24]

The first includes the medical encyclopaedias, the most famous of which are *al-Kitāb al-Manṣūrī fī 'l-ṭibb* ('Manṣūr's Book on Medicine') and *Kitāb al-Ḥāwī fī 'l-ṭibb* ('The Medical Compendium') by al-Rāzī (d. 925; Lat. *Rhazes*);[25] *Kitāb Kāmil al-ṣinā^c^āt al-ṭibbiyya* ('Complete Book of the Medical Art') – also known as *al-Kitāb al-malakī* ('The Royal Book') – by ^c^Alī Ibn al-^c^Abbās al-Majūsī (d. late tenth century; Lat. *Haly Abbas*); *al-Qānūn fī 'l-ṭibb* ('Canon of Medicine') by Abū ^c^Alī al-Ḥusayn Ibn Sīnā (d. 1037; Lat. *Avicenna*); *al-Tadkhirat ulī al-albāb wa 'l-jāmi^c^ li 'l-^c^ajab al-^c^ujāb* ('Memorandum for Those Who Have Understanding and The Collection of Wondrous Travels') by Dā'ūd ibn ^c^Umar al-Anṭākī (d. 1599); and ^c^*Umdat al-iṣlāḥ fī* ^c^*amal ṣinā^c^at al-jarrāḥ* ('Manual of Surgery') and *al-Shāfī fī 'l-ṭibb* ('The Healer in Medicine') by Abū 'l-Faraj Ibn al-Quff (1233–86).[26]

Hygiene literature devoted attention to sexual hygiene practices, including their possible therapeutic functions – for example, Ibn al-Khaṭīb's *Kitāb al-wuṣūl li ḥifẓ al-ṣiḥḥa fī 'l-fuṣūl* ('Book on Preserving Health') and the *Taqwīm al-Ṣiḥḥa* ('Almanac of Health') by Ibn Buṭlān (eleventh century).[27]

Sexual hygiene was also dealt with in dedicated treatises, including Qusṭā Ibn Lūqā's *Kitāb fī 'l-Bāh wa mā yuḥtāju ilayhi min tadbīr al-badan fī istiᶜmālihi* and *Kitāb fī 'l-Bāh* ('Book on Coitus and The Regimen that Is Necessary to Practise It'); al-Rāzī's *Kitāb al-Bāh wa manāfiᶜihi wa maḍārrihi wa mudawātihi* ('Book on Coitus, Its Benefits, Harmful Effects and Remedies').

Sexuality, particularly sexual health, appears frequently in religious literature, in hadith literature (the sayings of the Prophet) and, especially, as part of the so-called 'Prophetic medicine', which refers to a voluminous body of literature that provides therapy based on a combination of herbal medicine and tradition.[28] The most celebrated works in this category include *al-Ṭibb al-nabawī* ('Prophetic Medicine') by Ibn Qayyim al-Jawziyya (d. 1350) and Shams al-Dīn al-Dhahabī (d. 1348); *al-Manhaj al sāwī wa al-manhal al rāwī fī 'l-ṭibb al nabawī* ('The Correct Method and Refreshing Source for the Medicine of the Prophet'); *Mukhtaṣar al-ṭibb al nabawī* ('Abridgement of the Prophet's Medicine'); *al-Raḥma fī 'l-ṭibb wa 'l-ḥikma* ('Compassion in Medicine and Wisdom'),[29] by Jalāl al-Dīn al-Suyūṭī (d. 1505); and *Kitāb shifā' al-*ālām *fī ṭibb ahl al-Islām* ('Book on The Treatment of Pain in the Medicine of the Believers in Islam'), by al-Surramarrī (d. 1374).

Treatises devoted to sexual diseases may also be considered a subgenre, and concentrated on the characteristics and treatment of sexually transmitted illnesses – especially syphilis. Their authors included the Tunisians al-Bājī al-Masᶜūdī (d. 1879) and Aḥmad al-Dihmānī (d. 1835), and the Moroccan ᶜAbd al-Wahhāb Muḥammad Adarrāq (d. 1746). It was, in fact, through this 'imported' sexual disease – which subsequently became known as *ḥabb al-Ifranj* ('the Frankish chancre'), and was first referred to in Arabic medical literature as early as the fifteenth century – that Muslims developed a perfunctory interest in European medicine.[30] This was a major development since, until the nineteenth century, it was deemed devoid of merit. Generally speaking, the Arab-Muslim world showed little interest in European sciences, due to an unwavering conviction of the completeness, self sufficiency, and indeed superiority, of Muslim achievements in this field. This was particularly true for medicine, as medieval Muslim scholars were far ahead of their Christian counterparts.

Another category comprises literature that deals with sexual ethics, of which the most famous exponents are Abū Ṭālib al-Makkī (d. 996), *Qūt al-qulūb* ('Nourishment of the Hearts'); Abū 'l-Faraj Ibn al-Jawzī (d. 1200), *Dhamm al-Hawā* ('The Condemnation of Love'); al-Ghazzālī (1058–1111), *Iḥyā' ᶜulūm al-dīn* ('The Revival of the Religious Sciences');[31] Ibn Qayyim al-Jawziyya, *Rawḍat al-muḥibbīn wa nuzhat al-mushtāqīn* ('The Garden of Lovers and Excursion of the Longing'); al-Aqfahsī (d. 1406), *Rafᶜ al-janāḥ ᶜammā huwa min al-mar'a al-mubāḥ* ('The Raising of the Wing on What Is the Permissible Woman'); ᶜAbd Allāh al-Mawṣulī (tenth century), *al-Ikhtiyār li-taᶜlīl al-mukhtār* ('Selecting the Distraction of the Chosen').

Travel has always played a large part in Islam, not only as a means of seeking knowledge – as witnessed by the famous hadith *uṭlub al-ᶜilm wa law bi 'l-Ṣīn* ('Seek knowledge even in

China!') – but also because of the injunction on all believers to perform the pilgrimage (*ḥajj*) to the Muslim holy site of Mekka. This gave rise to a distinct subgenre of travellers' medical manuals addressing specific health issues facing travellers, especially pilgrims, and contained specific advice on matters relating to sexual hygiene. Examples include Ibn al-Jazzār's *Zād al-musāfir wa qūt al-ḥāḍir* ('Provisions for the Traveller and Nourishment of the Sedentary')[32] and Qusṭā Ibn Lūqā's *Risāla fī tadbīr safar al-ḥajj* ('Treatise on Organizing the Pilgrimage Journey').[33]

The rich Arabic pharmacological tradition dealt with all aspects of human well-being, including sexual health – in particular, how to enhance and treat it. Examples of these works include compendia like *al-Jāmiᶜ li mufradāt 'l-adwiya wa 'l-aghdhiyya* ('The Comprehensive Book on Simple Drugs and Foods') by Ibn al Bayṭār (d. 1248), and formularies such as the *Aqrābādhīn* by Sābūr Ibn Sahl (d. 869),[34] and the thirteenth-century *Minhaj al-dukkān* ('The Running of an Apothecary's Shop') by al-Kūhin al-ᶜAṭṭār.

Finally, as love is sometimes said to go through the stomach, it is very common for medieval Arabic culinary books to include information on the medicinal properties of certain foods and condiments, such as *Kitāb al-Ṭabīkh* ('Cookery Book') by al-Baghdādī (d. 1240) and the tenth-century *Kitāb al-Ṭabīkh* by Ibn Sayyār al-Warrāq.

Questions that arise from this overview include why and how sexuality, eroticism and erotology became such a significant element in Arabic literature, whether scientific or belles-lettres. Although there is no single ready-made answer to this question, it is true to say that a number of elements initially combined to form the basis of Arabic sexual literature.

Firstly, sexual enjoyment, as opposed to procreative intercourse, has been recognized in Islam since the very beginning. For instance, while in Christianity coitus interruptus is condemned as 'the sin of Onan', in Islam it is viewed as an acceptable sexual outlet without the goal of procreation.[35] It is also against this background that one should interpret the lawfulness (for some time at least) of the so-called *nikāḥ al-mutʿa*, the 'marriage of enjoyment', which was a temporary marriage (especially for soldiers and pilgrims), in which the believer could lawfully practise his sexuality in a short-term relationship that was religiously endorsed. Also, the famous Qur'ānic verse, 'Your wives are a tilth for you, so go to your tilth as you will' (II: 231) is often interpreted as meaning that the man may exercise his conjugal right whenever and *however* he pleases, which for some – but by no means all – legal authorities includes anally (*fī duburihā*).

This distinction is also evidenced in the use of terminology, with *nikāḥ* being the term reserved for sexual intercourse during marriage and, by extension, also denotes marriage itself. The act of coitus is more commonly referred to as *bāh* (which also means potency) and *jimāʿ*, with *waṭ'* being employed in Islamic law (*fiqh*).[36] When not practised within a lawful context of marriage (or a bond of ownership: master–slave/concubine), coitus is considered unlawful (*ḥarām*) and falls within the remit of fornication (*zinā'*).

The second key element, to some degree an extension of the first, was the attention given to the subject of sexuality in medicine, where it was an integral component of the holistic approach to physical well-being – a concept that ultimately went back to the Greek medical tradition. The influence and significance of medicine may be summarised as follows: 'Medicine ... and the sexual script it produced provided the scientific basis for most sex-oriented discourses in Muslim Middle Eastern societies. Its injunctions and prohibitions, believed to originate in scientific knowledge, were subsumed by other discursive arenas, from literature to sacred law, almost intuitively, as part of their basic assumptions about the world.'[37]

Although the erotic was present as far back as pre-Islamic poetry,[38] it was the sophistication and hedonism of the first centuries of the ᶜAbbāsid caliphate (750–1258) that would provide the breeding ground for the creation of both erotic and erotological literature.[39] Possibly the oldest known (but unfortunately lost) work is that by the Persian-born Ibn Bukhtīshūᶜ (late eighth to early ninth century). The ninth century witnessed a boom in the number of such works (see below). To some extent, this may be explained by the fact that they responded to a trend that was also visible in belles-lettres; alternatively, it may point to a development in the genre, rather than its starting point. Some indications are provided in one of the earliest sources: Ibn al-Nadīm's bio-bibliographical encyclopedia *Fihrist* ('Index'), which dates from the tenth century. It contains the names of a number of erotological and erotic works, revealing the substantial output in the field. In addition to details of individual authors (al-Ṣaymarī and al-Ṭahirī),[40] the text contains extensive lists of anonymous works, arranged in various categories: 'passionate lovers during the pre-Islamic period';[41] 'loving and fickle girls';[42] 'passionate lovers from the rest of the people, about whose traditions books were written';[43] 'passionate lovers whose traditions enter into the evening stories'.[44] As none of the titles mentioned are found anywhere else, it is impossible to trace the growth of the genre prior to the ninth century, when it suddenly appears.

Sources

Erotology in all of its aspects – views on male and female sexuality, coital practices, illnesses and treatments – was entirely subsumed within the medical system of medieval Islamic medicine. This owed much to the ancient Greek tradition, represented in particular by Rufus of Ephesus (Rūfūs al-Afsīsī),[45] Galen of Pergamon (Jālīnūs, 131–200),[46] Aristotle (Aristū, Arisṭūṭālīs, fourth century)[47] and Hippocrates (Buqrāṭ, ca. 460–ca. 375 BCE).[48]

It was ᶜAbbāsid rulers such as Hārūn al-Rashīd (766–809) and his son al-Ma'mūn (813–33), the founder of the famous 'House of Wisdom' (Bayt al-Ḥikma), who provided the impetus for the first translation movement in Muslim history, when many Greek scientific works were translated into Arabic, usually via Syriac.[49] Key actors in this movement included Nestorian Christian physicians, such as Ḥunayn Ibn Isḥāq[50] and Ibn Māsawayh (d. 857, known in Latin as Mesue).[51] Nestorians were renowned for their medical knowledge, and many served as physicians to the ᶜAbbāsid rulers. In some cases, this resulted in veritable dynasties; eight generations of the Ibn Bukhtīshūᶜ family, for example, acted in this capacity.[52]

When they were in turn translated into Latin from the eleventh century onwards, these texts, and the medical scholarship that was influenced by them, would have an impact that went beyond the Muslim empire. In many cases, it is thanks to the Arabic versions that Greek the originals have survived. This is of particular relevance to authors like Rufus and – especially – Galen, nearly all of whose works were translated into Arabic, and whose theories would be extremely influential in medieval and Renaissance Europe. From the point of view of historical scholarship, the translations provide invaluable clues for the reconstruction of the original Greek texts that survived only in later versions, as well as an insight into the history of medical terminology.[53]

In the field of erotology and sexology, the Greek influence was often direct. Firstly, all of the above-named scholars make an appearance in many erotological works, either through quotation or reference. The thirteenth-century author Ibn Māssa even devotes a chapter of his book to a paraphrase of the pseudo-Aristotelian *Problemata Physica*.[54] Finally, views on women's sexuality and medicine in the Arabic tradition can also be traced back to Greek texts.[55]

As Greek erotic handbooks were a prolific genre in Greek literature, it is tempting to posit a link and/or influence in this field, too. Any discussion of this question is complicated by the fact that only fragments of the Greek works have been preserved. One isolated piece of evidence is a reference by the tenth-century author al-Kātib to a Greek erotica book that included 'almost all the subjects to be found in Indian books'.[56] But the author does not specifically mention his having used – or even seen – this work. Upon closer examination, a Greek influence here would seem unlikely in light of the significant differences in both format and content. Firstly, the Greek works were all attributed to (fictional) women (usually *hetairai* – 'courtesans'), on whose professional experience they were putatively based; 'restricted primarily to a tabulation of schemata for intercourse',[57] the manuals were intended as a guide to an art or skill (*technê*).

What the Arabic and Greek works also have in common is the fact that the female protagonist is of a lower social status; equally, there is a 'close connection [with] other genres, principally medical writings, and other encyclopedic, scientific and culinary works'.[58]

The translation movement provides us with a second reason for the emergence of the erotological literature, which also played a role in the development of Greek sex manuals. The Greek medical and philosophical work, with its emphasis on taxonomy and analysis, held a powerful attraction for Muslim scholars, whose propensity for classification covered all fields and lay at the heart of the hadith literature, with the Prophet's sayings being methodically and meticulously arranged and ordered. In this sense, the genre may be seen as a 'continuance of the Aristotelian ... tradition of analysis and classification, wherein the contiua of the world are broken into discrete, nameable and hence controllable quanta'.[59]

One of the core elements of medieval Islamic medicine was the theory of humorism, which had originated with the Hippocratic school but was expanded by Galen. It was the latter's version of it that was imported.[60] Within this framework, human beings were seen as the microcosm of nature, subject to the interaction of the four elements (*arkān*) that make up all things: air, water, fire and earth.[61] Each of these was associated with two of the 'primary qualities' (hot, *ḥārr*/cold, *bārid*; moist, *raṭb*/dry, *yābis*): fire was hot and dry; air, hot and moist; water, cold and moist; earth, cold and dry. The basic elements were thought to be concentrated in one of the four so-called 'humours' (< Gr. *khumos*; Ar. *khilṭ*, pl. *akhlāṭ*, 'mixture'), essentially the bodily fluids: air in blood (*dam*); water in phlegm (*balgham*, < Gr. *phlegma*); fire in yellow bile (*mirra ṣufrā'*); and earth in black bile (*mirra sawdā'*). As a result, each of the humours was endowed with the primary qualities associated with the element: blood was hot and moist; phlegm was cold and moist; yellow bile was hot and dry; and black bile was cold and dry. The humours were also associated with a season: blood with spring, yellow bile with summer, black bile with autumn, and phlegm with winter. This may be illustrated as in Figure 1.[62]

According to Galenic theory, a human being's physical health relied on the balance in the mixture (Gr. *krasis*; Ar. *mizāj*) of the humours, i.e. the temperament (or 'complexion') and equilibrium (Ar. *iʿtidāl*) between the qualities, a state which was known in Greek as *eukrasia* or *symmetria*. For instance, if black bile was predominant, this resulted in a cold and dry (or melancholic) temperament, making the individual prone to sadness (melancholy). Similarly, sanguine temperaments were characterized by a predominance of blood, choleric ones by yellow bile, and phlegmatic ones by phlegm, each of which was associated with differences in character.[63] Another crucial

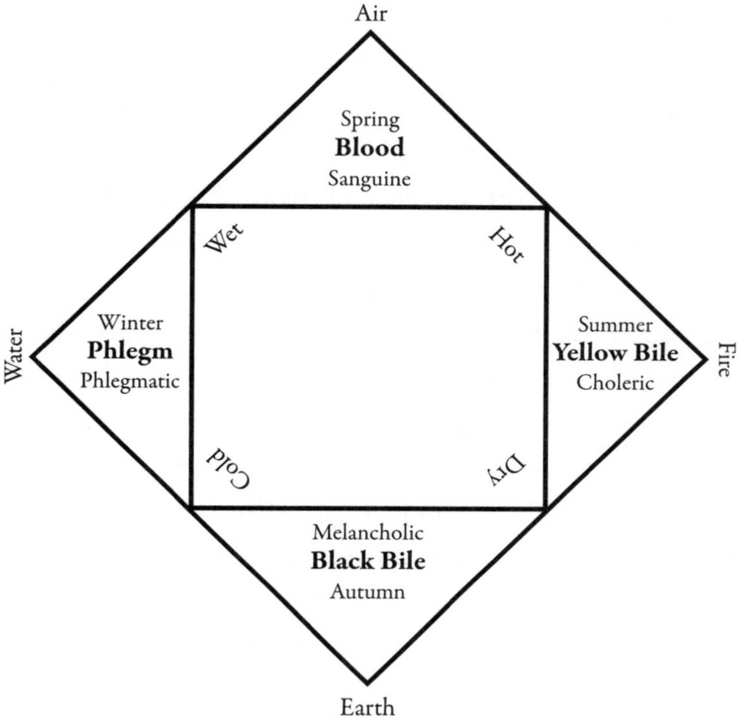

Figure 1

component of the Galenic system was the view (originally Aristotelian) that men and women shared a common reproductive system, with that of women being essentially a mirror-image of men's.[64]

The treatment of ill health was aimed at making the temperament balanced (*mu*ᶜ*tadal*) through therapies, medication or diet, to counterbalance the humours or qualities causing the disequilibrium (Gr. *dyskrasia*; *sū' al-mizāj*).

Spices and other foods were also associated with humours and with (varying degrees of) the above-mentioned qualities, and prescribed accordingly. For instance, cardamom was hot and dry, whereas cucumbers were said to be cold and moist.

Whether a fruit or plant was dried or fresh could also affect its qualities: for instance, fresh figs were hot and moist in the second degree, whereas dried ones were hot in the first degree, but moderately moist and dry.

A related concept was that of living beings' 'innate (or vital) heat' (Gr. *emphuton thermon*, Lat. *calidum innatum*; Ar. *ḥarāra gharīziyya*), which was said to be created by the heart and circulated through the body by blood, with its amount determining the place of a species within the biological hierarchy. Human beings were said to have the greatest innate heat, and were thus at the top of the pyramid. Similarly, men were considered 'hotter' (and 'drier') than women – and thus superior to them – which explained, for instance, the fact that the former's genital organs were on the outside.[65]

It has been claimed that the medieval Arabic medical scholars did not aim 'to discover new knowledge, or to reinterpret the processes which go on in the human body, or to develop new and more adequate therapies', and that 'the literature of the ancients [was] both example and authority'.[66] The implicit argument is that they made few original contributions. However, the Greek theories were not only borrowed, digested and assimilated, but also expanded and developed. The erotological literature includes a number of examples not only of innovation but also of empirical research. For instance, Ibn al-Jazzār refers to recipes invented (and tested) by both his predecessors[67] and himself – and when discussing the effectiveness of a pill for the retention of menstrual blood, he adds that he has 'tried it and approved of it'.[68]

The next question is that of whether authors drew on an existing pool of traditions and conventions. Although it is difficult to address this issue in the absence of a complete picture, there are a number of clues. The first are the references by some authors to predecessors in the genre (for example, al-Tīfāshī and al-Kātib).

The first mention of non-Arabic sources can be found in the famous *Kitāb al-ḥayawān* ('The Book of Animals'), by the poet al-Jāḥiẓ, where a number of Arab poets are mentioned, as well as an unnamed Indian (*Hindī*) author (*ṣāḥib*) of *Kitāb al-Bāh* ('Book on Coitus') – which one may speculate is a reference to the Kama Sutra – who is quoted as the source for the claim that the elephant has the biggest penis of all animals, and the gazelle the smallest.[69] However, the Indians' reputation in sexual matters was not based on this solitary author, as: 'the Indians are like the Arabs in all respects, except for the circumcision (*khitān*) of women and men, but they were driven to it by their pursuit of sexual prowess, for which they took medicines; they wrote books on the art of sex (*ṣināʿat al-bāh*) and instructed their sons.'[70]

Further references to an Indian connection are given by other authors, such as the poet Abū Tammām (788–845),[71] the legal scholar Ibn al-Jawzī (508–97),[72] Ibn al-Nadīm,[73] Ibn Abī Uṣaybiʿa (1200–79),[74] and, of course, in erotological works, such as al-Kātib's erotological compendium, *Jawāmiʿ al-ladhdha* ('Encyclopaedia of Pleasure').[75]

Among the Indians there was, it seems, one woman who was known as *al-alfiyya* ('The Thousander'), in reference to the number of men she had had intercourse with. Her expertise turned her into an oracle on matters sexual – a Dr Ruth *avant la lettre*. Her legend was transmitted by al-Jāḥiẓ and others, including al-Tīfāshī, who relates that

> groups of women gathered to visit her. They would say to her: 'Sister, tell us what is required and we will do it. What is it that makes women settle in men's hearts, what gives them pleasure and what morals do they abhor? What should we do in order to arouse their love and affection?'
>
> She replied: 'The first thing is that the look of a man should be on a body that is healthy, not smelly but fragrant, in which case [the woman's] beauty will be enhanced.'
>
> 'What does a man have to do in order to capture a woman's heart?'
>
> 'He should be playful prior to coitus and shudder before ejaculation (*firāgh*).'
>
> 'What is the reason for mutual love and concord [between a man and a woman]?'
>
> 'Their simultaneous orgasm.'[76]

While no translation of the *Kama Sutra* into Arabic has ever been found, or is even known to have existed, a number of Indian medical texts were translated into Persian and/or Syriac (and thence into Arabic) very early on by scholars in Gondēshāpūr, which was known for its physicians, and Indian medical knowledge thereby filtered through into Arabic-Islamic medical thought.[77] One may cite the famous *Ladhat al-Nisā* ('The Pleasure of Women'), which was a Persian translation of a Hindi text called *Kok-shastar* (or *Kokasara*), attributed to a certain Koka (Koka pandit) and based on a Sanskrit text entitled *Ratirahasya* ('On the Art of Love')[78]. In Arabic medical literature, there are a number of Indian references. For instance, the last chapter of the famous *Firdaws al-Ḥikma* ('Paradise of Wisdom'), by the Persian ʿAlī Ibn Rabban al-Ṭabarī (ninth century), is devoted to Indian medicine, with quotations from a number of works. While it is possible that al-Ṭabarī was able to access the original Sanskrit, it is more likely that he based himself on Syriac or Persian translations. The encyclopaedias by Ibn Qutayba (d. 885),[79] Ibn al-Nadīm[80] and Ibn Abī Uṣaybiʿa[81] also include references to Indian physicians (such as Cāṇakya/Shānāq[82] and Maṅka) and works, whereas al-Rāzī quotes a number of (unnamed) Indian sources.[83] Indian medical knowledge was highly respected, and it is said that Hārūn al-Rashīd called for Maṅka when he was ill and, together with a compatriot by the name of Ibn Dham, the latter translated a medical text on poisons.[84]

The second clue regarding the construction of the erotological genre involves similarities in approach and/or content in the various works. Examples include the 'comparatist' approach in some of al-Jāḥiẓ's and al-Suyūṭī's works, discussions of sexual positions[85] and sexual frequency related to sexual age,[86] and the lists of substances that invigorate coitus which many of the authors have in common, and whose creator is sometimes identified.[87]

Indirectly, the above question regarding the existence of an established tradition and corpus is inextricably linked to the extent to which the works spread across the Muslim world. When talking about a time when manuscripts were the currency, this is a particularly thorny issue and can only be addressed tangentially.

There are indications that, at least in some cases, the spread took place not only between genres, but also between languages. An example combining the two movements involves stories on homosexual prowling (*dabb*), which can be found in al-Tīfāshī, Abū Nuwās and, more surprisingly perhaps, the work by the sixteenth-century Turkish author Deli Birader, whose discussion of the various positions of anal intercourse is redolent of those found in other passages by al-Tifāshī.[88] And at least one author (al-Kātib) acknowledges a Persian source.[89]

This case leads us to another indication regarding the spread of the works, namely the translations into other languages, which also attest to the popularity – perceived or imagined – of the source text. In the case of al-Ṭūsī's work, there were translations into both Turkish[90] and his native Persian.[91]

Features

The list of 125 titles in the appendix to this volume is the most extensive bibliography to date of literature devoted wholly, or for the most part, to erotology. It is worth pointing out that it is by no means exhaustive, since it is more than likely that other works are held in collections that cannot be readily explored. As has been noted, the list does not include erotic poetry, which continued to be produced (and/or collected) in the post-classical age by, for instance, Khalīl Ibn Aybak al-Ṣafadī (1297–1363),[92] Ṣafī al-Dīn al-Ḥillī (1279–1348)[93] and Shams al-Dīn al-Nawājī (1386–1455)[94].

A number of elements merit discussion, including the authors, themes, formats, sources, and so on. A. Jarkas classified what he called 'erotic books' into the following categories, according to the topics they deal with:

- 'books dealing with the ethics, art, kinds, time and condition of coition;
- books dealing with the sexual capacity of men and women; kinds of invigorating food and drugs that keep sexual capacity normal; different kinds of medicinal prescriptions, consisting of tablets, powders, suppositories, ointments, and so on;
- books which deal with the subjects of former categories so that benefits may be more general;
- books dealing with one specific subject, such as prostitution, sodomy, lesbianism, masturbation, and the like.'[95]

However, the multitude of overlapping genres, intersecting fields of application and levels of discourse means that any classification of this type will be at once too narrow and too broad, as far too many exponents of the genre defy simplistic compartmentalization.

It makes more sense to view the works along a continuum in relation to the approach their authors take and the extent to which certain elements are present. On one end of the spectrum, for example, one may put belles-lettres (*adab*) works in which the erotic fictional component predominates, as in the works of al-Jāḥiẓ or al-Suyūṭī. On the other end, we find treatises that deal with erotology from a scientific (medical) perspective, such as those by Ibn Sīnā, al-Jazzār, Qusṭā Ibn Lūqā, Maimonides, or the author of the work that is presented here, al-Ṭūsī.

Neither of these subgenres exists in a 'pure' form, and varying elements associated with the other are present in both. For instance, even the 'fictional' type often deals with medical issues attendant upon sexuality – enhancing libido and performance, recommended practices, sexual positions, aphrodisiacs, and so on. In the case of al-Tīfāshī's *Rujūʿ al-shaykh ilā ṣibāh fi 'l-quwwa wa 'l-bāh* ('Return of the Old Man to his Youth and Coital Vigour'), this results in a neatly compartmentalized construction, with the 'medical' prefacing the fictional.

As for the 'scientific' type, it does not eschew the more frivolous and/or literary features associated with its counterparts' output. It might also include, for instance, some lines of relevant poetry – but generally no erotic stories.

In the middle of this continuum are texts distinguished by their form rather than their content. This category includes erotological works with high literary aspirations, expressed either in their use of poetic quotations or by the composition of the treatise itself in verse (for example, Ibn Kannān, Ibn Sīnā), or those with a lexicographical and taxonomical focus, such as al-Suyūṭī's *al-Wishāḥ fī fawā'id al-nikāḥ* ('The Sash in the Advantages of Sexual Intercourse'), which contains a veritable thesaurus of terms denoting the sexual organs, intercourse, and so on. This may be presented diagrammatically as in Figure 2.

What all of these works have in common, to a lesser or greater degree, is their didactic aim: irrespective of the genre

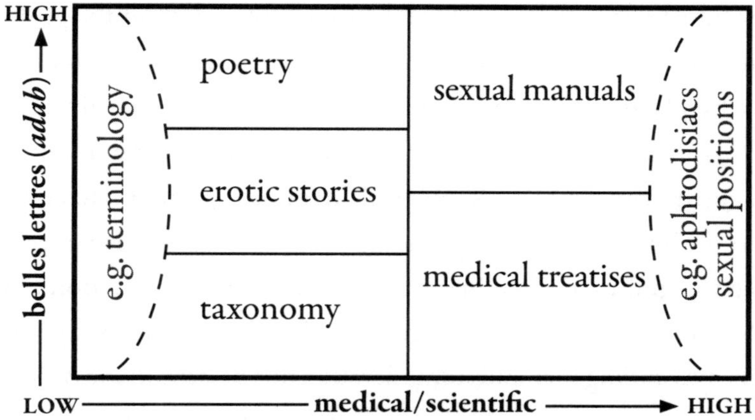

Figure 2

or medium (poetry or prose), the aim and tone are avowedly pedagogic, practical and scientific. In this sense, the books serve as teaching manuals or handbooks; even the ribald stories and obscene poetry (some of which would put Catullus to shame!) regarding past *roués* contain lessons – often 'morals' of sorts – deemed useful to the reader. The intended readership also merits some attention. It has been claimed that the authors' motive was to 'write sexual instructions that mothers gave their daughters on their wedding day'.[96] This is highly unlikely, however, not least because the books were written *for* men, *by* men.

In fact, the typical reader would be a fellow medical scholar or, as some authors inform us, a member of a courtly audience (often the ruler himself), whereas the medical treatises might also be used as self-medication manuals, as is the case for al-Ṭūsī's work. It is likely that a number of the works – or appropriate parts of them (stories, poems, and so on) – would be read at social gatherings of the elite, which would be exclusively male and, as such, would 'tend to spread information – one might say in certain cases a kind of initiation – by placing their science in the service of an art of living'.[97] This also underlies the link between sexuality and food as another constant in erotological literature – while references to the aphrodisiacal properties of food were, as we have seen, an integral part of culinary manuals. A similar connection can be found in classical Greek erotic works, albeit as part of a spirit of over indulgence and immoderation not present in the Arabic tradition, the 'association between the ethics of sex and ethics of food [being] a constant factor in ancient culture'.[98]

Another dimension of variation is the number of topics covered, ranging from the encyclopaedic to texts that focus on only one area (such as aphrodisiacs). The erotological corpus runs the full gamut of sexuality and erotology, generally combining *ars amatoria* and *scientia sexualis*: types and positions of intercourse, penis size, homosexuality, lesbianism, pederasty, hermaphroditism, impotence, nocturnal emissions, priapism, anilingus, cunnilungus, voyeurism, bestiality, sadomasochism, hymen restoration, contraception, prostitution, fetishism, and so on. Interestingly enough, the extant works do not contain any discussions of fellatio, which was prominent in the Greek and Roman traditions (which also included *irrumatio* – forced fellatio), both in literature (Catullus) and pictorial art, where it is often represented both between men and between men and women. Many of these themes also formed the object of the (pure) medical literature – though devoid of the fictional narrative content – which further consolidates the link between the medical and the erotological/erotic.[99]

It is difficult to overstate the importance and relevance of erotological literature for what it teaches us about various aspects not only of Islamic medicine but also, and more importantly, of Muslim society, gender relations and sex-power relations. Most of all, it provides a unique vantage point on the experience of sexuality – that is, 'the correlation between fields of knowledge, types of normativity, and forms of subjectivity in a particular culture', to use Michel Foucault's words.[100] Though Foucault was discussing sexual discourse in the West from the seventeenth century onwards, this comment is equally applicable to medieval Arabic sexual discourse. One of the questions that lies at the heart of his framework is deceptively simple: 'What were the effects of power generated by what was said?'[101]

Like Greek erotic literature, Arabic erotology is decidedly phallocentric in that the emphasis is on (active) male penetration. The role of women is entirely subordinate to the penis, with remedies including the tightening and narrowing of the vagina 'like that of a virgin'; women are often unnamed and invisible, as secondary characters. As one author put it, coitus is 'the greatest pleasure given to *men*'.[102] The terminology, too, is inscribed into this discourse, as the words for coitus (see above) tend to identify the male rather than the female as the 'primary' actor.

And yet, perhaps surprisingly in light of this, both the Arabic erotological and medical works paid attention to female pleasure; Ibn Sīnā, for instance, clearly placed the onus of pleasuring a woman on the man: 'If a man can't make her orgasm, some [women] turn to lesbianism (*musāḥaqa*)'.

Furthermore, female coital pleasure does not result from male ejaculation, but from her own ejaculation and the movement of her womb.[103] A revolutionary notion, indeed – and one that was entirely absent from the Greek and Roman traditions, in which Ovid is the only author to discuss a woman's pleasure during coitus.[104] The more active role of women – albeit with concomitants of predatoriness and deviousness – is also evidenced by the many stories about the wiles of women in seeking out and securing the amorous affections of invariably well-endowed men.[105] The same notion emerges from belles-lettres, in both poetry and prose, with a number of examples in the *Thousand and One Nights*. It has been argued that this view of a female sexual aggressiveness combined with artfulness runs throughout Muslim culture, and has contributed to the spread of the veil.[106]

The erotological works have a number of things in common, the most important of which is the varying proportions of pedagogic and literary intent in the discussion of sexual behaviour outside the 'norm', whether it be homosexuality or bestiality, which tend either to be presented without judgement[107] or treated as *medical* 'deviations', and worthy of study as such.

Use of the word 'norm' in this context does not in any way imply a moral judgement, and the same was broadly true in the Greek and Roman traditions, whose 'moral reflection concerning the pleasures was not directed towards a codification of acts, nor towards a hermeneutics of the subject, but towards a stylization of attitudes and an aesthetics of existence. A stylization, because the rarefaction of sexual activity presented itself as a sort of open-ended requirement.'[108]

However, as Holt Parker has pointed out, this statement does not apply to all Greek erotic texts, and sex manuals were considered to be 'shameless'[109] – a perception absent from Arabic erotological literature, which, it seems, bears out the aphorism: *lā ḥayā' fī 'l-ᶜilm* ('there is never any shame in science'). That is not to say, however, that the concept of (il)licitness did not exist in Arabic erotological literature. In order to discuss this, it is useful to introduce the Foucauldian contrast between 'moral code' and 'moral behaviour'. The former denotes 'a set of values and rules of action that are recommended to individuals through the intermediary of various prescriptive agencies',[110] whereas the latter, which is equated with 'morality', involves the actual behaviour of individuals 'in relation to the rules and values that are recommended to them', and 'thus designates the manner in which they comply more or less fully with a standard of conduct, the manner in which they obey or resist an interdiction or a prescription; the manner in which they respect or disregard a set of values'.[111] The 'moral code' is sometimes implicit, and sometimes – as in al-Tīfāshī's statement regarding the aims of his work – explicit:

> In the writing of this book I did not aim to increase corruption, to encourage sin, or assist those seeking pleasure and sinfulness by trying to make lawful what Allah the Almighty has made unlawful; rather, my aim is to help those whose passion is reduced to achieve pleasure in a lawful context (*fī 'l-ḥalāl*), which is the basis of civilized society and procreation.[112]

This passage provides us with a great deal of food for thought. Seemingly, it sets out the contours of the subject: the individual's relation towards sexuality, particularly the part that is divinely endorsed, and the aims of the sexual experience. Most saliently, it pre-emptively guards against accusations of irreligiousness due to the inclusion of topics that may arouse censure. This applies to sex that is considered illicit by religious precept – outside the confines of marriage or an ownership bond – and to homosexuality (and pederasty), the treatment of which provides a particularly good case in point.

Several verses of the Qur'ān[113] mention sexual actions between men in relation to the People of Lot (*qawm Lūṭ*), which gave rise to the word *liwāṭ* (< 'to attach oneself, to join oneself to'), with the active male homosexual being known in Classical Arabic as *lūṭī*, *lā'iṭ*, or *mulāwiṭ*.[114] Lesbianism (*musāḥaqa*, *siḥāq*) is not mentioned in the holy text.

The Qur'ān refers to homosexual intercourse as a depravity (*fāḥisha*), and it is equally condemned in various hadiths, the most famous one stating, 'Anyone finding those committing the act of Lot, kill both the active and passive party' (*man wajadtumūhu yaᶜmal ᶜamal qawm lūṭ fa-uqutulū al-fāᶜil wa 'l-mafᶜūl bihi*). Though *liwāṭ* is often equated with 'homosexuality' in its contemporary (Western) acceptation, it is important to state that the modern concept had no equivalent in Islamic society, law or language.[115] Similarly, there was (and still is) no word in Arabic for 'heterosexual(ity)'. For the purposes of punishment, homosexuality tended to be equated with *zinā'* in law (*fiqh*), with varying penalties, depending on the school of Muslim of jurisprudence.[116] The association with *zinā'* is based on the fact that, like heterosexuality, homosexuality was viewed as a binary construct involving an active/penetrating and passive/penetrated partner.[117] The same notion underlay views of the lesbian sexual experience, which, in addition to entailing friction, as the terms for it indicate (*siḥāq*, *musāḥaqa*, < *saḥaqa*, 'to grind'), was thought to be penetrative, by means of dildos.

Homosexual intercourse took place within a hierarchical relation, with the 'passive' partner (or 'bottom', to use the modern jargon) being invariably subordinate in age (with a preference for the *amrad*, the 'beardless youth') and/or status (as in the case of a servant or slave). It is because of this inequality that the passive partner, known as *ma'būn* (compare the *cinaedus* of Roman times), comes in for greater criticism, whereas a predilection for it (*ubna*) was commonly classified as a disease.[118]

Despite the censure embedded in the 'moral (religious) code', the erotological (and erotic) literature demonstrates that male sexual intercourse, within the above constraints, was part of 'moral behaviour' inasmuch as it derived from the established sexual script. In other words, disobedience to the established code was endorsed by socially accepted practice. As a result, the immanent contradiction of al-Tīfāshī's prefatory claims and the ostensible breaches of religion in the course of the book are superseded by what was considered 'moral behaviour'. Al-Kātib is one of the few erotological authors to discuss anal intercourse from a religious point of view – but only as a preamble to extolling the virtues of the rectum over the vagina![119]

In other texts, particularly medical treatises, the legal aspect was clearly divorced from the pursuit of science. Ibn Sīnā, for instance, simply stated that intercourse with youths (*ghulmān*) 'is reprehensible to the masses (*al-jumhūr*) and prohibited under the shariah',[120] before discussing it from a purely physical point of view. No author links homosexuality with a lack of 'morals' (*akhlāq*), or immoral behaviour.

The treatment of homosexuality and pederasty in erotic poetry and erotology reinforced the Victorian view that the practice had been historically condoned, and even encouraged, in Arab-Muslim society, as it was said to have been in ancient Greece.[121] Despite being thickly tarred with an Orientalist brush, this is a view that has some merit, albeit with the provisos mentioned above. In recent times, this perception has been rejected in its entirety on the grounds that, for instance, the severe legal constraints on proof of homosexuality (a confession, or four witnesses to the act) explain the absence of legal action against individuals in the pre-Modern period.[122]

Just as there is no single type of erotological work, there is no 'typical' author. Irrespective of the often raunchy contents of the works, the authors should by no means be considered seedy pornographers driven by scurrilous licentiousness. For a start, nearly all of the known authors were scholars (mainly physicians), many of whom became part of the canon of Islamic science for their activities in other fields – for example, Qusṭā Ibn Lūqā, Ibn Sīnā, al-Rāzī, Ibn al-Jazzār and Maimonides in medicine; al-Tīfāshī in mineralogy; al-Suyūṭī in jurisprudence; and al-Ṭūsī in astronomy. Secondly, the importance of the subject as a scientific field of study to these (and other) scholars is further demonstrated by the fact that they also addressed it in their specialized medical works – this was true of Ibn Sīnā,[123] Maimonides[124] and al-Rāzī,[125] for example.

A second factor that often emerges is the authors' association with the rich and powerful of the day, often their patrons. They not only dedicated their works to such figures, but also received commissions from them to produce treatises on the subject.[126] This relationship of patronage served a twofold purpose. On the one hand, it confirmed the writer's status within the establishment and, on the other, neutralized any accusations of immorality, shamelessness or frivolousness. It is also within this context that one should interpret the references to past scholars, especially Greeks, in order to corroborate statements, while anecdotes and erotic stories are sometimes 'defictionalized' by reference to past historic characters or unnamed dignitaries, such as judges, princes and the like.

Finally, it is striking that, except in some of the medical works, the authors do not appear as *actors*, but variously as *narrators* and/or diagnosticians. When they do appear as actors (as in the case of al-Jazzār), it is to endorse this or that remedy of their own making and attest to its efficaciousness.

The list allows us to draw up some interesting statistics. Firstly, of the 125 titles identified, 29 have been lost and 51 remain in manuscript form to this day. The remaining 45 texts are available in either editions (often incomplete) or translations. Finally, 21 of the entries are anonymous.

A number of the authors wrote several works: Ibn Sīnā, al-Kātib, al-Rāzī, Ibn Lūqā, al-Namlī, and al-Nafzāwī each wrote two; al-Tīfāshī and al-Ẓāhirī produced three; and al-Saymarī wrote six. But by far the most prolific in the field was the Egyptian polymath al-Suyūṭī, who wrote no fewer than 23 treatises on various aspects of erotology.[127] If periods of

Table 1

Century	al-Andalus[128]	Bilād al-Shām	Egypt	Iraq	Morocco	Persia	Sudan	Tunis	Turkey	Yemen
9th		1		6		2				
10th				2		1				
11th				2		2		1		
12th	1		2		1			1		
13th						2		2		
14th		2	3							1
15th			3		1					
16th								3		
17th		1			2					
18th							1			
19th			1							

emergence of these texts are correlated with the origins of the authors, the picture is also revealing (see Table 1).

The data demonstrate that the heyday of erotological literature fell between the ninth and fourteenth centuries, after which it tapered off considerably, with a few isolated works in the seventeenth, eighteenth and nineteenth centuries. The nineteenth century also marks the end of Arabic erotological literature. While, as we have seen, the dawn of the genre is cloaked in mystery, its demise is less enigmatic, as it coincides with increasing Western influence on Muslim societies and, through missionary movements, the importation of a Western-style morality – Victorian or otherwise.

The authors' origins are also of interest, with seven of Persian origin, both geographically and linguistically, while one is Turkish. Secondly, although I have been referring to the 'Islamicness' of the works, this should be taken to refer to a broad cultural tradition that the authors were a part of, rather than to their religious affiliation, as five of them were Christians and three Jews. Finally, certain regions – Tunis and Iraq – were clearly dominant in terms of output, which may be explained by the importance of these two places as cultural centres during certain periods.

When East Meets West

We have seen that at least some of the works spread throughout the Arabic-speaking world, and sometimes even as far as Turkey. Thanks to the effects of Latin translation movement on Arabic works in the eleventh and twelfth centuries, the Arabic medical tradition (both original and borrowed from the Greeks) would go on to influence not only medicine in Christian Europe, but also its views on sexuality.[129]

Greek medicine arrived in medieval Europe either via translations into Latin from the Greek source texts, or via Arabic. The earliest results of the former activity emerged in the fourth and fifth centuries in North Africa,[130] where some of the works (including one on gynaecology) of Soranus of Ephesus (*fl.* 100)[131] were translated. Over the next few centuries, the centre of activity moved north across the Mediterranean, to Ravenna in northern Italy.[132]

But it was in the south of the country, in Salerno, which became a centre of medical training in the tenth century, that the first translations of Arabic medical works into Latin were carried out.[133] The protagonist was a Muslim convert from Carthage by the name of Constantine the African, who arrived in Salerno in 1077, but became associated with the monastery of Monte Cassino through the offices of Alphanus (d. 1085), the archbishop of Salerno and abbot of the monastery, who was also a physician.[134] Constantine had brought a number of manuscripts from his native land, and during his translation career he rendered some 20 Arabic works into Latin, often with the help of his assistant (and fellow Muslim convert), Johannes Afflacius. The first was the *Isagoge*, a translation of Ḥunayn (known in Latin as *Johannitius*) Ibn Isḥāq's *Masāʾil fī 'l-Ṭibb* ('Medical Questions'), an abridgement of an introduction to Galen's *Techne iatrike* ('The Art of Medicine'), known in Latin as *Tegni* (also *Ars parva* and *Ars medica*). The *Isagoge Ioannitii ad Tegni Galieni* ('Johannitius's Introduction to the Art of Galen'), to give it its full title, is the earliest known Latin translation of an Arabic medical text, and subsequently became the core of the *Articella*, a collection of medical writings on the basics of Hippocratic and Galenic medicine that would become a core textbook at medical schools across Europe for many centuries.[135] Constantine's translation of Ibn al-Jazzār's *Zād al-Musāfir* (*Viaticum peregrinantis*) and, especially, of al-Majūsī's *Kāmil* (*Liber Pantegni*)[136] gained equal authority and currency among students of medicine.

An additional avenue opened up in the twelfth century, at Toledo, where a circle of translators applied themselves to the rendering of Arabic scientific works – including many on medicine – into Latin.[137] The leading light in the Toledan group was the Italian-born Gerard of Cremona (d. 1187),[138] to whom over 70 translations in various fields were ascribed, among them Ibn Sīnā's *Qānūn* (*Canon Medicinae*)[139] and al-Rāzī's *Kitāb al-Manṣūrī*, the ninth book of which became particularly popular in the paraphrase by the founder of modern anatomy, Andreas Vesalius (1514–64), which was published in 1537.[140] The distribution of the new scientific output was further ensured through the foundation during the same period of medical faculties in a number of cities – including Montpellier, Paris, Bologna, Naples and Padua.[141]

With the translations of Arabic medical texts, their views (and knowledge) of sexuality – which, it is worth remembering, was routinely coupled with erotology – entered the consciousness and work of European scholars. This influence, which manifested itself in a number of guises, developed at an interesting time, when perceptions of sexuality could not have been more different between the Christian European West and the Muslim East. In the West, Christian dogma condemned all sexual activity that was extramarital and non-procreational. What is more, even if conception was the aim, taking pleasure in the act was considered sinful.[142] As we have seen, this attitude was completely absent from – and indeed alien to – the Islamic tradition and its treatment of sexuality. Equally significant was the gap in gynaecological knowledge between the two medical traditions.

The translations of Arabic medical works would profoundly alter the perceptions and study of sexuality and women's medicine. Firstly, Constantine's translation of al-Jazzār's *Zād al-Musāfir* included a lengthy section on sexual matters, including aphrodisiacs and contraceptives.[143] Another treatise ascribed to Constantine was *De Coitu* ('On Coitus'), which would inspire a number of homonymous works.[144] Another *De Coitu* was a thirteenth-century translation of Maimonides' *Fi 'l-Jimāᶜ* by John of Capua, an Italian Jewish convert, who also translated Maimonides' work on hygiene (*De regimine santitatis*)[145] and *Kitāb al-Taysīr fi 'l-Mudāwāt wa 'l-Tadbīr* ('Book of Simplification of Medication and Regimen') by the Andalusian physician Ibn Zuhr (Lat. *Avenzoar*, 1094–1162).[146]

In addition to translations, original work was soon produced dealing with all matters sexual in ways that would have been unthinkable prior to the introduction of the Arabic tradition. Two examples may be cited. The first is *Thesaurus Pauperum* by Peter of Spain (d. 1277), the future Pope XXI, who included a large number of fertility and contraception prescriptions, emmenagogues (some of them being abortifacients), and aphrodisiacs.[147] The second is a Catalan work, entitled *Speculum al foderi* ('A Mirror for Fuckers'), which bears a strong resemblance to some of the Arabic erotological works.[148] Of particular interest is the fact that, from the outset, the author acknowledges a debt to an Arabic original – which, however, would seem to be a fictional device intended either to absolve the author or to add authority to the content. Whatever the case may be, it highlights the reputation of Muslims in the field.

Another direct Arabic influence, in terms of both content and format, can be observed in the so-called 'Secrets' literature (*Secretum Secretorum*, Ar. *Sirr al-asrār*), which can be traced back to Aristotle's advice to princes, and is of course part of the 'Mirrors for Princes' tradition. Taking the form of a dialogue (usually between two clerics or a cleric and a layman), it discussed how men should behave with women, but also contained medical information, for instance on physiognomy and regimen. An offshoot of this genre was the 'Secrets of Women' literature, which provided some semblance of sexual education.[149]

By the end of the thirteenth century a profound change, driven by the 'new' Arabic tradition (especially Ibn Sīnā, whose *Canon* had become the standard reference), had taken place in female medicine, the understanding of the female body and, concurrently, the medical ideas of maleness and femaleness, as shown by the works of European doctors between the twelfth and fourteenth centuries.[150] Among them was a female doctor of the eleventh–twelfth century from Salerno, called Trotula – the first female professor of medicine, to whom a number of treatises have (spuriously) been ascribed that show a clear influence from Arabic medicine.[151] Though it would take a few more centuries before the anatomy of the female sexual organs would be described and their functions understood, this could not have happened without the impetus provided by the Arabic texts.

A related development was the upheaval in the perceptions of sexuality and eroticism. Here, too, there was an undeniable influence from Ibn Sīnā, in particular – not least in making 'Arabic erotic lore ... a component of the didactic message'.[152] Ibn Sīnā, in effect, paved the way for the emergence of an erotic art with a medical preoccupation – a science offering a way out of the religious constraints that had hampered any clear perception, let alone discussion, of sexual matters.

This resulted in a split between theology, with its focus on reproduction within a marital context, and medicine, within which the sexual act and experience became a physiological necessity that was both beneficial and pleasurable. As we have seen, the latter was a key component in Arabic sexology and erotology.

The new ideas on sexual positions and, more importantly, of pleasure during sex – most of them passed on in Ibn Sīnā's *Canon* – filtered through very early on into European writings, including literary texts, in troubadour poetics and Capellanus's *De Amore*.[153] The focus on the importance of female pleasure during coitus and the benefits of kissing was at the heart of another innovation attributable to the Arabic tradition: foreplay.[154]

In the area of medical terminology, too, the Arabic works made substantial contributions; Latin translators were forced to grapple with new concepts for which new terms had to be coined, necessitating a quest for precision. In the field of sexuality, a particularly apt example is the translation of the word 'clitoris' (Ar. *baẓr*), which had eluded even some of the Arabic physicians; it was translated by Constantine the African as *badedera* and by Gerard of Cremona as *batharum*.[155] Though neither of these withstood the test of time, others did, with research into terminology resulting in new insights into the human body.

Is there any evidence of Arabic erotological works (other than Maimonides' *De Coitu*) having travelled to the West? The simple answer would appear to be 'no'. However, the chronology provides some interesting clues. First, the period of the Latin translations coincides with considerable erotological output taking place in the Muslim world. Second, we know that a number of the works were widely disseminated. Third, it is hardly far-fetched to speculate that 'bestsellers' such as those by an al-Tīfāshī – who was active in Tunisia, which had significant trading links with Italian territories – would have found their way across the Mediterranean, together with other Arabic science manuscripts.

The influence of Arabic sexology and erotology would endure beyond the Middle Ages; as a way of presenting a 'carnal technique',[156] it is difficult to ignore its impact on the erotica of the Italian Renaissance, with authors like Pietro Aretino (1492–1556) – whose name lives on in one of the favourite topics in Arabic erotology: sexual positions (*modi*) – even though he merely wrote the sonnets accompanying the engravings by Marcantonio Raimondi (d. 1534).

CHAPTER TWO

The Author

The thirteenth century marks a dramatic turning point in Arab-Islamic history. It witnessed the end of the great ᶜAbbāsid caliphate, which had been founded by descendants of ᶜAbbās Ibn ᶜAbd al-Muṭṭalib, the Prophet's paternal uncle, in 750, following the defeat of the Umayyad dynasty that had succeeded the four 'Rightly-Guided Caliphs' (*al-khulafā' al-rāshidūn*), who were at the head of the Muslim community (*al-umma*) after the Prophet Muḥammad's demise in 632 AD. The period of the ᶜAbbāsid caliphate, which soon after its establishment moved the centre of power from Damascus to Baghdad, built by al-Manṣūr (754–75), is commonly considered the Golden Age of Islam, during which culture, literature, philosophy and the sciences flourished.

That is not to say that the ᶜAbbāsid caliphate constituted a monolithic empire between 750 and 1258, or that its cultural and scientific advances continued with unabated vigour throughout its reign. Relatively early on, ᶜAbbāsid dominion was successfully challenged across its expansive empire, with the creation of several powerful dynasties, such as the Fatimids (in northern Africa, including Egypt) and the Seljuqs (in Persia and Central Asia).[157]

It was in the Seljuq-controlled Tus (Ṭūs)[158] – close to Meshed in Khorasan province (northeastern Iran), high in the valley of the Kashaf River – that Abū Jaᶜfar Naṣīr (also sometimes Nāṣir) al-Dīn Muḥammad Ibn Muḥammad Ibn al-Ḥasan al-Ṭūsī (al-Shīᶜī), usually known as Naṣīr al-Dīn al-Ṭūsī[159], was born on 11 Jumādā I 597 AH (17 February 1201).[160]

The name of Tus was famous in Arab history as the place where Hārūn al-Rashīd died, though it was eclipsed in importance by the much more famous Nishapur, which had been the capital of the Seljuq dynasty. In the year of al-Ṭūsī's birth, the city was going through a particularly difficult time. Less than a year before it had been a victim in the struggle between the Khwarezmid dynasty (which ruled Tus) and the Ghūrid empire, which conquered Khorasan. In the process, Tus was besieged and, after surrendering, sacked.

Al-Ṭūsī received his early education under his father's guidance in his native area, and at first focused on the Arabic language and religion, as was common for all scholars of the age. He concentrated in particular on Imāmism, the largest branch of Shīᶜa Islam, followers of which are also known as 'Twelvers', in reference to their belief in 12 divinely decreed leaders (imams). In his early teens, he left for Nishapur, which was a centre for medicine, and was instructed in mathematics, philosophy, natural science and medicine by former pupils of two of the most famous scholars in the whole of Muslim history – al-Rāzī and Ibn Sīnā.

It was during al-Ṭūsī's stay in Nishapur that he acquired first-hand experience with those who would eventually destroy Baghdad and establish an empire that stretched across the whole of Asia – the Mongols – when their forces, headed by Genghis Khan's generals Jebe and Sübetey, arrived in the city. As we shall see, this was not the last time that al-Ṭūsī would have direct contact with the Mongols.

After Nishapur, al-Ṭūsī travelled to Iraq, where he completed his training in Islamic (Shīᶜī) jurisprudence, followed by mathematics and astronomy in Mosul. In 1233, he went to Sartakht, in Persia's southwest Khuzistan province, and joined the court of the Ismaili governor Muᶜtaṣam Nāṣir al-Dīn ᶜAbd al-Raḥīm Ibn Abī Manṣūr. It was here that he would start composing his first major works, among them a treatise on ethics, titled *Akhlāq-i Nāṣirī* ('Nāṣirī Ethics'), in honour of his patron, and an autobiography, *Sayr wa-sulūk* ('The Path and Behaviour'), which outlines his spiritual journey towards Ismāᶜīlī esoteric philosophy.

In the mid-1240s, al-Ṭūsī appeared in Alamūt – the stronghold of the Ismaili community of the Assassins (*ḥashāshīn*) in the Alburz mountains of northern Iran that had been founded by Ḥasan al-Ṣabāḥ (d. 1124). The reasons behind his journey remain open to debate, but al-Ṭūsī ended up staying there for two decades, and in 1255 was sent to Hulago, the Mongol khan, who was about to attack Persia. The Assassin fortress fell to the Mongols a year later, as they swept through the region and headed west towards Baghdad. Al-Ṭūsī joined Hulagu's entourage on his campaigns, and was present at the capture of the capital of the Sunni caliphate – and the murder of the caliph – in February 1258. Al-Ṭūsī enjoyed the favour of the Mongol ruler, and it was thanks to the scholar that many of the Shīʿī sanctuaries were spared destruction. However, even before the sacking of Baghdad, al-Ṭūsī had been given a number of official duties, including those of court astrologer, and was put in charge of the religious endowments (*waqf*) and finances – duties he continued to discharge under Hulagu's son and successor, Ābāqā (1265–82).

In 1259, al-Ṭūsī oversaw the construction of an observatory (*raṣadkhāneh*) in Marāgha (currently in Iran's East Azerbaijan Province), which Hulagu had made his capital. The observatory, which also comprised a large library and school, became a hugely important scientific institution and centre of learning that attracted many leading scholars of the day, including Chinese astronomers. In addition to heading the observatory, al-Ṭūsī compiled astronomical tables (*al-Zīj al-Īlkhānī*, 'Ilkhanate Tables') for calculating the positions of the planets. Astronomy earned him great fame for many centuries to come, as did his work on planetary theory, which would later inform the work of Copernicus and others. Extracts of the tables were translated into Latin by John Greaves (1602–52), who was then the Savilian professor of astronomy at Oxford, as well as an accomplished Arabic and Persian scholar. The text was published in 1648, together with the astronomical and chronological tables of Timurid scholar-sultan Ulugh Beg (1394–1449).[161] Although the observatory was short-lived (it remained in operation for about 50 years), it would have a large impact on astronomy in both China and Europe in subsequent centuries.

Shortly before his death, al-Ṭūsī left Marāgha for Baghdad, and died a few months later, on 18 Dhū 'l-Ḥijja 672 AH (25 June 1274), at the age of 72, in Kadhimain. His body was laid to rest near the tomb of Mūsā al-Kāẓim (744–99 AD), the seventh of the Twelve Imams (and son of the sixth, Jaᶜfar al-Ṣādiq).

A prolific polymath, al-Ṭūsī, who has been called the most important Shīᶜī scholar of his age, built up a huge oeuvre (in excess of 150 works in both Arabic and Persian) across a wide range of fields, including mathematics, physics, geometry, mineralogy, astronomy, medicine, philosophy, ethics, mysticism and Islamic law (*fiqh*). In addition to composing original works, he prepared editions and wrote commentaries on Greek and Arabic mathematical works (including Euclid, Archimedes and Thābit Ibn Qurra), which became crucial resources in the spread of the Greek sciences in the Muslim world.

In the field of medicine, al-Ṭūsī wrote three other works besides the one treated here: *Qawānīn al-ṭibb* ('Medical Regulations');[162] *al-Risāla al-dhahabiyya fī tadbīr ḥifẓ al-ṣiḥḥa* ('Golden Treatise on the Regimen of Health');[163] and *Sharḥ qawl al-shaykh al-ra'īs anna 'l-ḥarāra tafᶜalu fī 'l-raṭab sawādan wa fī ḍiddihi bayāḍan* ('Commentary on the Statement by the Great Master [Ibn Sīnā] that Heat Causes Blackness in Moistness and Whiteness in the Opposite').[164]

Al-Ṭūsī's reputation spread very quickly throughout Islamic territories, and his commentary on Ibn Sīnā's *Kitāb al-ishārāt wa-l-tanbīhāt* ('Book of Hints and Pointers'), entitled *Ḥall mushkilāt al-ishārāt* ('The Solution to the Problems in the

Ishārāt'), was singled out for praise by none other than the Tunisian historian Ibn Khaldūn (1332–1406), who applied the Qur'ānic verse (XII, 76) *wa fawqa kulli dhī ᶜilmin ᶜalīmun* ('and over every lord of knowledge there is one more knowing') when comparing al-Ṭūsī's work to that of others.[165]

Later on, others bestowed equally grand epithets on the Persian scholar, such as 'the teacher of mankind' (*ustādh al-bashar*), 'the third teacher' (*al-muᶜallim al-thālith*) – the other two being Aristotle and the philosopher al-Fārābī (d. 950) – or, simply, *al-khwāja* ('Master').[166]

CHAPTER THREE

The Sultan's Potions

Contents and Structure

The text translated here was the only book written on the subject by al-Ṭūsī, and is modest in its aims inasmuch as it treats only aphrodisiacs. The title, *Kitāb albāb al-Bāhiyya wa 'l-tarākīb al-sultāniyya*, literally translates as 'The Book of Choice Sexual Stimulants and the Sultan's Mixtures'.[167] Dedicating the text to 'the Sultan of Qāzān' (Ābāqā Khan), al-Ṭūsī mentions that the book was written at the Sultan's request, since he had a child suffering from paraplegia. The link between the child's illness and a book on aphrodisiacs remains unexplained, however.

As for the intended readership, the author recommends his treatise as a self-study manual, as 'Anyone reading this treatise will no longer need a physician for medical treatment as it contains all the reader requires to treat ailments and diseases.' In the introduction the author states that the book is a compendium of existing knowledge, which raises the question of sources. In addition to Greek authors (Galen, Hippocrates, Aristotle), the only Arabic physician named is al-Rāzī, whereas the author's Shīᶜa affiliations are revealed by a quote from ᶜAlī Ibn Abī Ṭālib. Other sources are referred to, simply, as 'past scholars'. In none of these cases, however, is there a mention of the works from which the information was allegedly culled.

Despite its declared focus on aphrodisiacs, the treatise touches upon many of the topics addressed in erotological literature, and may therefore be put at the scientific/medical end of the continuum discussed in Chapter 1, above. Like other works in this category, it combines the fields of medicine, dietetics, hygiene and erotology, but is devoid of anecdotes, poetry and stories intended for titillation. The author's approach appears by then to have become firmly established, as it is shared by many other authors.

The text comprises an introduction and 18 chapters of uneven length, with some very brief ones alternating with more extensive ones. As is customary for many manuals of the period, the introduction outlines the reason for writing the treatise and the author's expert credentials in the field. It also provides a table of contents, which includes not only the titles of the chapters (or variants thereof) but also a brief description of their contents. This is followed by general information on key medical concepts – such as sperm, and the need, lawfulness and advantages of coitus, as well as the best seasons to engage in it. While there is 'no greater human pleasure than that of sexual intercourse', the author warns against excess, as this reduces innate heat. This was in line with the prevailing (Galenic) orthodoxy that frequent ejaculation resulted in a loss of *pneuma* (Ar. *rūḥ*) and its vitalizing power.

Chapter 1 addresses the link between sexual potency and lust for coitus on the one hand, and physiognomy and the individual's temperament, on the other. At the top end of the scale, it appears, are those with coloured skins, as well as some with white skins, though another section of the latter are incapable of having sex. This leads to a discussion of the reasons for the weakness of organs (including, of course, the penis), including descriptions of the symptoms and how each of them can be treated through syrups, electuaries and broths. The author identifies four *loci* which, when afflicted with weakness, cause limpness in the body's organs: the brain, heart, liver, penis and testicles. As for the weakness in the (male) genitals, this can be due to one of three factors: innateness, excess intercourse from an early age, or being over the age of 40. Despite the author's claim that the book purports to be a compendium, the information is sometimes tantalizingly compressed; the author refers, for instance, to a multitude of benefits for this or that concoction (for example, musk and spikenard electuaries) but omits them in order to restrict the size of the treatise.

Chapters 2 and 3 list simple foodstuffs that are used to increase libido and potency, whereas Chapter 4 concentrates on 'compounds' that serve the same purpose, in addition to restoring temperament imbalances and increasing innate heat. The various concoctions, ingredients and cooking methods are given in detail, including instructions on when to eat them. When it comes to their effects, hyperbole is never far away; the reader is advised that taking this or that dish will enhance his stamina to the extent that he is able to pleasure ten women every night!

The following three chapters plough the same general furrow, outlining syrups, electuaries and stomachics that, in addition to acting as aphrodisiacs, restore the temperament and purify the blood (Chapter 5); strengthen various organs, remove excess humours and open up blockages (Chapter 6); and eliminate various qualities and humours (Chapter 7). Enemas intended to increase potency, as well as remedying colic and back weakness, constitute the object of Chapter 8. Chapter 9 discusses the types of clothing fabric that should be worn in each of the seasons, and how they assist in preventing illness.

Chapter 10 devotes attention to the sexual positions that are to be preferred, which ones to avoid, and the possible harmful effects they may cause. The next four chapters are squarely phallocentric, enumerating ointments to be rubbed on the penis to stiffen and lengthen it (Chapters 11 and 12); or in between the fingers and toes in order to maintain an erection, even after having intercourse with ten women (Chapter 13).

Moving on from the question of penile prowess, Chapter 14 contains recipes for pleasure and potency enhancing pills. In Chapter 15, the woman is brought into the equation, with suggestions for various concoctions to ensure ecstasy during coitus for both partners. Chapter 16 turns its attention to the woman, albeit from the man's point of view, offering recipes aimed at narrowing the vagina and 'restoring' it to that of a virgin, which was in keeping with the prevailing – and religiously endorsed – gender orthodoxy. As well as suggesting potions for this same purpose, the final chapters provide recipes for concoctions for the purposes of contraception (Chapter 17) and conception; interestingly, the former recipe has gall as its main component, and the latter musk, which was also considered a highly potent aphrodisiac.

It is striking that the potions, drugs and therapies are 'gendered' in that they are mainly aimed at improving the man's coital performance and experience, while there is a focus on frequency of intercourse and penile strength. Coitus within marriage is conspicuous by its absence, as the sexual partners referred to are generally hierarchically inferior (servants) – which, as we have seen, is a prominent feature of both erotological and erotic literature.

How innovative was al-Ṭūsī? What was his influence, if any, on the genre and subsequent works? While some elements are similar to those of other treatises, others are peculiar to al-Ṭūsī. We have seen that the work was translated into Persian and Turkish, and this would suggest that it was held in high esteem, if only because of the reputation of its author – which he himself expounds upon at length at the beginning of his book, referring to himself as the '*shaykh* of the world', the 'king of scholars' and the 'teacher of scholars of all time'! It is therefore surprising to note that the extant erotological works do not contain any mention of the treatise or seem to have availed themselves of al-Ṭūsī's contribution. But it would be rash to exclude the possibility that he had any influence on the field, and a more detailed study of the erotological corpus will undoubtedly uncover new insights in this respect.

The Manuscripts

No autograph copy of the text is known to have survived. This critical edition is based on three manuscript copies, which are discussed below. It should be added that there is a fourth known manuscript of the text (Istanbul, Shahid Ali No 1/2068)[168] – which, however, had to be set aside in preparing this edition, since it has not been possible to consult it.

1. Berlin Staatsbibliothek 6383; dated 1208/1793; 35 folios (68pp), each counting 15 lines. This is the oldest surviving manuscript of al-Ṭūsī's treatise. Although the copyist is not mentioned in al-Ṭūsī's text, the name of Muṣṭtafā al-Kaftānī is included at the end of the second medical manuscript (an untitled translation of an anonymous Turkish treatise)[169] with which it is bound, and which bears the same date. The oriental *naskh* script of both texts is clearly identical, and thus one may confidently state that the same copyist also produced this version of al-Ṭūsī's text. The Berlin manuscript contains a number of errors, marginal additions and corrections (indicated in the Arabic and English texts by braces). Many of the errors involve interference from Egyptian Colloquial Arabic: *tānī* (for *thānī*), *kurrāt* (for *kurrāth*), *birisht, qizāz* (CA *zujāj*), *shuwayya* (CA *qalīl*), the consistent use of 'd' for 'dh' (for example, *idkhir/idhkir; yūkhad, aghdiyya, dālika/dhālika, sādaj/sādhaj*), *dīb* (CA *dhi'b*). In addition, there are also numerous misspellings: for example, *yaḥtarir* (*yaḥtariz*), *alif maqṣūra* (instead of *yā'*), and vice versa (for example, *ᶜalī* for *ᶜalā*),

omissions of hamza (for example, *ḥukamā*[ʾ], *mar*[ʾ]*a*, *al-māb*[*maʾāb*]), dotted *yāʾ* with superscript hamza, *yāʾ* for hamza, undotted *tāʾ marbūṭa*; *bāliᶜ* (for *bāligh*), *ḥawz* (for *jawz*), *jawz al-hindī* (for *al-jawz al-hindī*), *takhtaṭā* (for *takhtaliṭu*), *marr* (*marra*), *maṣṭilā* (for *maṣṭikā*), *ḥalwā* (for *ḥalwa*). There are frequent grammatical inconsistencies and mistakes, with errors in number agreement (for example, *al-adwiyat ... qawāmuhum*), dialectal clipping of the third person plural ending to *-ū* (CA of *-ūna*), and erratic alternation between verbs in third person plural, third person singular and second person singular, as well as between perfect and imperfect tenses. As it is the oldest and most complete of the three manuscripts, it has been chosen for the critical edition, which is represented here without emendations.[170] This manuscript is referred to as [A] in the present edition.[171] The page numbers in the English translation also refer to it.

2. Glasgow University, MS Hunter 144.4 (T.7.3), 11 folios (22pp), 27 lines per page. The manuscript is the fourth in a bound collection including three other treatises on medicine. The first is a commentary by Muḥammad al-ᶜAskarī, entitled *Ḥall al-Mūjiz* ('Solution of the Abridgement'), on the abridgement of Ibn Sīnā's *Qānūn* (*Mūjiz al-Qānūn*), composed by the Syrian physician Ibn al-Nafīs (d. 1288). The second is an Arabic translation of the famous epitome of the *Qānūn*, entitled *al-Qānūnja*, by the fourteenth-century Persian physician Maḥmūd Ibn Muḥammad Ibn ᶜUmar al-Jaghmīnī.[172] The third is

an Arabic translation of an (anonymous) Turkish work on colds (*Risālat al-Nāzila*). The Glasgow manuscript, whose date, copyist and origin are unknown, was copied in a tighter Farsi *nasta*ᶜ*līq* hand. It is almost identical with [A], save for a few minor variations and omissions. One may conjecture that it was copied after [A], which may have served as the original. It has far fewer language errors than [A]. The manuscript is referred to as [B] in the present edition.

3. Cairo, Dār al-Kutub, *Ṭibb* 582; dated 18 Rabīᶜ I 1224/03.05.1809; 11ff (20pp), 19 lines per page. This manuscript is incomplete, and is also the most recent. It is unclear whether it was copied from any of the others, and thus significantly emendated and/or poorly copied, or whether it should be traced back to another, hitherto unknown copy. Some of the passages are completed in the margin. In addition to substantive omissions, which include an entire chapter (4), there are a number of errors, many of which are 'Egyptianisms' (for example, final *–yā'* for *alif maqṣūra*). This manuscript is referred to as [C] in the present edition.

Notes

1. al-Nafzāwī n.d.: 28.
2. al-Nafzāwī (J. Colville trans.) 1999: 33.
3. al-Nafzāwī (R. Burton trans.) 1886: 34.
4. The passage is as follows in the original:

   > Et, lorsque la cessation de la jouissance aura mis un terme à vos ébats amoureux, gardez-vous de vous lever brusquement, mais restez près de la femme, couchez-vous sur le côté droit dans le lit témoin de vos plaisirs et retirez votre membre avec précaution; car c'est en agissant ainsi que vous trouverez le bien, et vous ne serez pas comme celui qui monte sur la femme ainsi qu'un mulet, sans avoir égard aux vrais principes de l'art, et qui, dès qu'il a éjaculé, s'empresse de se relever en retirant son membre. Une telle manière d'agir doit être écartée, car elle ne peut qu'éloigner tout bien des femmes. En résumé, il appartient au véritable amateur du coït de n'omettre aucune de mes recommandations; car, c'est de leur observation que résulte le bonheur de la femme, et ces règles comprennent tout ce qui convient en pareille matière. Dieu a tout fait pour le bien!

   Mohamed Lasly, ed., *Le jardin parfumé*, Paris: Philippe Picquier, 2002, pp. 155–6. The earliest preserved French translation dates from 1848 (mss Paris BN SG MS8-60 [1336]).
5. For background and a discussion of this term, which is often used in conjuncture with 'foreignization' and 'domestication' of the source text, see L. Venuti, *The Translator's Invisibility: A History of Translation*, London: Routledge, 1995.
6. Burton 1885–89: X, 173ff.
7. Ibid.: 205.
8. Ibid.: 206ff.
9. This term is used in preference to others, such as 'Arab' or 'Islamic', as the former would imply that the authors involved were ethnically Arabs, which was not the case. The term 'Islamicate' was coined by Michael Hodgson (1977: 59), who reserved 'Islamic' for 'pertaining to Islam *in the proper, the religious, sense*' (emphasis in the original), with 'Islamicate' referring 'not directly to the religion, Islam, itself, but to the social and cultural complex historically associated with Islam and the Muslims, both among Muslims

themselves and even when found among non-Muslims'.

10. Ṣ. al-Munajjid 1957, 1969, 1975; M. ᶜAbd al-Wāḥīd 1961; Y. El-Masri 1962; G. H. Bousquet 1966; R. Devereux 1966; L. Giffen 1971; A. Bouhdiba 1975; A. L. Al-Sayyid-Marsot 1979; B. Musallam 1983; D. Ze'evi 2006. To these, one may also add the 'popularizing' works on the subject by Malek Chebel (1984, 1986, 1988, 1995, 2004, 2006).
11. Rosenthal 1978; S. Murray and W. Roscoe 1979; A. Abu Khalil 1993; B. Nathan 1994; J. Wright and E. Rowson 1997; J. Dakhlia 2007; K. El-Rouayheb 2005; E. Rowson 1991b, 1997, 2003, 2004, 2006, 2008; P. Steckler 2007–8. Most of these centre on male homosexuality, with lesbianism being the focus in H. Samar 2007 and S. Amar 2009. An Iranian perspective on the issue is offered by A. Najmabadi 2005.
12. M. Cervulle 2008, 2009; M. Ghoussoub and E. Sinclair-Webb 2000; F. Lagrange 2000; O. Lahoucine 2006; A. Schmitt and J. Sofer 1992; M. Schildt 1988.
13. S. Amar, 'Cross-Dressing and Female Same-Sex Marriage in Medieval French and Arabic Literatures', in K. Babayan and A. Najmabadi 2008; E. Rowson 1991a.
14. P. Saunders 1991.
15. U. Wikan 1977 (in present-day Oman).
16. K. Ali 2006; N. J. Coulson, 'Regulation of Sexual Behavior under Traditional Islamic Law', in A. L. Al-Sayyid-Marsot 1979: 63–8. In this area, too, homosexuality has received a great deal of attention: H. El Menyawi; A. Shalakany 2008; S. Yep 2012; A. Schmitt 2001–2.
17. D. Hopwood 1999.
18. For a discussion, see J. Massad 2002.
19. This is the case, for instance, for a chapter on homosexuality and the reasons why some men prefer sexual intercourse with teenage boys to women in al-Isrā'īlī's *Nuzhat al-aṣḥāb fī muᶜāshirat al-aḥbāb* ('A Jaunt amidst Lovers' Copulation'): 2007: 49. A few pages down, the word *nayk* ('fucking') is emendated, while a footnote states: 'A word meaning "sexual intercourse", which we have preferred not to mention' (52).
20. J. Jumᶜa, ed., *al-Nuṣūṣ al-muḥarrama*, Beirut: Riad El-Rayyes, 1994.
21. For instance, al-Tīfāshī's *Tuḥfat al-albāb fīmā lā jūjad fī kitāb*, whose (abridged) English translation (Edward A. Lacey, *The Delight of Hearts: Or, What You Will Not Find in Any Book,* Los Angeles: Gay Sunshine Press, 1988) is based on the French text (R. Khawam, *Les délices des coeurs*, Paris: Jérôme Martineau, 1971; rev. eds, Paris: Phébus, 1981, 1988), rather than on the original Arabic.
22. al-Shayzarī, *Rawḍat al-qulūb wa nuzhat al-muḥibb wa 'l-maḥbūb*, ed. David Semah and George J. Kanazi, Wiesbaden: Otto Harrassowitz, 2003. See also D. Semakh, '*Rawḍat al-Qulūb* by al-Shayzarī: A Twelfth-Century Book on Love', Arabica 24 (1997): 187–206.
23. See also EI^2, s.v. 'muḳawwiyāt' (F. Sanagustin).
24. For an overview of Islamic medicine, see P. Pormann and E. Savage-Smith 2007.
25. The 'Compendium' was first translated into Latin as *Liber Continens* by the

Jewish physician and translator Faraj Ibn Sālim (Lat.: *Farraguth*) for King Charles of Anjou (1226–85) in the last quarter of the thirteenth century. It was printed for the first time in 1515, in Lyon.

26. *EI*[2], s.v. 'Ibn al-Ḳuff' (S. H. Hamarneh). For the part dealing with simple drugs, see H. G. Kircher 1967.
27. It was first translated into Latin in the thirteenth century, by the already-mentioned Farraguth, and published in 1531 as *Tacuinum Sanitatis* (Strassburg: J. Schott). It was a key medical text in Europe for many centuries.
28. cf. I. Perho 1995; F. Rahman 1989; W. Rasslan 1934; ᶜA. al-Sharīf 1990. On sexuality in this literature, see U. Weisser 1983; J. Bummel 1999.
29. al-Suyūṭī n.d.: 24–6, 159–67 (recipes of various aphrodisiacal electuaries).
30. See R. Serjeant 1965; O. Spies 1969.
31. See Madelain Farah (trans.), *Marriage and Sexuality in Islam: A Translation of Al-Ghazali's Book on the Etiquette of Marriage from the Ihya ᶜulūm al-dīn*, Salt Lake City, UT: University of Utah Press, 1986. Extracts from the erotological sections were also published separately, in *al-Jins ᶜinda 'l-ᶜArab*, vol. 3, 127–47.
32. The whole of Book 6 is devoted to the subject (see G. Bos 1997).
33. G. Bos [al-Jazzār] 1992: 23–7.
34. O. Kahl 2003.
35. For a discussion, see B. Musallam 1983; A. Bouhdiba 1975 (esp. 143ff); *EI*[2], s.v. 'ᶜazl' (G. H. Bousquet).
36. See *EI*[2], s.vv. 'bāh' (G. H. Bousquet), 'djins' (Ch. Pellat), 'nikāḥ' (J. Schacht et al.); 'zinā' (R. Peters); E. Lane 1863–74: I, 315; IV, 451; VIII, 102; al-Suyūṭī 2001: 119ff.
37. Ze'ev 2006: 16.
38. See for example J. C. Bürgel, 'Love, Lust and Longing: Eroticism in Early Islam as Reflected in Literary Sources', in A. al-Sayyid-Marsot 1977: 81–117.
39. See *EI*[2], s.v. 'djins' (C. Pellat).
40. See list at the end of the Introduction.
41. Ibn al-Nadim 1871–72: II, 306 (trans. II, 719–23) – 51 entries.
42. Ibid.: 307 (trans. II, 721) – 12 entries.
43. Ibid.: 306–7 (trans. II, 720–1) – 28 entries.
44. Ibid.: 307–8 (trans. II, 722–3) – 38 entries.
45. For the introduction of Rufus's works in Islamic medicine, see *GAS*, III: 64–8; M. Ullmann 1970: 71–6; *EI*[2], s.v. 'Rūfūs al-Afsīsī' (M. Ullmann). Ibn Lūqā 1974: 26 (trans. 34); 1973: 43 (trans. 29), 47 (trans. 31). For one of Ibn Lūqā's translations of Rufus, see Hakim Syed Zillur Rahman, ed., *Risalah al Nabidh' of Rufus by Qusta bin Luqa*, Aligarh: Ibn Sina Academy of Medieval Medicine and Sciences, 2007.
46. For the introduction of Galenic works in Islamic medicine, see M. Ullmann 1970: 35ff; *GAS*, III, 274ff; *EI*[2], s.v. 'Djālīnūs (R. Walzer).
47. For an overview and key bibliography, see *EI*[2], s.v. 'Arisṭūṭālīs or Arisṭū' (R. Walzer).
48. For Hipocrates in the Arabic tradition, see M. Ullmann 1970: 25–35; *GAS*, III, 23–47; *EI*[2], s.v. 'Buḳrāṭ' (A. Dietrich).
49. See D. Gutas 1998; R. Walzer 1962; D. Jacquart and F. Michaud 1990: 32–

3. For the developments in literature, see J. Ashtiany et al. 1990.

50. *EI*[2], s.vv. 'Ḥunayn b. Isḥāḳ al-ʿIbādī' and 'Isḥāḳ b. Ḥunayn' (G. Strohmaier). For Ḥunayn's biography, see G. Bergstrasser, 'Hunain ibn Ishaq, Über die syrischen und arabischen Galen-Übersetzungen', *Abhandlungen für die Kunde des Morgenlandes* XVII: 2 (1925), XIX: 2 (1932).
51. *EI*[2], s.v. 'Ibn Māsawayh' (J.-C. Vadet).
52. On Ibn Bukhtīshūʿ and his family, see *EI*[2], s.v. 'Bukhtīshūʿ' (D. Sourdel); A. Contadini, *A World of Beasts: A Thirteenth-Century Illustrated Arabic Book on Animals (the Kitāb Naʿt al-Ḥayawān) in the Ibn Bakhtīshūʿ Tradition*, Leiden: Brill, 2012.
53. *EI*[2], s.v. 'Djālīnūs (R. Walzer).
54. This work consists of 38 chapters each dealing with a particular medical subject in the form of questions and answers. Chapter X had previously inspired an earlier translation/adaptation by the physician Thābit Ibn Qurra (Chapter X), whereas Ibn Māssa (1971: 33–4) used Chapter IV (No. 31). For a discussion, see R. Kruk 1976.
55. P. Pormann and E. Savage-Smith 2007: 105–8.
56. al-Kātib 1977: 334ff.
57. See H. N. Parker 1992: 92.
58. Ibid.
59. Ibid.: 100.
60. For more details, see, for example: Dols 1984: 3–24; P. Pormann and E. Savage-Smith 2007: 41ff; M. Ullmann 1970: 97–100, 108–84; M. Green 1985: 323–7; Ibn Sīnā 1999: I, 28–35.
61. The theory was also an integral part of prophetic medicine; see, for example, al-Suyūṭī n.d.: 2–5.
62. Adapted from www.calvin.edu/academic/medieval/medicine/overview/overview.htm.
63. See Ibn Sīnā 1999: I, 19–23; R. M. Stelmack and A. Stalikas, 'Galen and the Humour Theory of Temperament', *Personality and Individual Differences* 12: 3 (1991), pp. 255–63.
64. D. Jacquart and C. Thomasset 1988: 36ff.
65. For a discussion of the Galenic view on sexual differences between men and women, see for example Gadelrab 2010, and M. Levey and S. Souryal, 'Galen's On the Secrets of Women and on the Secrets of Men: A Contribution to the History of Arabic Pharmacology,' *Janus* 55 (1968), pp. 208–19.
66. M. Ullmann 1978: 23–4.
67. G. Bos 1997: 135 (trans. 266) – Ibn Māsawayh; 136 (trans. 267) – Isḥāq ibn ʿImrān.
68. Ibid., 138 (trans. 267).
69. al-Jāḥiẓ 1938: VII, 226. See also, in the same work: II, 216 (wolves and dogs), V, 218–19 (on birds); and al-Kātib 1977: 365ff.
70. Ibid.: VII, 29.
71. Abū Tammām, *Diwan*, 172, 11.
72. Ibn al-Jawzī 1902: 142.
73. Ibn al-Nadīm 1871–72: II, 303.
74. Ibn Abī Uṣaybiʿa 1882: I, 34, 69.

75. Abū 'l-Hasan al-Kātib 1977: 216, 229, 251, 332ff, 370; 2002: 23, 29.
76. al-Tīfāshī 1892: 64; S. al-Munajjid 1975: 154–5; al-Kātib 1977: 75.
77. See P. Pormann and E. Savage-Smith 2007: 21–3; M. Meyerhof, 'On the Transmission of Greek and Indian Science to the Arabs', *Islamic Culture*, 1937, 11, pp. 17–29; *GAS*, III, 191ff. The traditional view regarding the importance of Gondēshāpūr (a former city in southwestern Iran) as a centre for medical care (including a hospital), training and scholarship has recently been called into question on the grounds that the earliest report on the hospital dates from the thirteenth century, in the work of the Egyptian historian al-Qifṭī. Even if this is true, the reputation of the town as a medical centre is less uncertain, as it is already referred to in the ninth century, by al-Jāḥiẓ. See *EI*[2], s.v. 'Gondēshāpūr' (Cl. Huart-Aydin Sayili); P. Pormann and E. Savage-Smith 2007: 20–1; M. Dols 1984: 5–6; R. Serjeant 1997: 86.
78. C. Storey 1972: 321–322.
79. Ibn Qutayba 1925–30: I, 24–5, 27–8, 30.
80. Ibn al-Nadīm 1871–72: II, 303.
81. The whole of Chapter XII is devoted to Indian physicians.
82. Ibn al-Nadīm (trans. B. Dodge) 1970: II, 738; *GAS*: III, 193–6.
83. al-Rāzī 1955–68: III, 210; V, 179; VI, 30, 47, 214; VIII, 205, X, 18, 133, 331; XII, 219.
84. Ibn al- Nadīm 1871–72: II, 245, 303.
85. vide post.
86. al-Tīfāshī 1970: 13ff (trans. 27ff) vs Ibn Sīnā (Cairo 519, fol. 5b).
87. For instance, Ibn al-Jazzār mentions a decoction of roots created by Ibn Māsawayh (G. Bos 1997: 135 – trans.: 266) and a powder composed by Isḥāq ibn ᶜImrān (ibid.: 136 – trans.: 267).
88. al-Tīfāshī 1892: 76ff/Deli Birader [S. Kuru 2000]: 208ff/al-Kātib 2002: 105ff – trans. 299ff (anal intercourse positions); A. Nuwās 1994: 71 (trans. P. Kenney 2005: 40–2)/Deli Birader [S. Kuru 2000]: 193; al-Tīfāshī 1992: 207ff./Deli Birader [S. Kuru 2000]: 202ff/al-Kātib 1977: 323ff (homosexual prowler).
89. al-Kātib 1977: 57, 330, 331.
90. Gotha 105; Gotha 124; Dresden 172.
91. For example, Bodleian 1622.
92. The most famous of his works is *Lawᶜat al-shākī wa damᶜat al-bākī* ('The Anxiety of the Complaining Lover and the Tears of the Weeper'). ᶜU. al-Kaḥḥāla n.d.: IV, 113; XIII, 385; *EI*[1], s.v. 'al-Ṣafadī' (F. Krenkow); *EI*[2], 'al-Ṣafadī' (F. Rosenthal); *GAL* II: 39–41, *GALS* II: 27–9.
93. *EI*[2], s.v. 'al-Ḥillī' (W. P. Heinrichs). His works include *Risālat al-ashwāq fīmā yataᶜalliqu bi 'l-ᶜushshāq* ('Treatise on Longings Connected with Lovers') – e.g. BN 3074.
94. *EI*[2], s.v. 'al-Nawādjī' (I. Kratschkowsky). He is most famous for his anthologies of erotic poetry, especially related to the love of boys, for example, *Khalᶜa ᶜidhār fī waṣf al-ᶜidhār* ('Throwing Off All Restraint in the Description of the First Growth of Beard' (BN3041), and *Kitāb ṣaḥā'if al-ḥasanāt* (BN 3041).
95. Al-Kātib 1977: 35.

96. Ibid.: 36.
97. D. Jacquart and C. Thomasset 1988: 126.
98. M. Foucault 1978–90: II, 50; H. N. Parker 1992: 98.
99. For example, Ibn Sīnā 1999: II, 746–7 (penis size), 746 (hermaphroditism), 730–1 (impotence), 728–9 (benefits of coitus), 744–5 (priapism), 745–6 (*ubna*), 745 (ʿ*udhaywiṭ*, involving orgasm-induced defecation).
100. M. Foucault 1978–90: II, 4.
101. Ibid.: I, 11.
102. al-Ghazlāwī (BN 3069): 1.
103. Ibn Sīnā 1999: II, 746.
104. H. N. Parker 1992: 96–7.
105. See, for example, the stories in al-Tīfāshī 1892: 70–9; al-Nafzāwī n.d.: 55–6, 45–50. See also Gadelrab 2010.
106. For example, Fatima Mernissi, 'The Muslim Concept of Active Female Sexuality,' *Women and Sexuality in Medieval Societies* (Istanbul: Women for Women's Rights/Kadinin Insan Haklan Projesi, 2000), pp. 19–35.
107. al-Jāḥiẓ 1938: I, 370–2; II, 203–4; IV, 117–18; al-Tīfāshī 1892: 90 (story of a woman having sex with a donkey), 92 (about a woman and a bear).
108. M. Foucault 1978–90: II, 92.
109. H, N. Parker 1992: 91, 98.
110. M. Foucault 1978–90: II, 25.
111. Ibid.: II, 25–6.
112. al-Tīfāshī 1892: 2.
113. Qur'ān, VII, 80, 81; XXVI, 165–8; XXVII, 54–6; XXIX, 28–9.
114. The usual contemporary term, *mithlī*, is a late-twentieth-century neologism.
115. For a full discussion, see K. El Rouayheb 2005.
116. See *EI*², s.v. 'liwāṭ' (ed.). For discussion of the views on male homosexuality in Islamic jurisprudence, see A. Schmidt 2001–2; Shalakany 2008.
117. The same was true in ancient Greece and Rome: see K. Dover 1984: 143–57; C. Williams 1999: 200.
118. See F. Rosenthal 1978 (on a treatise by al-Rāzī devoted to *ubna*).
119. Al-Kātib 1977: 237ff.
120. Ibn Sīnā 1999: II, 729.
121. See for example Abu Khalil 1993; K. El Rouayheb 2005.
122. A. Shalakany 2008: 51–2.
123. The *Qānūn* devotes a whole chapter to reproductive organs and the sexual instinct: Ibn Sīnā 1999: II, 725–47. See also E. H. Hoops, 'Die sexologischen Kapitel im '*Canon Medicinae*' des Avicenna, vergleichen mit der Schrift De coitu des Maimonides', *Aesthetische Medizin*, 1967, 16, pp. 305–8.
124. Maimonides, *Fī tadbīr al-ṣiḥḥa* ('Regimen of Health'), Chapter 4 (Ariel Bar-Sela, Hebbel E. Hoff, Elias Faris, 'Moses Maimonides' Two Treatises on the Regimen of Health: *Fī Tadbīr al-Sihhah* and *Maqālah fī Bayān Baʿḍ al-Aʿrāḍ wa-al-Jawāb ʿanhā*", *Transactions of the American Philosophical Society*, New Series 54: 4 [1964], pp. 3–50); *Fuṣūl Mūsā fī 'l-ṭibb* ('Medical Aphorisms of Moses'), Treatise 17 (English trans. F. Rosner and S. Muntner, *The Medical Aphorisms of Moses Maimonides*, New York: Yeshiva University Press, 1973; G. Bos, *Medical Aphorisms. Treatises 16–21*,

Chicago: Chicago University Press, 2013).

125. See the chapter on coitus in *al-Rāzī, Kitāb al-Murshid aw al-fuṣūl.*

126. For example, Maimonides dedicated his work to Sultan al-Muẓaffar ʿUmar Ibn Nūr al-Dīn of Hama; al-Isrāʾilī to Nūr al-Dīn Muḥammad Ibn Qārā Arslān of the Artuqid dynasty; al-Nafzāwī to Muḥammad al-Zawāwī, grand vizier of the Ḥafṣid ruler of Tunisia; ʿAbd al-ʿAzīz al-Hafṣī, Ibn Raqīqa to the Ayyubid ruler al-Ashraf; and al-Ṭūsī to Ābāqā Khan.

127. For a discussion of al-Ṣuyūṭī's erotological and erotic works, see H. Jughām 2001.

128. This term is used for the area covered by the historical Greater Syria, which includes present-day Jordan, Syria, Lebanon.

129. For general overviews, see H. Schipperges 1964 and 1976; D. Jacquart 1996.

130. M. Green 1985: 134–40.

131. On this physician's work, see ibid.: 91–101.

132. Ibid.: 140ff.

133. See ibid.: 195–413; Green 2002: 3–7; V. Nutton, in L. I Conrad et al. 1995: 139–46; D. Jacquart and F. Michaud 1990: 87–130.

134. Green 1985: 218ff; 2002: 10–11; D. Jacquart and F. Michaud 1990: 96–107; V. Nutton, in L. I. Conrad et al. 1995: 140–1.

135. See, for example, Jon Arrizabalaga, *The 'Articella' in the Early Press, c. 1476–1534,* Cambridge: Cambridge Wellcome Unit for the History of Medicine, 1998. For an extensive and erudite analysis of the *Isagoge*, which confirms Constantine as the translator, see Francis Newton, 'Constantine the African and Montecassino: New Elements and the Text of the *Isagoge*', in C. S. F. Burnett and D. Jacquart 1994: 16–40.

136. For background, see the various contributions in C. F. S. Burnett and D. Jacquart 1994. Constantine's translation was in fact incomplete, and a few decades later the Pantegni was retranslated in its entirety by Stephen of Antioch (*Liber regalis dispositionis*), who had studied in Salerno.

137. For an overview, see C. Burnett 2001.

138. D. Jacquart and F. Michaud 1990: 147–52.

139. The first three books of the Latin *Canon* were printed in 1472 in Milan, with the complete edition appearing one year later. The book would remain the authoritative medical text until the seventeenth century.

140. Gerard's translation, *Liber Medicinalis ad al Mansorem*, was published for the first time in Milan in 1481; other printings followed in Venice (1497) and Lyon (1510). Vesalius's redaction was entitled *Paraphrasis in nonum librum Rhazae medici arabis clariss: ad regem Almansorem, de singularum corporis partium affectuum curatione* (Basel: Robert Winter), and remained a core textbook in European medical faculties for many centuries. For the influence of al-Rāzī on Vesalius's thought and oeuvre, see A. Compier 2012.

141. See D. Jacquart and F. Michaud 1990: 167ff; D. Jacquart 1996; C. O'Boyle 1998; P. Pormann and E. Savage-Smith 2007: 164–7.

142. D. Jacquart and C. Thomasset 1988: 89, 90, 93.

143. See G. Bos 1997. For discussion of the impact of the *Viaticum*, see H. Schipperges 1964: 40–3; idem 1976: 106–8; Mary E. Wack, *Lovesickness in the Middle Ages: The Viaticum and its Commentaries*, Philadelphia:

University of Pennsylvania Press, 1990.

144. It is now accepted that *De Coitu* was in fact an adaptation of the work of al-Jazzār. See D. Jacquart and C. Thomasset 1988: 116–20, 221; E. Montero Cartelle, ed., *Constantini Liber de Coitu. El tratado de andrologia de Constantino el Africano,* Santiago de Compostella: Universidad de Santiago de Compostella, 1983.

145. Dedicated to Pope Bonifacius VIII, it was first printed in 1480. For Maimonides in Latin, see Hasselhoff 2002; and G. Hasselhoff, 'Medieaval Translations of the Maimonidean (Medical) Oeuvre', in G. Tamer, ed., *Die Trias des Maimonides. Jüdische, arabische und antike Wissenskultur / The Trias of Maimonides. Jewish, Arabic and Ancient Culture of Knowledge*, Berlin/New York: Walter De Gruyter, 2005, pp. 395–410.

146. D. Jacquart and C. Thomasset 1988: 120–1; C. F. S. Burnett, 'The Latin Versions of Maimonides' *On Sexual Intercourse (De Coitu)*', in F. E. Glaze and B. K. Nance, eds, *Between Text and Patient: The Medical Enterprise in Medieval and Modern Europe* (Micrologus' Library, 39), Florence: SISMEL/Edizioni del Galluzzo, 2011, pp. 467–80.

147. D. Jacquart and C. Thomasset 1988: 91–2.

148. Ibid.: 135ff.

149. Ibid.: 126–8. The first *Secrets Secretorum* was translated by John of Sevillem (who also translated one of Qusṭā Ibn Lūqā's works on the soul and the spirit, *De differentia spiritus et animae*) around 1120, and dedicated to the first ruler of the kingdom of Portugal, Queen Teresa – daughter of the Spanish king Alfonso VI. See Steven J. Williams, *The Secret of Secrets: The Scholarly Career of a Pseudo-Aristotelian Text in the Latin Middle Ages*, unpublished PhD dissertation, Northwestern University, Evanston, IL, 1991.

150. For detailed discussions of this, see for example D. Jacquart and C. Thomasset 1988: 7–8, 12–14, 22–40; J. Cadden 1993; A. Lindgren 2005; Helen Rodnite Lema, *Women's Secrets: A Translation of Pseudo-Albertus Magnus' De Secretis Mulierum with Commentaries*, Albany, NY: State University of New York Press, 1992; Sarah Alison Miller, *Virgins, Mothers, Monsters: Late-Medieval Readings of the Female Body Out of Bounds*, unpublished PhD dissertation, University of North Carolina at Chapel Hill, 2008.

151. The 'Trotula texts' comprise three treatises: the 'Trotula major', known also as *De passionibus mulierum curandarum* ('Diseases of Women') or by the *incipit* 'cum auctor', which is devoted to gynecological medicine; the 'Trotula minor' ('ut de curis'), on medical matters and cosmetics; and *De ornatu mulierum*, on cosmetics. See Benton 1985; M. Green 2002: 51–115. The texts have been translated by M. Green (2002). On the Arabic medical influence, see D. Jacquart and C. Thomasset 1988: 121–2, 132.

152. D. Jacquart and C. Thomasset 1988: 133.

153. Ibid.: 96–110.

154. Ibid.: 130–5.

155. Arab physicians like Ibn Sīnā and al-Rāzī were unclear about the clitoris, whereas al-Majūsī confused it with the labia. It would take until the mid-sixteenth century for its function to be 'discovered' – at least by men! The same confusion existed about the female genitals in general, with the word

'vulva', for example, signifying the vagina, the womb, or both, until the late Middle Ages. See D. Jacquart and C. Thomasset 1988: 44ff; A. Lindgren 2005: 95; T. Laqueur 1992: 64ff.

156. D. Jacquart and C. Thomasset 1988: 137.
157. See P. M. Holt 1992.
158. See *EI*², s.v. 'Ṭūs' (C. E. Bosworth).
159. The author's name is also sometimes given as Naṣīr al-Dīn Abū Jaᶜfar Muḥammad Ibn Muḥammad Ibn al-Ḥasan al-Ṭūsī (M. Sharif 1963–66, I: 564) or Naṣīr al-Dīn Muḥammad Ibn Muḥammad al-Ṭūsī (C. Storey 1972, II: 2, 216).
160. For biographical details, see the following, from which the information in this section has been drawn: *EI*², s.v. 'al-Ṭūsī' (al-H. Daiber/F. J. Ragep) (with extensive bibliography); *GAL* I: 670–6; *GALS* I: 924–33; *GALS* III, 1,245–7, 1,314–5; Storey 1972, II: 1, xl, xlii–xliv, 6–7, 52–60, II: 2, 216–17; ᶜU. Kaḥḥāla n.d.: XI.
161. Ulugh Beg, *Binae tabulae geographicae una Nassir Eddini Persae, altera Ulug Beigi Tatari*, London: J. Flesher, 1652.
162. *GALS* I: 932.
163. Ibid.
164. Ibid.
165. F. Rosenthal 1986, III: 148 (where al-Ṭūsī is also called 'an Iraqi', i.e. one hailing from non-Arab Iraq).
166. Originally derived from the Turkish and Persian words for teacher (*khōja*), it was a title used for a variety of people, including scholars, teachers, merchants and ministers. It also became a term of reference for non-Muslims, especially Europeans, in which sense it is still used in modern Egypt (*khawāga*). *EI*², s.v. 'khwādja' (ed.).
167. *GAL* I: 676 refers to the book '*albāb al-bāhiyya fi 'l-tarākīb al-sultāniyya* as a health manual (*Gesundheitsbuch*), 'the last part of which deals with coitus and aphrodisiacs'.
168. A. Ihsanoglu 1984: 378.
169. This manuscript is much longer (104 folios) and includes 61 chapters (besides an introduction and conclusion) on a wide variety of medical conditions.
170. This includes misspellings, which are indicated by underscore in the edited text.
171. This was the manuscript used by Ghassan Ammari for his edition (unpublished PhD dissertation, Universität Erlangen–Nürnberg, 1974).
172. *EI*², s.v. 'al-Djaghmīnī' (H. Suter [J. Vernet]); *GAL* I: 473; II: 213; C. Storey 1958, II: 1, 50, 219. The Glasgow catalogue misspells the author's name as 'al-Yaghmini'.

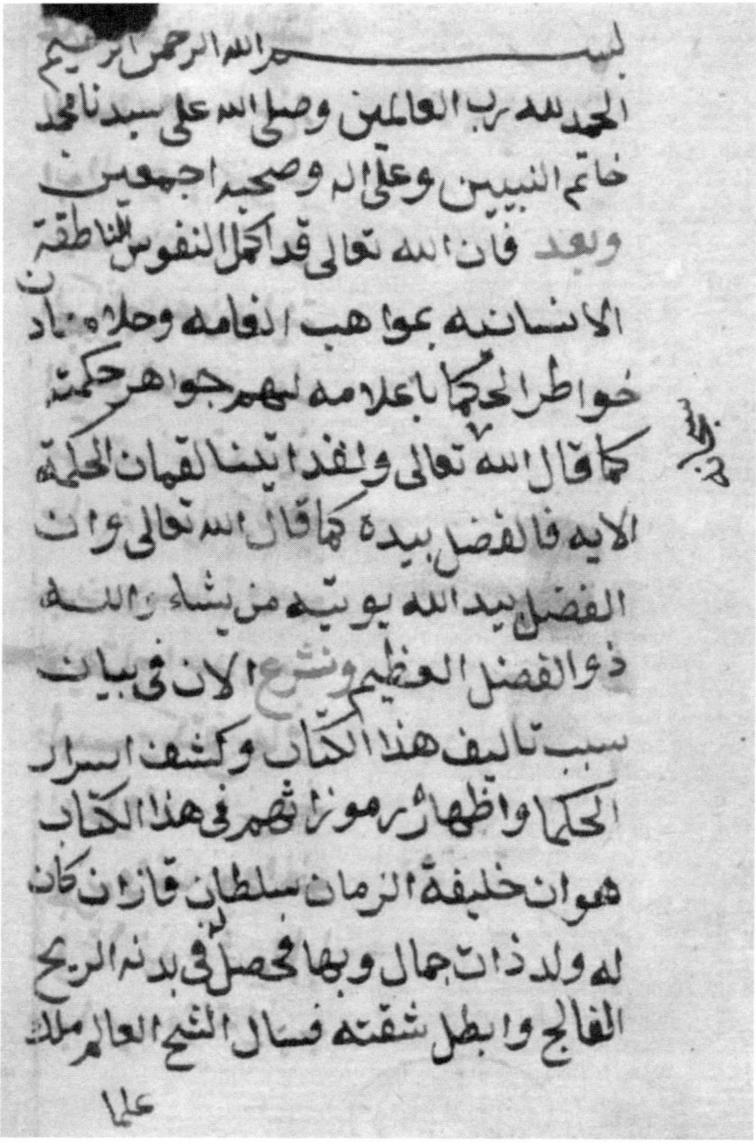
بسم الله الرحمن الرحيم
الحمد لله رب العالمين وصلى الله على سيدنا محمد
خاتم النبيين وعلى اله وصحبه اجمعين
وبعد فان الله تعالى قد اكمل النفوس الناطقة
الانسانية بمواهب انعامه وجلا [illegible]
خواطر الحكما باعلامه ليفهم جواهر حكمته
كما قال الله تعالى ولقد اتينا لقمان الحكمة
الاية فالفضل بيده كما قال الله تعالى وان
الفضل بيد الله يوتيه من يشاء والله
ذو الفضل العظيم ونشرع الان في بيان
سبب تاليف هذا الكتاب وكشف اسرار
الحكما واظهار رموزاتهم في هذا الكتاب
هو ان خليفة الزمان سلطان غازان كان
له ولد ذات جمال وبها فحصل في بدنه الريح
الفالج وابطل شقته فسال الشيخ العالم ملك
علما

Illustration 1: Facsimile of first page of Berlin Mss 6383

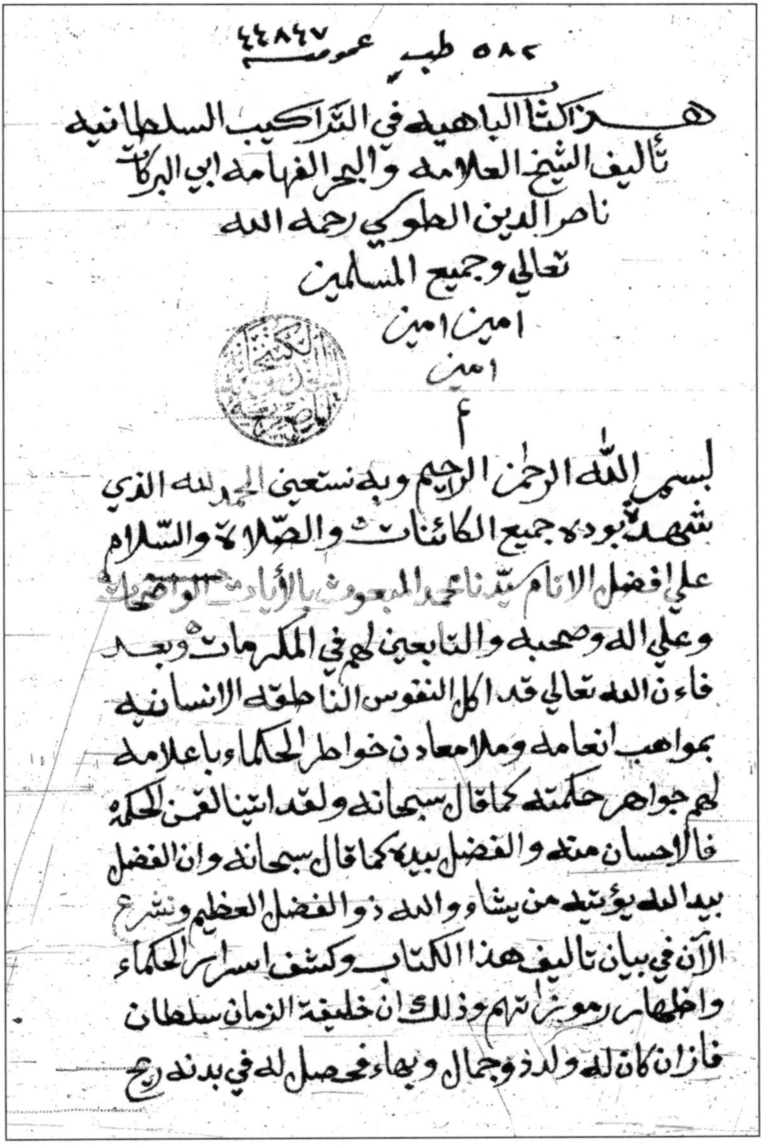

٥٨٢ طب عمومية ٤٤٨٦٧

هذا كتاب الباهية في التراكيب السلطانية
تاليف الشيخ العلامة والبحر الفهامة ابي البركات
ناصر الدين الطوخي رحمه الله
تعالي وجميع المسلمين
امين امين
امين

بسم الله الرحمن الرحيم وبه نستعين الحمد لله الذي
شهدت بوجوده جميع الكائنات والصلاة والسلام
علي افضل الانام سيدنا محمد المبعوث بالايات الواضحات
وعلي اله وصحبه والتابعين لهم في المكرمات وبعد
فان الله تعالي قد اكمل النفوس الناطقة الانسانية
بمواهب انعامه وملا معادن خواطر الحكماء باعلامه
لهم جواهر حكمته كما قال سبحانه ولقد اتينا لقمن الحكمة
فالاحسان منه والفضل بيده كما قال سبحانه وان الفضل
بيد الله يؤتيه من يشاء والله ذو الفضل العظيم ونشرع
الآن في بيان تاليف هذا الكتاب وكشف اسرار الحكماء
واظهار رموزاتهم وذلك ان خليفة الزمان سلطان
فازان كان له ولد ذو جمال وبهاء فحصل له في بدنه ريح

Illustration 2: Facsimile of first page of Cairo Mss No. 582

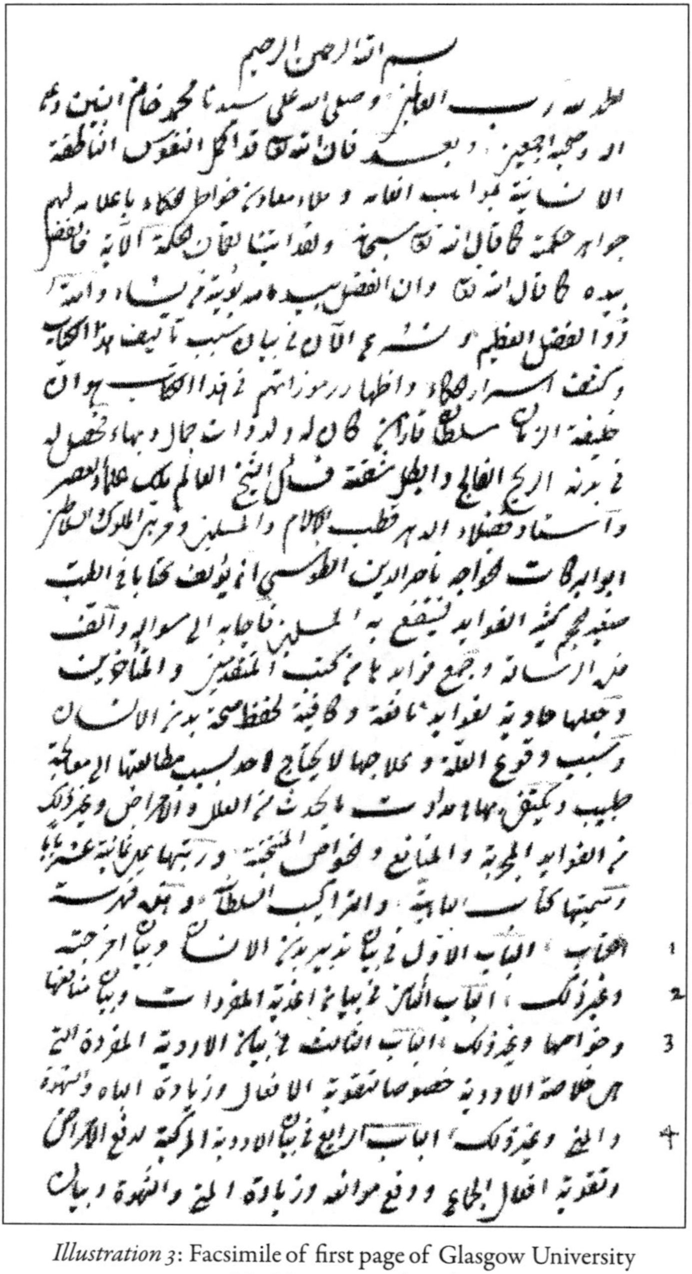

بسم الله الرحمن الرحيم
الحمد لله رب العالمين وصلى الله على سيدنا محمد خاتم النبيين وعلى
آله وصحبه أجمعين، وبعد فإن الله تعالى قد أكمل النفوس الناطقة
الإنسانية بمواهب أنعامه ومنّ على معادن خواطر الحكماء بإعلامه لهم
جواهر حكمته كما قال الله تعالى سبحانه ولقد آتينا لقمان الحكمة الآية فخص بفضل
بيده كما قال الله تعالى وإن الفضل بيد الله يؤتيه من يشاء والله
ذو الفضل العظيم، ومنه ما الآن في بيان سبب تأليف هذا الكتاب
وكشف أسرار الحكماء وإظهار رموزاتهم في هذا الكتاب هو أن
خليفة الزمان سلطان قازان كان له ولد ذوات جمال وبهاء فحصل له
في بدنه الريح الفالج والبطن شفقة فسأل الشيخ العالم ملك علماء العصر
وأستاذ فضلاء الدهر قطب الإسلام والمسلمين ومربي الملوك والسلاطين
أبو البركات الخواجه ناصر الدين الطوسي أن يؤلف كتابا في الطب
صغير الحجم كثير الفوائد ينتفع به المسلمين فأجابه إلى سؤاله وألف
هذه الرسالة وجمع فوائد بالغ من كتب المتقدمين والمتأخرين
وجعلها حاوية لفوائد نافعة وكافية لحفظ صحة بدن الإنسان
وسبب وقوع العلة وعلاجها لا يحتاج أحد بسبب مطالعتها إلى معالجة
طبيب وتحقيق مهماته ما يحدث من العلل والأمراض وغير ذلك
من الفوائد المجربة والمنافع والخواص المنتخبة ورتبها على ثمانية عشر بابا
وسميتها كتاب الباهية والتراكيب السلطانية وهذه فهرست
الكتاب: الباب الأول في بيان تدبير بدن الإنسان وبيان أمزجته 1
وغير ذلك، الباب الثاني في بيان الأغذية المفردات وبيان منافعها 2
وخواصها وغير ذلك، الباب الثالث في بيان الأدوية المفردة التي 3
هي خلاصة الأدوية خصوصا لتقوية الأفعال وزيادة الباه والشهوة
والمني وغير ذلك، الباب الرابع في بيان الأدوية المركبة لدفع الأمراض 4
وتقوية أفعال الجماع ودفع موانعه وزيادة المني والشهوة وبيان

Illustration 3: Facsimile of first page of Glasgow University Mss Hunter 144 (T.7.3)

TRANSLATION

The Book of Sexual Stimulants and the Sultan's Potions[1]

[1][2] In the name of Allah, the Compassionate, the Merciful.

Praise be to Allah, Master of the Two Worlds. May He bless our lord Muḥammad, the seal of the Prophets, his family and companions.[3] Allah the Almighty has perfected the human spirit through His beneficences and embellished the depths of scholars' hearts through the revelation of His pearls of wisdom, as He said: 'And verily We gave Luqmān[4] wisdom'[5] and the bounty is in His hand. The Almighty also said 'that the bounty is in Allah's hand to give to whom He will. And Allah is of Infinite Bounty.'[6]

We begin by explaining the motive behind the writing of this book, the discovery of scholars' secrets and the revelation of their lucubrations. The caliph of Qāzān[7] had a beautiful son, whose body was struck by paralysis which incapacitated [the movement of] the lips. The caliph asked the *shaykh*[8] of the world, the king [2] of scholars of the age, the teacher of scholars of all time, the pillar of Islam and all Muslims, preceptor of kings and sultans, one who is full of blessings, Master[9] Nāṣir[10] al-Dīn al-Ṭūsī – may the Almighty have mercy on him! – to compile a book on medicine that is small in size but has many benefits that will be useful to Muslims. He acceded to the request and compiled the present book, in which he has gathered the wisdom culled from the works of past scholars and made it a compendium including that which is most useful and beneficial for the preservation of a healthy body, and the causes for the appearance of illnesses and their treatment. Anyone reading this treatise will no longer need a physician for medical treatment as it contains all the reader requires to treat ailments and diseases that are described in terms of tried and tested benefits and selected specialist remedies.

I have divided the book into 18 chapters and named it 'The Book of Choice Sexual Stimulants and the Sultan's Potions'. Here is the index [3] of the book for reference purposes:

Chapter 1: explanation of the organization of human beings, their temperaments, etc.;

Chapter 2: description of simple remedies, their benefits, properties, etc.;

Chapter 3: description of simple drugs,[11] which are the main medicines, especially for the strengthening of bodily functions, sexual potency, lust, sperm, etc.;

Chapter 4: description of compound drugs[12] that ward off illnesses, strengthen performance during coitus, protect against obstructions, increase sperm and lust; description of compound remedies and sweets that are beneficial for the human temperament and restore it, remove paralysis in the body and limpness of the limbs, and increase sexual potency;[13]

Chapter 5: description of syrups that remedy spoiled

temperaments, purify the blood and body, invigorate coitus and are of great benefit; [4]

Chapter 6: description of stomachics[14] that raise the spirits and ward off restlessness, are highly beneficial for the stomach and strengthen it; remove jaundice and phlegm; cut short melancholy; are beneficial for the brain; open up blockages in organs; reduce foul wind; strengthen the lungs; protect against headache and catarrh; and strengthen innate heat and all bodily actions;[15]

Chapter 7: description of the remedies[16] that extract and expel wind and coldness arising from the hip, back and organs; that remove moistness, yellow and black bile[17] from the stomach, intestines and other parts of the body;

Chapter 8: description of enemas which remove joint ache; protect against foul wind and expel it from the body and lungs; cure sciatica; remove back pain, colic; strengthen the back [5] and hip, and all functions;[18]

Chapter 9: description of the bandages that are tied around the hip during the four seasons and of everything that is appropriate for each season in order not to upset human nature and cause illness;[19]

Chapter 10: description of the conditions and manner [of coitus] so as to avoid harm and impotence;[20]

Chapter 11: description of medicines to rub on the penis so that it becomes strong, long, and erect;

Chapter 12: description of medicines to rub on the penis so that it becomes erect and long, as is desirable;[21]

Chapter 13: description of medicines that are rubbed in between the fingers and toes so that they are useful during coitus, strengthen it, and prevent impotence resulting from frequent intercourse;[22]

Chapter 14: description of pills that are placed in the mouth during coitus to increase the individual's pleasure;

[6] Chapter 15: description of the positions during coitus that provide pleasure to both the man and the woman, as reported by physicians;[23]

Chapter 16: description of medicines which, if used by women, colour their faces and cheeks pink, with intercourse becoming highly pleasurable, to the extent that no one can have sex with them anymore due to their hotness and [their vaginas'] narrowness;[24]

Chapter 17: description of medicines that prevent pregnancy in a woman so that she remains like a virgin forever;[25]

Chapter 18: description of the medicines that make a woman become pregnant, if Allah the Almighty wills it.[26]

This concludes the index of chapters,[27] which we have provided to make it easier for the user who is looking for something to find it without effort or difficulty. I seek help from Allah. 'Allah is Sufficient for us! Most Excellent is He in Whom we trust!'[28]

[7] Know, student,[29] that Allah grants us success in achieving obedience to Him and that Allah, praise be to Him, the Sublime, has created animals and brought them into being out of nothing. He has created them in pairs and given them a soul so that they need and yearn for each other in pairs.[30] He has given preference to human beings over all others and favoured them with intellect, adorned them and bestowed His honour upon them; as Allah the Almighty has said – and He is the most truthful of utterers:[31] 'Verily, We have honoured the children

of Adam. We carry them on the land and the sea.'[32] He made their food the finest of all animals. We have extended the discussion in this chapter because there is no more awful cause[33] for the destruction of the soul than sexual intercourse. Every disease can be treated, except those that are caused by frequent intercourse, which douses the innate heat, for which there is no treatment or therapy that can offer solace. May Allah save us from that!

Sperm, when it flows, comes from the principal organs and from all [8] extremities;[34] as ᶜAlī[35] (may Allah be pleased with him!) said[36]: 'Your sperm is your soul, the light of your eyes, the brain in your head and legs. If you want to, conserve it.' When you have learned about intercourse and practise it as it should be, you will acquire 24 benefits;[37] for instance, it cures melancholy, protects against yellow bile and phlegm illnesses, and causes happiness and high spirits, as described by past scholars, sages and physicians, who based themselves on their experiments and experience.[38]

As for the view held by a number of scholars that sexual intercourse is bad and harmful, and that it is not necessary for anyone to practise it, but rather that it should be abandoned, this is devoid of foundation, and erroneous because [a person's] dignity and beauty is rooted in five things – namely, the five faculties: hearing, sight, smell, taste and touch.[39] Taste mostly refers to taste in sexual intercourse and lust.

[9] The result of pleasure during sexual intercourse is the creation of living beings and, thus, the reproduction and propagation of the human species. Hence, any talk about the inadmissibility of sexual intercourse is a falsehood.

It is clear that this statement is nonsensical and only applies to those who engage in coitus while being ignorant of the time and circumstance when it should or should not take place, of the conditions and regimen it requires. When coitus takes place in these cases, it results in the above-mentioned ailments and the individual's destruction, in contrast with those who know how to manage coitus and its conditions. In the latter case, sexual intercourse does not cause any harm; rather, it is hugely beneficial,[40] as we have mentioned, whereas there is no greater human pleasure than that of sexual intercourse. It is part of the natural disposition and it is mixed into the make-up of human beings and all other animals. It is rooted in their very being, which is why there is no animal in whose soul and brain such lust is not present, except if it has [10] a defect in its temperament, limpness in the limbs, or its libido has died.

Know that a man grows weak, becomes afflicted by illness and pain, only if the principal organs are aching. As long as the principal organs remain strong because of medicines and treatments by avoiding wrong conduct and guarding against harm, the limbs will remain sound and free from defects and illness, and will not be afflicted by pain until the moment of death, if Allah the Almighty wills it. Death cannot prevent anything; its verdict cannot be changed and its judgement cannot be opposed.[41]

The principal organs are the brain, heart, liver and testicles, together with their organs [*sic*]. Some scholars also count the lungs among the principal organs; others include the kidneys.[42] Human beings should strengthen these organs and the stomach with medicines, electuaries, syrups and unguents, [11] whose properties and preparation will be explained later, Allah the Almighty willing, in line with what was said about this by the ancient philosophers and physicians, who relied on their experiments and experience, in their books. They include Plato, Aristotle, Hippocrates, Palladius,[43] Aristo[44] and scholars like them.[45]

Description of the benefits and harmful effects of sexual intercourse during the four seasons, which are spring, summer, autumn and winter.

Note that spring is the best and most beneficial season for sexual intercourse, as it is the most temperate[46] and its air the most agreeable.[47] It purifies the blood, restores balance and increases the pneuma in the veins, which strengthens the innate heat, enhances vitality and taste, removes weakness in the penis and makes it powerful. If this is the case,[48] sexual intercourse in this season is not harmful, does not make the body sluggish or cause illness and pain, regardless of whether sexual intercourse occurs after taking medicines, electuaries, [12] and so on.[49] Sexual intercourse in any other season is harmful, except with the use of medicines since, in truth, passion is derived from the potency of the latter as it does not come from within the individual. So, sexual intercourse during summer, autumn and winter requires treatment through medication and electuaries for it to be beneficial and not harmful.[50]

CHAPTER 1

The regimen required for each person and a description of the signs referring to the temperament of each individual.

Know that those with brown or wheat-coloured skin, with either strong or limp flesh,[51] wide veins and black hair, who are temperate and clean, with bluish-black eyes, thick eyebrows and powerful testicles, are endowed with a hot and dry temperament. Those who fall into this category are eager [13] for sexual intercourse[52] and are not spoilt by it. Those who have a yellow colour, red face, white skin and big belly, have a cold and moist temperament. Those with a moist temperament desire to engage in coitus but are not sufficiently strong to do so. If such a person increases the frequency of intercourse, it weakens him.[53] Those with a black colour, a clean skin and body, of lean and slight build,[54] with small eyes and very red gums, have a hot temperament and a strong desire for sexual intercourse. As for those who are white-skinned, they come in two categories: either they have a clear colour and beautiful eyes, or the whiteness of the skin tends towards yellow, with yellow hair.[55] The second group have a high libido. Those who have a white colour and a phlegmatic temperament have flaccid limbs and are not strong enough to have sexual intercourse.[56] If they practise it to excess [14] they will die, and so have to take great care when engaging in coitus.[57]

The weakness in limbs and the limpness of organs derives from a weakness in the brain, which is called 'brain weakness'. Its signs are as follows: vertigo, sunken eyes, poor eyesight,[58] weak physical strength, variable colour, increased shame at having a limp penis, and feeble coital activity, without experiencing ecstasy. If such a person has intercourse, he has no strength to repeat it a second time due to the weakness of his limbs. Someone like this should remedy these ailments by strengthening the brain, the treatment for which is sugar syrup because the defects arise from increases in moistness; it dissolves superfluities, strengthens the sperm and invigorates coitus. Sugar syrup has many other benefits, whose explanation would take too long.[59]

Recipe for sugar syrup: take ginger[60] and cinnamon bark[61] [15], two-fifths of a *dirham* of each,[62] two *dirhams* of cardamom[63] and two *dirhams* of clove.[64] Pound all of these separately and then mix everything together. Put the mixture in a pot, add seven times the amount of fresh water and boil over a small fire until the strength of the medicines is extracted and the required substances have been cooked thoroughly. Then, strain the water and throw away the sediment. Take four times the weight of the mixture in sugar, which amounts to 32 *dirhams*, and boil all the ingredients so that everything becomes mixed, without thickening. If you want to reduce it, add half a *dirham* of saffron.[65] Remove from the fire and take a spoonful each day on an empty stomach. Wait until dawn before eating it. It is beneficial and curative, Allah the Almighty willing.[66]

The second cause for the weakening of limbs and limpness of organs, which leads to [16] sexual impotence, is weakness of the heart. The sign of a weak heart is that during forceful movement or walking, as when crossing a threshold; when being angry with someone; when good news is received; when gazing upon the object of one's desire; or by being in a large group, the individual will experience the following symptoms:[67] heart palpitations, trembling hands and knees, anxiety, shortness of breath and a change in colour. Anyone suffering from this will experience weakness during coitus, after which there will be palpitations.

{People like this should guard against these ailments by strengthening the limbs and the limpness of organs with apple syrup so as to remove the symptoms,}[68] increase stomach secretions, heat up and proliferate the sperm. This syrup has many other benefits, but a description of this would take too long, and this is sufficient.

The apple syrup is made as follows: [the author] says take an apple,[69] peel and core it. Pound it and strain its juice through a thin piece of cloth or a fine sieve, [17] add the same measure of rosewater[70] and mix it with the apple juice. Take the same weight of purified bee honey[71] from which the froth has been skimmed.[72] Place the honey in a pot together with a small quantity of the rosewater and apple mixture. Add half a *dirham* of saffron, half a *dirham* of peppercorns,[73] a *dirham* of ginger and two *dirhams* of clove. Boil everything until the strength has been brought out of the ingredients, then strain and use when needed, at which time add[74] double the quantity of the mixture in rain water, blend it all with the water you have boiled with the seeds; pour into the pot, place on a low fire, and stir the mixture until it thickens. Before it becomes thick, add a *qirāṭ*[75] of pure musk.[76] Remove the pot from the fire and let the contents cool down.[77] Drink one or one-and-a-half spoonfuls each day on an empty stomach. It is beneficial.

The third reason for the limpness of organs, and [18] the weakness of limbs and coitus is a weakness in the liver, which is characterized by a yellow colouring of the face, as in jaundice, the drying up of the tongue and lips, sunken eyes, emaciation and a loss of appetite.[78] When a person afflicted by this eats anything, he is unable to digest the food. When he gets up, his legs will tremble, whereas he finds it difficult to stand and is weakened. He is incapable of coitus, and when he is able to, it gives him no enjoyment or pleasure. His sperm is cold, as are the hands and feet. If a man like this engages in sexual intercourse to excess, he will be struck by one of the following three illnesses: hemiplegia, impotence, or the dissipation of his innate heat, which results in sudden death[79] – may Allah protect us from that! This ailment should be treated with syrup of spikenard,[80] which heats up the stomach, strengthens the liver,[81] [19] innate heat and potency. It has twenty-six other beneficial properties, which, if we were to mention them all, would make the book too long. As for the recipe of spikenard syrup:[82] take one *dirham* each of cinnamon bark, cardamom and Indian aloewood,[83] and half a *dirham* of clove. Pulverize all the ingredients and, if needed, add five times the measure of water, then boil the liquid until the substances have been cooked thoroughly and half of the water remains. Afterwards, strain it, add skimmed honey in an amount equalling that of the water and cook for one hour, until everything is mixed. Add half a *dirham* of saffron dissolved in rosewater and mix. The use of this remedy will be beneficial, as we have mentioned.

The fourth cause for weakness in sexual potency, the penis and testicles, and their limpness, comes in three types.[84] Firstly, the limpness of the penis and testicles is innate and is already present in the mother's womb; secondly, [20] excessive sexual intercourse from a young age;[85] and, thirdly, frequent sexual intercourse above the age of 40. The sign for the first of these – weakness that is already present in the mother's womb – is the inability to obtain an erection of the penis. In spite of this, the individual has a longing for sexual intercourse, without having any lust, but is impotent. This is to be treated with moderation over a long period of time. As for the second type – the high frequency of sexual intercourse in youth – it is characterized by the fact that the penis is erect only at the start and end of the night, only in the morning, or only in spring. This condition can be treated quickly, as will be described elsewhere, Allah willing. When the condition is caused by frequent sexual intercourse in adulthood, above the age of 40, the penis is erect only rarely, and on certain days.[86] Coitus is performed without energy and the individual either ejaculates cold sperm [21] or the ejaculation is accompanied by a burning sensation. Someone who suffers from this will not be able to produce offspring. The cause for this coldness lies in the back and loins; the individual is overcome with coldness.[87] This should be treated with a musk electuary, which removes the coldness and moistness[88] from his back and loins. It purifies the bladder, causes the sperm and blood in the veins to flow, and opens up blockages.[89] The person should guard against eating food that counters this action so as to ensure a speedy recovery and prevent the disease from worsening. We shall discuss the beneficial foodstuffs with which the individual can protect himself, Allah the Almighty willing. This electuary has 33 benefits in addition to the ones that we have mentioned.[90]

The recipe for the musk electuary is as follows: take a *qīrāṭ* of musk; two *dirhams* each of cinnamon,[91] spikenard, malabathrum[92] and Greek gentian,[93] three *dirhams*[94] each of saffron, cumin,[95] carrot[96] seeds and mastic,[97] [22] and half a *dirham* each of aloewood,[98] clove[99] and Turkish myrrh.[100] Pulverize all the ingredients, strain, and take three times the measure of the mixture in bee honey, and knead into an electuary.[101] Use one *mithqāl*[102] daily. It is beneficial, Allah the Almighty willing.

Here is another treatment: take some cockerels,[103] before they start crowing, slaughter them and collect ten *dirhams* of their gall. Add a sufficient measure of litharge[104] to enable you to knead the collected gall into a fine paste.[105] Then, leave it out in the sun so that the gall and litharge become mixed. Take care that the paste does not dry out and become hard.[106] Have a bath, and upon getting out,[107] rub the paste into the penis, armpits and buttocks. This should be done on an empty stomach. Then use with the musk electuary.[108] Cook the slaughtered cockerels, whose galls have been collected, with the same weight in onions.[109] [23] Sprinkle radish[110] and peppergrass[111] seeds[112] on the mixture and eat it. It is beneficial, Allah the Almighty willing.

It is advisable to eat it, as required, and it lends itself to being used like *harissa*,[113] with pullets or mutton[114] and unleavened bread, whose dough is made from coarse flour and chickpea water, in the manner of the sages. This is made as follows: take white chickpeas,[115] soak them, peel them, and cook them in a pot until they are cooked thoroughly and their essence has infused in the water.[116] Then, strain and remove the sediment. Collect some plump house sparrows,[117] slaughter and clean them, and cut them into pea-sized pieces. Place in a pot with the chickpea water and cook everything together with the lid on so that the steam cannot get out. Cook over a low fire so that it does not burn, that is, before you start noticing [24] the smell of grilled meat. Then, remove the pot from the fire and add the following ingredients:[118] five *dirhams* of ginger, two-and-a-half *dirhams* of long pepper, and ten *dirhams* of cinnamon bark. Pulverize all of them and add to the pot or sprinkle on top, as we have mentioned, before eating the dish. Whenever you eat this dish sprinkle these spices on. If you cannot find any sparrows,[119] use young pigeons to use in their stead. You can also eat *taqliyya*[120] with carrots and the meat of a one-year-old lamb,[121] chicken, or cockerels before they have started to crow. After the carrots have been washed, peeled and cut into small pieces, cook them with the meat, as we have mentioned. Then, sprinkle the aforementioned spices[122] on and eat the mixture. This is drunk with cow's milk in which dried dates[123] have been cooked [25] in order to sweeten it. It can also be eaten with grilled fish[124] and white onions. If you eat it in a broth, then add garlic.[125] It is beneficial.

Recipe for making garlic broth:[126] take fresh Syrian garlic and peel the cloves. Take beef fat, clarify and strain it, and take some of the meat in which it was cooked. Pulverize the garlic, mix it with the fat, and cook everything through. Place in a bowl[127] and forcefully knead with the hands until it is smooth and thin.

Put on a low fire until it is slightly thickened, and then add the grated garlic, mix everything, and beat it until it has thickened. Remove from the fire and sprinkle the aforementioned spices on top.[128] One may also add half a *dirham* of saffron in a glass vessel.[129] Take three *mithqāls* of the mixture each day. It is said that [26] this garlic broth removes coldness from the back and loins, clears phlegm from the stomach and chest, and superfluities from the chest, expelling all illnesses from the body, Allah the Almighty willing.[130]

One can also use roses preserved in bee honey jam, the recipe for which is as follows: take roses and place them in a glass container in the sun. Add the honey and let both dry. Whenever the honey dries out, add some more until it reaches the required consistency. This should be eaten with unleavened bread spread with fresh cow ghee[131] and a ripe sweet apple, as we have mentioned. One should avoid eating all acidic foods, dairy produce and jerked meat strips[132] made from fresh beef, and guard against goat meat and black raisins.[133] One should only drink sweet beverages and avoid acidic and bitter ones. [27] Master al-Ṭūsī transmitted the accounts he has heard about Hippocrates, Aristotle, and others, so that those treating themselves with the foodstuffs and acidic syrups we have mentioned will remain free from harm, pains and illnesses. It will remove all weakness and invigorate the individual, especially during coitus; when, Allah willing, he has sexual intercourse, he will not grow weak, his face will not change [in colour], he will never get bored, and his condition will be improved. His condition will be enhanced.

CHAPTER 2

Description of simple foodstuffs that benefit, strengthen and restore the human body and nature.[134]

Among them, there is Persian halva,[135] the flour for which has to be very fine, moderately salted and ripe. The physician Master al-Ṭūsī – may Allah the Almighty have mercy on him – recounts a report from the ancient philosophers that those who from earliest childhood [28] eat dry bread without anything will not be afflicted by disease at the end of their life. Disease is the result only of increases in humours, which are the result of various foodstuffs, including beneficial food such as roasted sheep's meat, which does not disturb the stomach and is quickly digested. The natural foodstuffs that are most appropriate for human nature, and more agreeable than the former two, are:[136] the meat of pigeons,[137] squabs,[138] goslings,[139] chickens,[140] pullets,[141] cockerels before they start crowing, fresh fish,[142] and soft-boiled[143] chicken and goose eggs (but note that the eggs of other animals are harmful).[144] One should also eat fish roe,[145] the meat of house sparrows[146], their brains,[147] fresh cow's and sheep's milk,[148] half-cooked white onions, carrots, turnips,[149] [29] chickpeas, leek,[150] sugar, honey, cow ghee,[151] almonds,[152] hazelnuts,[153] pistachios,[154] fresh ripe dates,[155] green figs,[156] grapes,[157] sweet local pomegranates,[158] sweet ripe[159] local apples, and sweet ripe quince[160] which do not contain any trace of bitterness any more. All of the things that we have mentioned strengthen sexual potency, the brain and organs. There are many others but this selection is sufficient.[161]

CHAPTER 3[162]

Description of simple remedies, and a summary of medicines that are beneficial for all illnesses that are treated with them, heighten sexual performance, increase sperm and strengthen potency.

These are the following: musk, amber,[163] saffron, parsnip,[164] centaury,[165] cubeb,[166] pepper, ginger, clove, [30] anchonium,[167] lac,[168] cinnamon bark, aloewood, common ash,[169] lemon peel,[170] anise,[171] pistachio, cucumber,[172] long pepper,[173] costus,[174] marshmallow,[175] red and white tar,[176] galingale,[177] pellitory,[178] lion's fat,[179] goatsbeard,[180] Greek pitch,[181] poppy,[182] carrot seeds, turnip seeds, peppergrass seeds and fruit, walnuts,[183] mace,[184] Indian spikenard, poppy, cardamom, Armenian borax,[185] unbored pearls, zerumbet,[186] malabathrum, chebulic myrobalan,[187] belleric myrobalan,[188] the fruit of emblic myrobalan,[189] silk, black cumin,[190] coconut[191] and flatsedge.[192] All these ingredients strengthen coitus and potency, increase sperm, and cure illness.[193] It is especially the medicines that are beneficial that we have mentioned. Commit them to memory so you will remember when any of them are mentioned [31] elsewhere in the book when this is required.

CHAPTER 4

Description of compound remedies and foodstuffs that ward off illnesses; sweets that restore human temperament and remove paralysis, limpness of the limbs, strengthen coitus and potency.

Take two white onions, peel and cut them up. Cook in a small amount of olive oil[194] and water until they are cooked thoroughly. Then cook two squabs with rock salt,[195] and when they are cooked through add the onions that have been cooked in oil, and fry everything until it is mixed well. Take a *dirham* each of cinnamon bark, galingale and peony.[196] Pound all of these condiments and sprinkle them on top of the cooked onions.[197] Eat with unleavened bread and drink the gravy. It is very beneficial, remedies foul temperament, brightens the face, purifies the colour and blood, and strengthens [32] coitus. This dish has 17 other beneficial properties in addition to the ones we have mentioned, but it would take too long to enumerate them all. The benefits will become apparent to you during use, Allah the Almighty willing.[198]

Here is another recipe: take lamb meat that is neither too fat nor too lean, i.e. average. Chop it into small pieces and cook with an identical amount of onions until everything is cooked thoroughly. Afterwards, take a little coconut oil and pour on it cardamom, a *dirham* of cinnamon bark, half a *dirham* of clove and a *qīrāṭ* of musk. Pulverize these ingredients,[199] mix with coconut oil, pour on the meat in the pot, and stir until everything is mixed. Stew for a little while and then remove from the fire while keeping the lid on the vessel so that the steam does not escape. Leave for an hour to cool down and settle. This should be eaten at lunchtime. It remedies foul temperament, removes weakness, strengthens sexual potency, increases sperm, and invigorates coitus, when necessary. It has many benefits that will become apparent [33] when it is used.[200]

Another recipe: take some pullets; slaughter them; dry, wash and cut them up into slices. Sprinkle rock salt on the sides and grill on live coal, turning them over on each side, until they are cooked. Then take five *dirhams* of black cumin, three *dirhams* of goatsbeard, four *dirhams* of common ash and half a *dirham* of coconut. Pound[201] all of these and sprinkle on the meat. This dish is eaten for supper. It strengthens the principal organs, increases innate heat, removes coldness from the back and loins, expels moistness and superfluities from the body, reddens the face, and purifies the blood. It also strengthens coitus to the extent that even when one has intercourse for three days running, one need not worry about growing weak. One is able to pleasure ten slave girls and freewomen [34] every night, without any trouble or discomfort, as stated by the ancient philosophers and physicians. They also said that one should only divulge these secrets to one's own family. Anyone who uses this recipe for longer will observe its advantages and benefits in a short period of time.

Section containing a description of sweets which, when used by human beings, remedy the temperament, cure paralysis, remedy limpness, strengthen the principal organs, increase innate heat, invigorate coitus and increase sperm.[202]

Take 100 *dirhams* of white skimmed bee honey and the same quantity of white onions that have been peeled and cut into small pieces. Cook the two ingredients together and add a little water until they are cooked thoroughly. Add some olive oil, stir through, transfer to a pot, and heat[203] on a low fire until it is semi-thickened. Strain [35] and wait a little while until it cools down. Then sprinkle the grounds of five *dirhams* of cinnamon bark, five *dirhams* of lemon peel,[204] two *dirhams* of Indian aloewood and half a *dirham* of saffron on top. Pulverize everything, strain through a silk cloth and add to the onions and honey. Beat the mixture with a spoon and transfer to a glass jar. Eat it every evening before going to sleep. You will see that it works wonders.[205]

Here is another recipe. Take yellow chickpeas, soak in water, peel and fry in cow ghee until they turn red. Take care that they do not get burnt and turn black. Then, pulverize everything, add the same weight in ground Syrian pine[206] kernels and mix with white skimmed bee honey. Sprinkle the following ground mixture on top: half a *dirham* of saffron, five *dirhams* of lemon peel, one *dirham* of cinnamon bark, half a *dirham* of Indian aloewood, and ten [36] *dirhams* of Chinese cinnamon.[207] Pulverize all the ingredients and sprinkle them on the dish. Use every day before going to sleep. It is effective and you will see it works wonders. Even if you had ten slave girls you would be able to pleasure them without any trouble or a change in temperament. It has been tried and tested.[208]

CHAPTER 5

Description of syrups that remedy spoiled temperaments, purify the blood, invigorate coitus, and strengthen potency.

Note that a sweet or red syrup is known as garnet syrup. It is beneficial. A syrup whose colour tends towards yellow is called Yazdi[209] syrup and is sweet, white and beneficial. Syrup made from squeezing ripe white grapes is referred to as fragrant syrup and is also beneficial. However, the best syrup is mixed and cooked syrup.

Syrup can be harmful and should be cooked three times [37], in accordance with the customs of sages, with ingredients that are natural and provide benefits, as is known from experiments.

Here is a recipe for a syrup cooked three times, according to the custom of the sages. Take any of the syrups you like from the ones mentioned above and place them in a pot with three times the amount of fresh water and cook it until two-thirds of the fluid has evaporated and only one-third remains. Take the weight of 300 *dirhams* from the cooked mixture and add 50 *dirhams* of white bee honey,[210] or white sugar, and cook until the froth appears. Then take[211] two *dirhams* each of ginger and Chinese cinnamon, and one *dirham* each of Indian aloewood, amber and Indian spikenard. Crush all of these into dust, strain through a silk cloth, and add to the syrup. Boil it for a second time for one hour over a low fire, until everything is mixed together. [38] Remove from the fire, wait until it cools down, and transfer to a glass container. To eat the syrup, take 40 *dirhams* and mix it with the same amount of water, and drink.

This is beneficial, Allah the Almighty willing. It strengthens the stomach, heats the liver, brightens the face, purifies the blood, strengthens innate heat and invigorates coitus. Even if you were to have intercourse with ten slave girls, you would be able to pleasure them all without fatigue, weakness or discomfort. Your energy will be increased. However, wait two hours before coitus and do not eat anything until afterwards. You will see the wonders it does, Allah the Almighty willing.[212]

CHAPTER 6

Description of stomachics that raise the spirits and ward off restlessness, strengthen the stomach, remove[213] *phlegm and black bile, open up blockages in the brain and organs, purify the blood, dissolve foul wind, strengthen* [39] *the principal organs, cure headache, catarrh and innate heat,*[214] *and invigorate coitus to such a great extent that if you were to have intercourse with 20 women, these stomachics would enable you to do so tirelessly, without the member becoming weak. These substances have innumerable benefits, especially when it comes to sexual potency.*

As for the recipe for a cardamom stomachic, the author, may Allah forgive him, says:[215] take four *dirhams* each of frankincense pellets,[216] cardamom and mace; eight *dirhams* of long pepper and ginger; one *dirham* each of amber and Indian aloewood; and ten *dirhams* of saffron. Crush these ingredients as finely as kohl,[217] and strain. Then add the same amount – or half – of skimmed honey to the mixture, and transfer. Use when necessary, and you will see that it works wonders.[218] [40]

The recipe for an Indian spikenard electuary is as follows: take half a *dirham* each of Indian spikenard, mace, walnuts,[219] clove, black cumin, cardamom and Chinese cinnamon, and sixty *dirhams* of white hulled sesame seeds.[220] Pulverize all of these, except the sesame, into fine dust.[221] Pound the sesame separately and then mix with the other grounds. Knead the mixture with half the amount of skimmed bee honey. Use when needed three *dirhams* and you will see wonders, especially during coitus.

A recipe for a caltrop[222] electuary: take the prickles of the chosen amount of caltrop, cut them finely, place into a pot and boil in water until the active ingredients of the plant have been extracted. Strain the water so that the peels remain, then take out the peels and leaves. Leave the water outside in the sun on hot summer's days. Whenever it dries out, stir it [41] so that it becomes syrupy and remains unctuous and smooth. Take one *dirham* of the infusion and add one *dirham* of pellitory, half a *dirham*[223] of ginger, and ten *dirhams* of house sparrows'[224] brains. Thoroughly pound the herbs and then mix with the sparrows' brains. Add the same amount of sugar and skimmed bee honey, and knead everything together into an electuary.[225] Place into a glass container and use when needed. Whenever you wish to engage in coitus, drink two or three glasses of the 'threefold syrup' whose recipe we have provided here. You will see that it works wonders, to the extent that even if you had intercourse with ten women in one night, you would be able to satisfy them all.[226]

The recipe for an electuary of *iṭrīfal*[227] has great benefits and innumerable advantages. It strengthens the intellect,[228] clears the brain from all pains and catarrh,[229] sharpens the eyesight, increases [42] its brightness, opens blockages in the head and eyes;[230] improves hearing; purifies the blood; thickens and strengthens the principal organs and innate heat; strengthens potency; tautens the nerves[231] and veins in the penis and testicles; heats the kidneys, bladder and sperm; and greatly invigorates coitus to the extent that one can have sex whenever one wants without growing bored, weak or limp, or suffering any harm.

The recipe is as follows:[232] take three *dirhams* each of the peel of yellow (chebulic) myrobalan, the unripe fruit of belleric myrobalan, the fruit of emblic myrobalan,[233] and long pepper; four *dirhams* of the peel of mace and ginger; one *dirham* of parsnip; five *dirhams* of common ash; seven *dirhams* of Chinese cinnamon; and 20 *dirhams* of hulled white sesame. Pulverize everything, strain through a thin cloth, and add half the amount of white sugar [43] or skimmed bee honey. Knead all the ingredients and decant to a glass vessel, which should be covered with the lid. Bury it in barley[234] for 40 days. When needed, take three *mithqāls* of the mixture and drink with water.[235] It is beneficial, Allah the Almighty willing, and has been tried and tested.[236]

CHAPTER 7

Description of medicines that expel moistness from organs; remove coldness from the back and hip;[237] *extract phlegm, yellow bile and black bile; and greatly strengthen coitus.*

As for the recipe: take five *dirhams* of white sugar, two *dirhams* of ginger and one *qīrāṭ* of pellitory, and finely pound everything so that it becomes like kohl powder.[238] Add the same amount of skimmed bee honey, knead it together with the grounds, and eat the resultant mixture before going to sleep. It is beneficial, Allah the Almighty willing.

Another recipe that is beneficial: take the brains of three sparrows and one *qīrāṭ* of pellitory; pound the two finely [44] together, strain, and knead with bee honey to make the medication. Take it before going to sleep. It will achieve the desired result and is beneficial.[239]

Another recipe: take three *dirhams* each of cotton seeds[240] and colchicum,[241] pulverize the two, and knead together with lion's fat to make the medication. Take before going to sleep with cotton. When the two are brought together, you will see its wondrous effects, especially during coitus. It is beneficial, Allah the Almighty willing.

CHAPTER 8

Description of enemas which protect against joint ache, sciatica, back and hip aches; expel foul wind; remove colic; tauten the back and strengthen coitus.

Take the testicles of two lambs,[242] crush them, and place in a pot. Add the same amount of red wheat and a handful of turnip seeds, and place everything in an earthenware pot. Pour water over it until it has covered the mixture [45], cover the vessel with a lid, and put in the oven[243] overnight until it is cooked thoroughly. Remove it from the oven in the morning. Take 30 *dirhams* of the water and pour two *dirhams* of coconut oil over it. Administer the enema in the morning, after bathing and on an empty stomach. Put a cushion underneath the hips so that the head is positioned low and the legs high in order for the water to penetrate the belly and flow through the bowels. You will see that it does wonders when the enema is administered twice a year, once[244] in spring and once in autumn. It will protect from all illnesses and ailments, Allah the Almighty willing.

Here is another type of enema: take three *dirhams* each of carrot seeds, gourd[245] seeds, dill,[246] onion seeds, leek seeds, cinnamon bark, ginger, pepper,[247] long pepper; a handful of peeled chickpeas and ground wheat; [46] a thin piece of meat; the fat and testicles of a lamb. Place the preparation in a pot with the lid on and leave overnight in a hot *tannūr*[248] or oven until everything is cooked thoroughly. Then, take it out and make an enema, which is known as the 'aperient enema'.[249] It has 27 benefits. If it is administered once a year, in spring, it protects against all illnesses and ailments until the next spring, Allah the Almighty willing.

CHAPTER 9

Description of the bandages and clothing that are appropriate for human nature when they are tied tightly during the four seasons.

If the bandages run counter to human nature according to the seasons, the individual may become afflicted with diseases, and so it is necessary that the bandages and clothes are appropriate for the period of the year [47] during which they should be worn to ensure that the organs are tightened and remain strong, and that their temperament does not get spoilt.

The most appropriate bandages and clothes for spring, which is the best of all seasons because of its temperate heat and coldness, are those made of cotton, since it has an average temperature and does not disturb the temperament.

As for the second season, summer, in which the heat intensifies, the bandages and waistbands should be woven out of silk and linen, or only linen, but not just silk.

In autumn, the bandages and clothes should be made out of wool, woven fabric, or patches.[250]

As for furs, they should be [48] sable, ermine, grey squirrel, or white and black sheepskin. Bandages can also be made from camel wool or sable pelt, which has to be purified in the manner known in Turkish as *kamar qashāq*.[251] Anyone who proceeds in this way will be protected from a weakening of the principal organs, ache in the joints, palpitations, colic, and various other illnesses,[252] Allah the Almighty willing.

CHAPTER 10

Description of the conditions of coitus and how to conduct it so as to as to avoid weakness, harm, premature old age and grey hair.[253]

Know that having sexual intercourse standing up harms human beings and causes palpitations, pleurisy, sciatica, pneumonia, gout and headache[254] – may Allah protect us from all of this![255] These are all dangerous diseases [49] that are difficult to treat. Most of them occur as a result of having coitus standing up. Some people do not heed these words, claiming that they have always had intercourse standing up, without being afflicted by any of these illnesses. However, we say that these illnesses caused by coitus while standing up occur either immediately, or result in a weakness of the innate heat or of the temperament. How can those who subscribe to this view say that they are free from these illnesses when they may occur gradually? We say that this only applies to those who perform sexual intercourse standing up to excess, not once or twice in their lifetime, out of passion or love in their youth. Perhaps protection against this kind of pain [50] and harm is offered by great innate heat and strength of the principal organs. Some of these people also experience harm due to a lack of knowledge about themselves or about their strength. This should suffice for the intelligent.

As for coitus practised sideways, it is also extremely harmful and causes heart and liver pains, colic and urinary incontinence.[256] Allah protect us from this! Sexual intercourse on the right-hand side, in particular, is more harmful than that on the left.[257]

Coitus from behind, with the woman lying on her stomach, causes bladder pain, inhibited urination,[258] urine dribbling or a burning sensation when urinating, gall pains with blood and pus in urine, or both, whether urinating or not. Allah protect us from that!

[51] An intelligent man should be wary of engaging in coitus in the aforementioned harmful positions, so as to avoid the illnesses we have described.

These illnesses can be cured as follows: take ripe black nightshade[259] and squeeze the juice out. Then take ripe juniper,[260] extract the juice from it by cooking, and add the same amount of cane sugar.[261] Mix both liquids together and cook the mixture over a low fire. Use in a quantity of one spoonful on an empty stomach, and one spoonful in the evening before going to sleep. It is beneficial, Allah the Almighty willing.

Know that the best and most appropriate position for coitus is when the woman is lying flat on her back.[262] Put a thin cushion underneath her hips, with the woman then lifting her thighs by herself, rather than the man doing it, since this will cause him hardship [52] during coitus and be harmful. The man should be on all fours until he is close to ejaculation. When he is close to ejaculation, he places his knees on the floor and lies down on the woman, who embraces him with both arms and legs, clutching him tightly to her chest until ejaculation has been completed and the sperm goes straight to the uterus. The man should not get up so that the sperm is not wasted, since this will lead to non-conception, while also causing harm to the man. Coitus that takes place in this manner and under the conditions that we have just described leads to the benefits that we have mentioned and protects the man against the illnesses listed.

CHAPTER 11

Description of the medicines that are rubbed on the penis in order to thicken and harden it and making it stand up without any limpness.

Especially if a man [53] is unable to ingest hot substances, he is treated with medicines that are rubbed onto the penis. Take identical measures of narcissus bulbs,[263] pellitory and seedless red raisins, and pulverize them with one-quarter the amount of coconut so that everything is finely ground. One hour prior to coitus, wash the penis with hot water, massaging it vigorously when doing so. Then, rub the mixture onto the penis. You will see that it works like fire and will make the penis thick, powerful and sturdy, as required.

According to another preparation, you should take half a *dirham* of cottonseed kernels, two-and-a-half *dirhams* of cyperus, half a *dirham* of Syrian carob kernels and one *qīrāṭ* of coconut. Pulverize all the ingredients, add the juice of grapes or Rāziqī[264] raisins, and cook over a low fire until everything is mixed and the juice has thickened. Remove the decoction from the fire and rub on [54] the penis, when required.

Another recipe, which works on those whose organs and penis are limp, leaving them impotent after coitus or when they have not had it, or for whatever other reason. This is treated by[265] taking ten *dirhams* of goat gall and pellitory, which is finely ground and mixed with the oil of fragrant flatsedge. Leave it outside in the sun for three days, until everything has been mixed together, and then add one-and-a-half *dirhams* of ground coconut. Rub the decoction on the penis several times a day for three days prior to coitus. It will restore and strengthen the penis. Galen stated that it improves the condition of those who treat themselves by using this preparation; it stiffens the limp penis and restores youth to old age, [55] whereas those who use it in their youth will never become impotent, and are able to perform like a 20-year-old. This is how the situation is resolved.

Description of the properties of aromatic oils, such as fragrant flatsedge oil and others.

If you wish to use an aromatic oil, take any one you like. For instance, take an aromatic herb and cut it up, or take cyperus and pulverize it. Put the ground substance in a flask, pour on double the measure of good olive oil, and cover with a lid secured with wax so that the container becomes airtight. Hang it outside in the hot sun for 40 days during summer. The sun should shine on it uninterruptedly from sunrise until sunset. Afterwards, strain the mixture through a fine-meshed sieve or a thin cloth, and take it out. This is the method by which oil of aromatics such as cyperus or sweet violet is extracted.

As for oil of cores, such as [56] pistachio oil, almond oil, hazelnut oil, cottonseed oil, walnut oil and other cores, and pomegranate blossom[266] oil and the like, these are made differently. They are extracted as follows: take the desired quantity of cores and pound them until you obtain something resembling a fine oil cake. Take a white copper plate and place it on live embers.[267] Wet your hands with tepid water and beat the grounds on the plate. Turn over and roll until all the oil has been extracted. Proceed in this fashion for all cores.[268]

CHAPTER 12

Description of the medicines that are rubbed on the penis so that it is lengthened and strengthened, as you desire.

Know that the penis consists of many veins and that it becomes longer during coitus and by massaging it. However, this is not similar to what happens when using an ointment, which is [57] stronger due to the medicines it contains, as mentioned by Plato, Aristotle, Hippocrates and Galen, who have written about this phenomenon based on their knowledge and experiments.

Muḥammad al-Dāmghānī[269] and the Imam al-Rāzī[270] – may Allah the Almighty have mercy on him – reported from Plato the following about lengthening the penis.[271] Take the root of a caltrop plant over one year old, clean it with water, dry it, pound it fine, and strain through a fine-meshed sieve. Get into the bath, massage the mixture into the penis and wash it with hot water until it grows red. Then, put the ground caltrop root on the penis with cyperus oil mixed with half a *dirham* of ground coconut. If you comply with this recipe and apply the oil onto the penis three times while in the bath, until it rises above the surface of the water, you will be astonished by its lengthening. It will only be effective [58] for ten days, but you may repeat the procedure.

Here is an unusual and strange recipe, which is one of the secrets of the wise, and doubles the length of the penis. Take fresh thick sheep dung and dry amber in an amount that is required for rubbing the penis, as well as one *qīrāṭ* of musk. Pound it and mix vigorously with two *dirhams* of very finely ground coconut. Get into the bath and forcefully massage your penis with the cyperus oil until your member becomes red. Then rub the ingredients mixed with the sheep dung on the penis in the way that you rub in a seal, and wrap it into a cloth from dawn till dusk. Afterwards, remove the cloth and wash the penis. You will see a wonder, since the penis will have grown twice in size. This effect only lasts for 20 days, and must be repeated.

CHAPTER 13

Description of medicines that are rubbed in between the fingers [59] *and toes in order to invigorate coitus and stiffen the penis so that one never becomes weak, tired or limp, no matter how much one engages in sexual intercourse.*

Take house sparrows before they have acquired their flight feathers, tie them up with a string and hang them from the entrance of a beehive. Then, agitate the bees so that they start stinging the sparrows. Once the birds have been stung several times, take them down quickly and slaughter them, making sure not to waste one drop of their blood. Put them in a pot and pour over the aforementioned aromatic oil until the birds are fully covered with it. Cover the pot and place on a fire until the sparrows are cooked thoroughly. Then, remove them, and strain the water with a cloth until the essence of the birds becomes infused in the oil. Then finely pound a *qīrāṭ* of resin spurge[272] until it has the texture of kohl, and mix thoroughly with the oil. Put the oil into a flask and cover. Place in the hot sun for three days. If required, pour some of the oil on a cotton cloth [60] and rub between your fingers and toes. You will see a wonder, as you will be able to engage in coitus as much as you like without ever becoming weak, limp or tired. Your penis will not go to sleep either, and will remain standing until you wash it several times with cold water.

Another recipe: take 100 small and black ants and put them in a flask. Pour on five *dirhams* of blue liquorice oil, which should cover the ants; close the flask and hang in the hot sun for 20 days. Then, vigorously pound everything until the mixture has fermented. At the time it is needed, take one *qīrāṭ* of Indian aloewood, crush it finely, put it in ten *dirhams* of hot water and wash the penis, hands, feet and armpits with the water. Take one drop of the ant oil from the glass [61], or another small quantity, without the water, and rub it on your fingers, teeth, armpits and elbows. Wait one hour before coitus. Even if you were to engage in coitus with ten women during the night, you would not be incapacitated or weakened.

CHAPTER 14

Description of pills, which, when used by a man, provide great pleasure during coitus.

Take a *dirham* of mastic, one-and-a-half *qīrāṭs* of musk, half a *dirham* of clove, five *dirhams* of sugar and half a *dirham* of coconut. Pound everything as finely as kohl powder, place in a flask, pour oil over it, covering the grounds, and hang in the sun for three days until everything has mixed with the oil. Then add the same amount of white skimmed bee honey and mix the ingredients. From the mixture, mould pills of one *dirham* in weight each. When needed [62] for coitus, place one pill in your mouth and you will see the wonders it does.

Another type of recipe: take unpeeled pistachios and roast them evenly on a fire, making sure that they do not get burnt. Once they are roasted and dried, crush an amount equalling one *dirham* and add clove, one *qīrāṭ* of musk, and one *dirham* of amber. Pound everything as finely as kohl and stir in the pistachio oil remaining from the roasting until it turns into a paste, and leave it out in the sun for three days. Make the pills with sugar or skimmed bee honey, in the usual manner. Each pill should weigh one *dirham*. When needed, put one pill in your mouth and then have sexual intercourse. You will see a miracle.

CHAPTER 15

Description of the position during coitus that provides great pleasure to both the man and woman, as stated by the ancient philosophers and physicians [63] *who gained knowledge of this from their experiments.*

Take one *dirham* of cinnamon bark, half a *dirham* of pellitory and one *qīrāṭ* of cardamom, and pound everything as finely as dust. Afterwards, mix it with Rāziqī grape juice and rub the preparation onto the whole penis. Wait one hour and wash the penis with hot water. Put half a *dirham* of Chinese cinnamon in your mouth and chew it. Take some of the saliva and rub it on the penis before engaging in coitus. Both the man and woman will experience wondrous rapture, without either of them suffering any disturbance.

Another type of preparation: take one *qīrāṭ* each of cubeb, pellitory, Chinese cinnamon, ginger and coconut. Pound everything together and knead with thick bee honey. Put some of the mixture in your mouth, and then rub some of the saliva on your penis prior to coitus. You will see the wonder of indescribable rapture experienced by both the man and the woman.

CHAPTER 16

Description of medicines which, if inserted by women, lead to a narrowing of their wombs and vaginas, increasing their heat and pleasure.[273]

[64] Take two *dirhams* of pyrethrum, five *dirhams* of goatsbeard, sixteen *dirhams* of myrtle fruit,[274] and pulverize everything. Place in a pot, immerse in water, and boil over a fire until one-third of the water and some of the syrup have evaporated. At that point, the woman should stand over the steam seven times, after which the pot is removed. When needed, the woman moistens a cloth with the decoction and inserts it [into her vagina]. This will make the vagina narrower and hotter than a virgin's.

Another preparation: take equal parts of myrtle fruit, pomegranate peels and pellitory. Crush everything and cook in pure aged wine.[275] The woman then moistens a wool cloth with it and inserts for one hour. This will make the vagina as narrow and hot as a virgin's.[276]

Another one: take equal measures of acorn,[277] safflower, cyperus, rosemary,[278] and houseleek.[279] Mix them all together [65] by coarsely grinding, then boil and strain. Afterwards, strain the weight of five *dirhams* of pellitory onto the mixture and boil everything over a high fire. Remove it and, when needed, the woman takes two or three portions, as a result of which her vagina will be as narrow and hot as a virgin's.

CHAPTER 17

Description of medicines that, when inserted by a woman, prevent pregnancy for as long as she uses them and make her vagina as tight and hot as a young girl's.

Take bear gall and mix thoroughly with Rāziqī grape juice. If the woman puts a very small amount of the mixture inside [her vagina], she will not conceive and will remain like a young virgin.

According to another recipe, take one *mithqāl* of cow gall and the same amount of wolf gall, place in a pot, and immerse in sesame oil. When a woman soaks a piece of cotton or wool in the mixture and wears it inside her vagina, she will become like a young virgin and will not conceive.

Another one: anyone who takes tar[280] and rubs it on his penis at the time of [66] coitus will experience the greatest pleasure, and the woman will not be able to conceive, unless she receives treatment.[281]

CHAPTER 18

Description of the medicines that result in a woman becoming pregnant, if Allah the Almighty wills it.

Take Indian aloewood, green myrtle, half a *dirham* of each, one *qīrāṭ* of musk, and pulverize everything. Then, wrap the mixture in a fine cloth and place in a pot. Pour over a little aged wine and boil on a low fire until the essence of the ingredients has infused in the wine. Then, strain with water and transfer to a flask. When needed, the woman inserts a piece of wool [soaked in it]. She will be like a young virgin and it will make her conceive, Allah the Almighty willing.

Another recipe: take green gallnuts,[282] Mekkan lemongrass,[283] two *dirhams* each, and one *dirham* of dates.[284] Pound everything finely until the essence of these ingredients has infused in the syrup. When necessary, a woman inserts a piece of wool [soaked in it]. This will make her conceive, [67] Allah the Almighty willing.

Another one: take four *dirhams* of raw camphor peel, two *dirhams* of red alum,[285] one *dirham* of cyperus, four and a half *dirhams* of crushed green gallnuts, and half a *qīrāṭ* of Mekkan soil. Coarsely grind all of these, except the gallnuts, and then boil in wine as usual, strain its water, and remove. When it is needed, the woman soaks a piece of wool in the decoction and inserts it, while lying down on her back for one hour prior to coitus. She will be like a young virgin, and conceive, Allah the Almighty willing.

Another recipe: take goatsbeard, pound and pulverize it

to extract its juice. Then, take green gallnuts, pomegranate peels, Indian aloewood and lemon peel, half a *dirham* each, four *dirhams* of red alum, and one *dirham* of cyperus. Pound everything and cook in aged wine until the essence of the substances has infused in the wine. When [68] the woman inserts it, she will become like a young virgin and conceive, Allah the Almighty willing.

Another recipe: take cardamom, half a *dirham*; gum Arabic[286] and black cumin,[287] one *qīrāṭ* of each; Isfahani kohl and lemon peel,[288] half a *dirham* each. Pound everything together and boil in aged wine, until the essence of the substances has infused in the wine. When needed, the woman puts some on a piece of cloth and inserts it. She will become like a young virgin, untouched by a man, and conceive, Allah the Almighty willing.

This completes the book, thanks to Allah, His assistance and His granting of success. Praise be to Allah for everything and may Allah bless our Master Muḥammad, his family and companions, and grant them salvation until the Day of Judgement, He is the Lord of the Worlds. In the Name of Allah, the Merciful, the Compassionate.[289] (1208[290])

Notes

1. [C] addition: 'This is the book of sexual stimulants and the sultan's potions written by the most erudite shaykh, freeborn and endowed with great understanding, holder of blessings, Nāṣir [*sic*] al-Dīn al-Ṭūsī, may Allah have mercy on him and all Muslims. Amen. Amen. Amen.' In [B], the title is missing.
2. The numbers in square brackets refer to the pages in [A].
3. [C] addition: 'and the one we seek assistance from, praise be to Allah, who demonstrates His love for all beings. Prayers and peace upon the finest of the human race, Master Muḥammad, the messenger of clear verses, upon his family and companions, and exaltations upon those who follow them.'
4. This character, commonly endowed with the epithet *al-ḥakīm* ('the wise') was known for his wisdom. The thirty-first *sūra* of the Qur'ān is named after him.
5. Qur'ān 31:12. The Qur'ān translations are those of M. Pickthall, *The Meaning of the Glorious Koran*.
6. Qur'ān 57:29.
7. See Introduction.
8. [A]: *shakhkh*.
9. *Khōja* – see Introduction.
10. This is how the name appears in all three manuscripts, rather than the more correct 'Naṣīr'.
11. *al-adwiya al-mufrada* or *al-basīṭa* (< Gr. φάρμακα ἁπλᾶ). In Islamic medicine, drugs (*adwiya*, sg. *dawā'*) were divided according to both origin (vegetable, animal, mineral) and composition ('simple' vs 'compound'), which, of course, went back to the Greek tradition (especially Galen and Dioscorides). The simples were subdivided into a number of categories, depending on their source: botanical (*nabātiyya*) – which were also called *ᶜuqqār* (pl. *ᶜaqāqīr*) – animal (*ḥayawāniyya*) and mineral (*maᶜdiniyya*). See *EI*^{2}, s.v. 'adwiya' (B. Lewin).
12. *al-adwiya al-murakkaba* (< Gr. φάρμακα σύνθετα), also known as *aqrābādhīn* (< Gr. γραφίδιον, 'small table'). The most famous treatises dealing with the 'compound drugs' were those by Sābūr Ibn Sahl (d. 869), Amīn al-Dawla Ibn al-Tilmīdh (d. 1165) and al-Rāzī. *EI*^{2}, s.vv. 'Akrābādhīn' (B. Lewin), 'Sābūr b. Sahl' (O. Kahl); Ibn Sahl (O. Kahl 2003); *GAL* I: 269, 642.
13. The passage 'obstructions ... sexual potency' is abridged in [C] to: 'on medicines beneficial for the temperaments, weakness of the organs, etc.'

14. *ja/uwārishāt*, sg. *ja/uwārish* (with *ja/uwārishn* being a common variant in medical texts) – compound medicines, which could come in the form of a paste ('electuary') or syrup, while some could even contain alcohol. They were recommended to be taken before meals to shrink the stomach. See al-Warrāq (N. Nasrallah 2010): 481–7, 753; E. Lev and Z. Amar 2008: 562; Ibn Sīnā 1999.
15. The description of this chapter appears as follows in [C]: 'The description of electuaries and stomachics that are beneficial for the stomach and the removal of yellow bile, phlegm, black bile, and the brain; to open blockages in the organs; reduce foul wind; and strengthen the innate heat.'
16. *ashyāf* (sg. *shiyāf*) – this term generally denoted eye medicines, collyrium. E. Lev and Z. Amar 2008: 568; E. Lane 1863–74, IV: 1,619.
17. [C] omits reference to yellow and black bile.
18. The passage 'lungs ... all functions' is omitted in [C].
19. The phrase 'in order not to upset human nature and cause illness' is omitted from [C], which simply has 'to restore [human] nature'.
20. [C] omits the reference to impotence.
21. [C]: 'on other benefits related to sexual potency and increasing lust [of medication] to rub on the penis'.
22. In [C], 'they are useful during coitus, strengthen it and prevent impotence resulting from frequent intercourse' is reduced to 'to strengthen coitus'.
23. The description of Chapter 15 in [C] is as follows: 'description of what happens to the man and the woman in terms of pleasure during coitus and the frequency of it'.
24. The passage 'if used by women...' is as follows in [C]: 'if women use it, their cheeks will become red and their vaginas will improve'.
25. [C]: 'description of medicines that prevent pregnancy and tighten the vaginas'.
26. [C]: 'description of drugs for conception and other benefits, Allah the Almighty willing'.
27. [B]: 'the index of the book and chapters'.
28. Qur'ān 3:173.
29. The passage 'which we have presented ... student' is as follows in [C], 'In order to make it easier for those who need it to obtain information without difficulty, in the Name of Allah who provides assistance and to Whom you pray. Know that He grants us success.'
30. The passage 'praise be to Him ... pairs' is as follows in [C]: 'Through His beneficence and generosity Allah has created animals and brought them into existence out of nothing. He has created them in pairs and given them souls as they need and yearn for each other as a pair.'
31. This phrase is omitted from [C].
32. Qur'ān 17: 70. This is only part of the verse, the remainder of which reads: 'and [We] have made provision of good things for them, and have preferred them above many of those whom We created with a marked preferment'.
33. The previous sentence and the part until 'no more awful cause' is missing from [C].
34. The notion of sperm (*minan*) in Islamic medicine went back to the Greek

(Galenic) tradition, and women were also thought to have sperm. There was a correlation between the amount of sperm and sexual potency in men. The concept of sperm was discussed by a number of authorities, both medical and philosophical, including Ibn Sīnā 1999, II: 726ff; D. al-Anṭākī 1999: 174ff; al-Ṭabarī 1928: 266. See B. Musallam 1983: 43–52; D. Jacquart and F. Thomasset 1988: 52–6; E. Anwar, in S. Joseph and Nağmābādī 2003: 31ff. For the Galenic view, see P. de Lacy 1992. For the Roman tradition, see J. Dugan, 'Preventing Ciceronianism: C. Licinius Calvus' Regimen for Sexual and Oratorical Self-Mastery', *Classical Philology*, 96: 3, 2001, pp. 400–28.

35. ᶜAlī Ibn Abī Ṭālib (600–61), cousin and son-in-law of the Prophet Muḥammad, and the fourth of the so-called 'Rightly Guided Caliphs' (*al-khulafā' al-rāshidūn*). The conflict surrounding the succession to the Prophet pitted two sides of the Muslim community against each other, with ᶜAlī's supporters considering him the only rightful heir to the Prophet, and thus the first caliph. This disagreement gave rise to the split between sunni (< *sunna*, 'sayings and deeds of the Prophet') and shīᶜī (< *shīᶜat ᶜAlī,* 'the party of ᶜAlī').
36. Instead of ᶜAlī, [C] has 'Prince of the Believers' (*amīr al-mu'minīn*), the title reserved for caliphs.
37. The preceding part of this sentence appears as follows in [C]: 'He who knows the circumstances and conditions of coitus is not harmed by it, but benefits from it.'
38. cf. al-Kātib 1977: 48–50.
39. cf. ibid.: 48.
40. The remainder of this paragraph and the whole of the next are mising from [C].
41. al-Ṭūsī's phrase *lā rāda li-qaḍā'ihi wa lā māniᶜ li-ḥukmihi* is a variant on the more common *lā rāda li-qaḍā'ihi wa lā muᶜaqqab li-ḥukmihi wa lā ghālib li-amrihi*: which is a quote from *al-ᶜAqīda al-Ṭaḥāwiyya*, by Imam Abū Jaᶜfar al-Ṭaḥāwi (d. 935).
42. This sentence is omitted from [C].
43. Gr. Παλλάδιος – in the text, the name is transliterated as *Bal(la)ṭiyūs*. This sixth-century Greek author was active in Alexandria, and is known to have written commentaries on some of Hippocrates' and Galen's works. Palladius was also quoted by al-Rāzī.
44. *Arisṭū* – this is somewhat confusing, as this is the usual rendition in Arabic texts of 'Aristotle' (alongside the more narrow transliteration *Arisṭūṭālīs*, a variant of which, *Arṭāṭālūs*, appears earlier in the sentence).
45. The last two sentences appear as follows in [C]: 'These organs are strengthened by medicines, electuaries, syrups and unguents, and by taking precautions against harm to ensure that the limbs remain safe from defects and illnesses.'
46. 'the most temperate' is omitted from [C].
47. For similar comments, see Ibn Lūqā 1973: 24 (transl. 16); Ibn Māssa 1971: 7–8 (though he is also favourable towards autumn, provided the nights and days are of equal length [*istiwā' al-layl wa 'l-nahār*]). In addition to seasons, frequency of sexual activity was also linked to age (see, for example, al-Tīfāshī 1970: 13–16).

48. 'If this is the case' is omitted from [C].
49. Part of the sentence ('does not make the body sluggish…') is missing from [C].
50. The last two sentences appear as follows in [C]: 'Coitus outside spring is harmful except if it is done with medication, [in which case] it does not cause any harm, Allah the Almighty willing.'
51. In [C], 'wheat-coloured skin, with either strong or limp flesh' is reduced to 'with strong flesh'.
52. [C]: 'and coitus does not harm them' (for 'Those who fall into this category are eager for sexual intercourse').
53. The last two sentences are missing from [C].
54. 'of and slight lean built' is omitted from [C].
55. cf. Ibn Lūqā 1974: 24.
56. According to al-Suyūṭī (n.d.: 24), sexual intercourse was harmful to those with choleric and melancholic temperaments (even if they practised it only once a year!), whereas phlegmatics and sanguines were endowed with a great capacity for coitus and should have intercourse two or three times a week (though not twice in one day or night). Ibn Sīnā (1999, II: 728) held that coitus was beneficial for the melancholic.
57. The whole passage on white-skinned individuals is missing from [C].
58. The first part of the sentence is as follows in [C]: 'weakness of the limbs arises from weakness for coitus and its signs are vertigo, weak eyesight and sunken eyes.'
59. This sentence is as follows in [C]: 'Its treatment consists of sugar syrup which dissolves superfluities, strengthens coitus and increases sperm; it has a number of benefits.'
60. *zanjabīl* (< Gr. ζιγγίβερι) – hot (in the third degree) and dry (in the second degree), only the root was used of this plant, which is also mentioned in the Qur'ān (76:17). In medicine and pharmacology, it was considered beneficial for digestion and as a sexual stimulant (especially in a preserve, *zanjabīl murabbā,* 'ginger jam'). E. Lev and Z. Amar 2008: 174–5; al-Bīrūnī 1973: 206ff; Ibn Sīnā 1999, I: 455–6, II: 734; al-Rāzī 1955–69, XX: 569–73; al-Tīfāshī 1892: 13, 14; Ibn Lūqā 1974: 16 (transl. 23); *Kitāb* (Tunis No. 20648[09]): fol. 86b; al-Shayzarī, *al-Īḍāḥ,* fol. 3a; D. al-Anṭākī 1952. I: 180; Ibn al-Bayṭār 1874, II: 167–8, and 1992: 183, 215; Ibn al-Jazzār 2004: 126–7; al-Dhahabī 1987: 185; al-Suyūṭī n.d.: 14; A. Dietrich 1988, II: 306; al-Warrāq (N. Nasrallah 2010): 678–9; Ibn al-Quff (H. Kircher 1967): 195.
61. *qirfa* (*Cortex Cinnamomi Cassiaei*) – the dried rolled bark of the cinnamon tree, which some authors credited with aphrodisiacal qualities. See al-Tīfāshī 1892: 14; *Kitāb* (Tunis No 20648[09]): fol. 86b; al-Shayzarī, *al-Īḍāḥ*, fol. 3a; al-Warrāq (N. Nasrallah 2010): 668; al-Rāzī 1955–69, XXI: 270; Ibn Sīnā 1999, I: 643, and II: 734; al-Bīrūnī 1973: 398; Ibn al-Bayṭār 1992: 230; Dietrich 1988, II: 127–8; J. Leibowitz and S. Marcus 1974: 233; Ibn Sahl (O. Kahl 2003) ('canella', *Canella winterana*). For a discussion of the terminology relating to 'cinnamon', see E. Lev and Z. Amar 2008: 143–6. See also the notes below on *salīkha* and *dār ṣīnī*.
62. 1 *dirham* = 3.125 grammes; Hinz 1970: 3; *EI*[2], s.v. 'Dirham' (G. C. Miles); S.

D. Goitien 1967–88, II: 267 (3.5 grammes).

63. *qāqulla* – in Arabic medicine and pharmacology, a distinction was made between 'large (male) *qāqulla*' (*haylabū*) and 'small *qāqulla*' (*hāl* or *hīl*). Hot and dry, this aromatic spice was used in cooking and as a digestive, anti-emetic, to relieve obstructions in the liver and kidneys, and as a remedy for colds. It should not be confused with *qāqullā* (saltwort, *Salsola fruticosa*), which was sometimes also known as *qilī* (the etymon for the English 'alkaline'), *mallūkha* and *qullām*. Some authors claimed it had aphrodisiacal properties. Ibn al-Bayṭār 1955–69, IV: 2; Ibn al-Jazzār 2004: 15, 21; D. al-Anṭākī 1952, I: 253–4; Ibn Sīnā 1999, I: 642–3; al-Tīfāshī 1892: 14; *Kitāb* (Tunis No 20648[09]): fol. 86b; al-Bīrūnī 1973: 299 (transl. 263); Ibn Wāfid 2000: 83ff; A. Dietrich 1988, II: 425–6, 488; al-Warrāq (N. Nasrallah 2010): 666–7.

64. *qaranful* (< Gr. καρυόφυλλον), *Syzygium aromaticum* – this herb (the unopened flower buds of evergreen trees from China and India) had a wide range of applications, and was used in perfumes and cooking, as well as medicine for all manner of ailments. In Arab pharmacology it was recommended for improving eyesight, breath, digestion and sexual potency, as an enti-emetic, and to treat diabetes. When taken by women, cloves could either aid or prevent pregnancy. According to Maimonides, it was an ingredient in an aphrodisiac pill for stimulating erection and increasing sexual pleasure. *EI*², s.v. 'ḳaranful' (E. Ashtor); E. Lev and Z. Amar 2008: 151–2; A. Dietrich 1988, II: 394; D. al-Anṭākī 1952, I: 255; Ibn al-Bayṭār 1874, IV: 7ff, and 1992: 229–30; Ibn al-Jazzār 2004: 73; al-Kindī (M. Levey 1966): nos 3, 106, 152, 213, 225–6; al-Warrāq (N. Nasrallah 2010): 667; al-Bīrūnī 1973: 302; Ibn al-Quff (H. Kircher 1967): 314–15; al-Suyūṭī n.d.: 15; Ibn Sīnā 1999, I: 642.

65. *zaᶜfarān* (*Crocus sativus*) – in addition to its uses in cooking, saffron (which was considered hot and dry) was said to have a number of medicinal properties (for example, as a stimulant for the nervous system, as a digestive, anaesthetic, diuretic and emmenagogue, and as an ingredient in collyria), as well as being an aphrodisiac. It is for this reason that, according to one hadith, the Prophet forbade the wearing of clothes dyed with saffron (or warras) for pilgrims who were in a state of ritual purity (*muḥrim*), and thus debarred from sexual activity. According to some scholars (for example, al-Qazwīnī), high doses of saffron were poisonous. The spice was also sometimes known as *ghumr*, *jasād*, *rayhaqān*, *jādī*, or even *kurkum* (which in fact denotes turmeric). *EI*², s.v. 'zaᶜfarān' (D. Waines and F. Sanagustin); E. Lev and Z. Amar 2008: 270–3; al-Bīrūnī 1973: 202–4 (transl. 166–8); Ibn Wāfid 2000: 146–7; al-Dhahabī 1987: 184–5; Ibn al-Bayṭār 1874, II: 162–3, and 1992: 216, 215; Ibn al-Jazzār 2004: 78–9; Ibn Sīnā 1999, I: 464; D. al-Anṭākī 1952, I: 178–9; al-Tīfāshī 1892: 14; *Kitāb* (Tunis No 20648[09]): fol. 87a; al-Kātib 2002: 36; al-Shayzarī, *al-Īḍāḥ*: fol. 2b; *Risāla* (Cairo 362): fol. 3a; Maimonides (M. Meyerhof 1940): No 135; E. Lev and Z. Amar 2008: 270, 272–3; al-Warrāq (N. Nasrallah 2010): 678; Qazwīnī 1849: 250; A. Dietrich 1988, II: 107–8; Ibn al-Quff (H. Kircher 1967): 193–4.

66. [C]: 'caradamom ...': 'clove and cardamom, two *dirhams* each; pour freshwater on until everything is covered and boil over a fire until the essence of the medicines is infused in the water. Strain and throw away the dregs. Add thirty-three *dirhams* of sugar, boil over a fire until everything is mixed and then remove it before use.'

67. [C]: 'During coitus, there is weakness of the heart, which manifests itself during foreceful movement, walking and anger in...'

68. [B]: '... heart and nerve palpitations, and when the nerves have subsided they will become weak and limp. If there is excess in these ailments during coitus the person will die. These ailments should be treated with apple syrup, which expels them, strengthens the heart ...'; [C]: 'the person's colour will change and this harms him during coitus. This should be treated with apple syrup as this expels ailments, strengthens the heart, removes superfluities from the stomach, and heats up and increases sperm. It has many benefits and its recipe is as follows: take an apple segment, peel it and throw ...'

69. *tuffāḥa*; *Malus sylvestris* (*Pyrus malus*), *Rosaceae* – the Syrian and Isfahani apples were traditionally considered the best variety. In medicine, apples (especially the skin), which were cold and dry, were used to relieve intestinal pains, as a lactation inducer, and as an antidote (especially the juice from the leaves) against poisons (especially scorpion bites). The mere smell of apples was said to be able to strenghten the heart and brain. As a treatment for eye diseases, apples were cooked in water, or even breast milk. Ibn Wāfid 2000: 123–4; *EI*[2], s.v. 'tuffāḥ' (A. Dietrich); E. Lev and Z. Amar 2008: 335–6; A. Dietrich 1988, I: 86–7, and II: 175–6, 631–3; al-Dhahabī 1987: 137; Ibn al-Bayṭār 1874, I: 138–9; D. al-Anṭākī 1952, I: 96; Ibn Sīnā 1999, I: 691–2; Ibn Sahl (O. Kahl 2003): nos 255, 279, 318, 327; al-Bīrūnī 1973: 115–16 (transl. 91); al-Warrāq (N. Nasrallah 2010): 640.

70. *mā' al-ward* – in addition to its primary uses in cosmetics (for example, as a deodorant) and cooking, rosewater (usually distilled from the damask rose) had a number of medical uses, mainly in ophthalmic treatments, such as ophthalmia and cataract, as well as against migraine and nausea. Frequent application of the substance to the hair allegedly accelerated grey hair growth. It was considered cold and dry in the first degree. *EI*[2], s.v. (F. Sanagustin); D. al-Anṭākī 1952, I: 339; Ibn al-Bayṭār 1874, IV: 136, and 1992: 239; Ibn al-Jazzār 2004: 9–10; Ibn al-Quff (H. Kircher 1967): 332–3; al-Dimashqī 1866: 195–8; E. Lev and Z. Amar 2008: 264–6.

71. *ʿasal naḥl muṣaffā* (i.e. strained of its wax and impurities) – the healing properties of honey are referred to on numerous occasions, both in the Qur'ān (16:68–9) and hadith, whereas 'rivers of purified honey' are one of the beneficences to be enjoyed in Paradise by the elect. In medicine and pharmacology, honey – which was hot and dry – was used as a diuretic and laxative, and a powerful antidote against poisons (as well as rabies). It also appears in compounds for the treatment of eye diseases (especially cataract). According to Maimonides (F. Rosner 1984:168), honey water helped erection. In cooking, honey was, of course, the core ingredient in a host of sweet dishes, pastries, syrups, and so on, as well as being a preserving agent. In botany, the termʿasal al-naḥl also denotes the lemon balm (*Melissa*

officinalis). *EI*², s.v. 'naḥl' (F. Viré); E. Lev and Z. Amar 2008: 185–7; A. Dietrich 1988, II: 238; al-Bīrūnī 1973: 264–6 (transl. 225ff); Ibn Wāfid 2000: 164–5; al-Warrāq (N. Nasrallah 2010): 592–5; *Risāla* (Cairo 362): fol. 4a; al-Kātib 2002: 36; al-Dhahabī 1987: 258; al-Suyūṭī n.d.: 12–13; Ibn Sīnā 1999, I: 619–20; D. al-Anṭākī 1952, I: 236–7; Ibn al-Bayṭār 1874, III: 121–3, and 1992: 183, 225; Ibn al-Quff (H. Kircher 1967): 274–6.

72. *ᶜasal manzūᶜ al-raghwa* – recipes calling for boiling honey usually require the skimming of the froth or scum that forms on top to remove the impurities and pollen that rise to the surface, and also to eliminate the acridity. Al-Warrāq (N. Nasrallah 2010): 593.

73. *fulful* – considered hot and dry, pepper (both white and black) was used extensively in medicine – for example, in the treatment of bladder stones, gum and throat inflammation and joint aches, as well as being an effective digestive, carminative and aphrodisiac (arousing desire, stiffening erection and increasing sperm). Other terms for pepper included *ḥabb Hindī* ('Indian seeds') and *bābārī* (< Gr. πιπέρι). E. Lev and Z. Amar 2008: 236–9; A. Dietrich 1988, II: 305–6; al-Warrāq (N. Nasrallah 2010): 651; al-Dhahabī 1987: 224; al-Suyūṭī n.d.: 14; ; Ibn al-Bayṭār 1874, III: 16–20, and 1992: 227; Ibn al-Jazzār 2004: 183, 195–6; Ibn Sīnā 1999, I: 626–7, and II: 734; al-Rāzī 1955–69, XXI: 235–9; al-Ṭabarī 1928: 395–6; al-Bīrūnī 1973: 292; al-Tīfāshī 1892: 14; Ibn Lūqā 1974: 16 (transl. 23); *Kitāb* (Tunis No 20648[09]): fol. 86b; al-Shayzarī, *al-Īdāḥ*: fol. 3a; *Risāla* (Cairo 362): fol. 3a.

74. 'thin piece of cloth ...'; [C]: strain then mix with the same measure of rosewater, add the weight of both in skimmed honey and boil over a fire. Sprinkle on it half [a *dirham*] of saffron and cardamom, a *dirham* of ginger, two *dirhams* of clove, strain, and then take ...'

75. 1 *qīrāṭ* = 0.195 grammes. Originally denoting the weight of a carob seed, it was one-sixteenth of a *dirham* and equalled four *shaᶜīra*, whereas its canonical (Iraqi) variant was one-twentieth of a *mithqāl*. L. Chipman 2009: 91; W. Hinz 1970: 27.

76. *misk* – considered hot and dry (in the third degree), musk was highly prized because of its rarity. It was used to strengthen the internal organs and heighten the senses, in the treatment of headaches, muscle spasms, palpitations, a gloomy disposition, and as a diuretic, emmenagogue, abortifacient, aperient, carminative and antidote (*tiryāq*) against venomous stings and bites. Its reputation as a powerful aphrodisiac was based on the fact that it is produced by a gland in the male musk deer (*Moschus*) to attract the female during the mating season. It was also recommended as a remedy for colds and as a deodorant. Arab scholars believed that the best musk came from a species of gazelle indigenous to China and Tibet (Ibn Wāfid, Ibn al-Baytār). The medicinal uses of musk were pioneered by al-Rāzī. In cooking, musk was used as an aromatic (*ṭīb*), whereas it was a key ingredient in perfumes as well. *EI*², s.v. 'misk' (A. Dietrich); E. Lev and Z. Amar 2008: 215–17; Ibn Wāfid 2000: 156–7; al-Dhahabī 1987: 259–61; Ibn al-Bayṭār 1874, IV: 155–7, and 1992: 182, 236; Ibn al-Jazzār 2004: 61; Ibn Sīnā 1999, I: 553, and II: 735; D. al-Anṭākī 1952, I: 297–8; al-Shayzarī, *al-Īḍāḥ*, fol. 3a; *Kitāb* (Tunis No

20648[09]): fol. 86b; al-Tīfāshī 1892: 14; al-Rāzī 1955–69, XXI: 516; H. Schindler and Frank 1961: 288–92; al-Warrāq (N. Nasrallah 2010): 664–5; Ibn al-Quff (H. Kircher 1967): 346–7.

77. The passage 'blend it with the water …' appears as follows in [C]: 'boil everything over a fire, sprinkle a *qīrāṭ* of musk on it, remove and use'.

78. This sentence has the following variant in [C]: '[it is useful] as has been mentioned. The signs are a weak liver, yellow face, dry tonge and lips, emaciation and a weak appetite.'

79. 'When a person …' is as follows in [C]: 'He cannot digest [food] and does not have the strength for coitus. When he does engage in sexual intercourse he does not experience any pleasure, while his sperm and limbs are cold. In addition, he flees coitus and baulks at it, lest he be afflicted by hemiplagia and a drop in innate heat because of it.'

80. *sunbul* (*Nardostachys jatamansi*, also known as *nardīn*) – one of the basic aromatic spices (*afwāh*, sing. *fūh*), it was synonymous with *nārdīn* in Arabic botanical and pharmacological works. There were three principal varieties: *sunbul hindī* (also referred to as *sunbul al-ṭīb, sunbul al-caṣāfīr*); *sunbul rūmī* (*Valeriana celtica*), which Ibn Sīnā equates with *nardīn*; *sunbul barrī* (*Asarum europaeum*). In the medical and pharmacological literature, the Indian variety was considered the most powerful; it was beneficial for the liver and stomach, colds, skin conditions, haemorrhoids, uteral tumours, to sweeten the breath, and as a diuretic, abortifacient, and sexual stimulant. E. Lev and Z. Amar 2008: 289–93; Ibn Wāfid 2000: 75–6; Ibn al-Bayṭār 1874, III: 36–8; Ibn al-Jazzār 2004: 26–7 (*sunbul hindī*), 27 (*sunbul rūmī*); D. al-Anṭākī 1952, I: 328; al-Rāzī, 1955–69, XXI: 579–82; *Kitāb* (Tunis No 20648[09]): fol. 87a; al-Shayzarī, *al-Īḍāḥ*: fol. 3a; A. Dietrich 1988, II: 91; al-Warrāq (N. Nasrallah 2010): 673; Ibn al-Quff (H. Kircher 1967): 220–1; Ibn Sīnā 1999, I: 575, 602–3.

81. This is missing from [B].

82. 'strengthens the liver …'; [C]: 'it increases coitus and there are other benefits, which would take too long to explain. The recipe is as follows …'

83. *ᶜūd hindī*, which also appears as *aghālūgh(/kh)un* (< Gr. ἀγάλοχον), *cūd liyyā*, *(y)alanjūj* and *alanj*, was used to make the breath smell sweet (by chewing on it), as a carminative and diuretic, to strengthen the stomach, to relieve obstructions and to cure liver defects and dysentery, all of which are also indications for *ᶜūd* (see below). Indian aloewood was considered the best variety of *ᶜūd*, Ibn Wāfid equating both with *bakhūr*. Like *ᶜūd*, it was recommended for its aphrodiasiac qualities. A. Dietrich 1988, II: 105–6 (Nos 19, 20); Ibn Wāfid 1987: 166–7; Ibn Sahl (O. Kahl 2003): nos 58, 65, 254, 265, 293 ('Indian lignaloes'); Ibn al-Bayṭār 1874, III: 143; D. al-Anṭākī 1952, I: 51, 241–2; al-Tīfāshī 1892: 14; *Kitāb* (Tunis No 20648[09]): fol. 86b; al-Shayzarī, *al-Īḍāḥ*: fol. 3a; al-Qazwīnī 1849: 260; al-Dhahabī 1987: 220; al-Bīrūnī 1973: 52 (transl. 34); al-Warrāq (N. Nasrallah 2010): 676–7.

84. The last three sentences are as follows in [C]: 'Add half a *dirham* of saffron dissolved in rosewater, remove and then use when needed. It is beneficial, as we have mentioned. As for the limpness and weakness of the penis, this comes in three types.'

85. The notion that a lack of moderation in sexual intercourse was harmful to health goes back to Galen – see for example P. de Lacey 1994: 138–41.

86. 'without having any lust…'; [C]: 'and there is no treatment for it. The second sign is that the penis is erect at the end of the night. This is remedied by the following medication and electuaries. The third sign is…'

87. 'ejaculates cold sperm…'; [C]: 'and his sperm is cold, whereas the ejaculaton is accompanied by a burning sensation, without lust. This is due to coldness in the person's back.'

88. 'and moistness' is omitted in [C].

89. *sudad* (sg. *sudda*), lit. 'obstruction', or, more specifically in this context 'a thing that obstructs the passage of the humours, and of the food, in the body' (E. Lane 1863–74, III: 1,329).

90. 'food that counters this action…'; [C]: 'bad bitter food in order to get rid of this illness. This electuary has thirty-three benefits.'

91. *salīkha* (*Cinnamomum cassia*); hot and dry in the third degree, the spice was an important simple and was said by Islamic medical authorities to strengthen the stomach, liver, womb and to relieve obstructions. The information for women was, somewhat contradictory; on the one hand it was said to strengthen the womb, provided a woman sits in a decoction of the herb, whereas it was also an emmenagogue and abortifacient. The term was often used interchangeably with *dār ṣīnī* (see below). In erotological literature it is frequently mentioned as an aphrodisiac. A. Dietrich 1988, II: 96–7; E. Lev and Z. Amar 2008: 143f; Ibn Lūqā 1974: 16 (transl. 23); J. Leibowitz and M. Shlomo 1974: 233; Ibn al-Bayṭār 1874, III: 25–6; Ibn al-Jazzār 2004: 135–6, and G. Bos 1997: 246, 265, 294, 307 ('cinnamon'); Ibn Sahl (O. Kahl 2003): 'cassia'; al-Tīfāshī 1892: 14; D. al-Anṭākī 1952, I: 196; Ibn Sīnā 1999, I: 603–4, 643; al-Rāzī 1955–69, XXI: 4ff; al-Bīrūnī 1973: 226–8 (transl. 186–7); al-Ṭabarī 1928: 319; al-Warrāq (N. Nasrallah 2010): 670; Issa Bey 1930: 49 (no 3); Ibn al-Quff (H. Kircher 1967): 228–9.

92. *sādaj* (a dialectal variant of the more common *sādhaj*) was said to be hot and dry in the second degree. A Persian borrowing, it was often wrongly equated with spikenard (*sunbul*) and sometimes appears as *sādaj hindī*. The identification of the plant is somewhat uncertain, and according to some it involves a member of the *Stratiotes* family (*Stratiotes aloides* or *Pistia stratiotes*), a cinnamon (*Cinnamonum citriodorum* [*Laurecae*]) or a laurel (*Laurus malabathrum*). In medicine, it was used as a diuretic, to strengthen the stomach or, in an unguent, for the treatment of tumors (especially in the eyes), and to combat flatulence. Due to its fragrance, it was also said to sweeten the breath (when chewed). See A. Dietrich 1988, II: 94–6; E. Lev and Z. Amar 2008: 444–5; Ibn al-Jazzār 2004: 97–8; Ibn Sīnā 1999, I: 585–6; Ibn Wāfid 2000: 76; D. al-Anṭākī 1952, I: 185; al-Rāzī 1955–69, XXI: 6; Ibn al-Bayṭār 1874, III: 2; E. Lev and Z. Amar 2008: 444–5; F. Steingass 1892: 639; Ibn Sahl (O. Kahl 2003): no. 366 ('laurel', *Laurus malabathrum*); al-Ishbīlī 1995, I: 259 (who states that *sādhaj hindī* is the term used in al-Andalus for *rand hindī*), 382 (= *nārdīn nahrī*); al-Warrāq (N. Nasrallah 2010): 670, 758 ('Indian leaf'); Dioscorides 2000: 17.

93. *janṭiyāna* (< Gr. γεντιανή), *Gentiana lutea*, which was used as a fortifier,

emmenagogue and abortifacient, and to treat digestive problems (appetite, gas, diarrhoea). A. Dietrich 1988, II: 344–5; D. al-Anṭākī 1952, I: 109; al-Rāzī 1955–69, XX: 230–2; Ibn al-Bayṭār 1874, I: 170–1; Ibn al-Quff (H. Kircher 1967): 142–3.

94. [C]: 'one *dirham*'.

95. *kammūn, Cuminum cyminum* – considered hot and dry, the seeds of this plant (whether wild or cultivated) were a highly popular aromatic for cooking, whereas in medicine it was used as a digestive, carminative, eructative, diaphoretic, emmenagogue, aphrodisiac (Maimonides adding that it stiffened the penis) and a cure for urinary, intestinal and eye diseases. Several varieties occur in the literature (for example, Persian, Syrian, Kirmani, Nabataean), whereas the term was also used as a generic to denote other plants: *kammūn rūmī/armanī* ('Byzantine/Armenian cumin' – caraway), *kammūn ḥulw* ('sweet cumin' – aniseed). The variety known as black cumin is referred to in Arabic as *ḥabba sawdā'* (see below). Confusingly, the Persian *zīre siyāh* ('black cumin') refers to caraway (Ar. *karāwiyā; Carum carvi*). *EI*², s.v. 'kammūn'(G. S. Colin); E. Lev and Z. Amar 2008: 159–60; A. Dietrich 1988, II: 408ff; al-Dhahabī 1987: 235; Ibn al-Jazzār 2004: 160–1; al-Warrāq (N. Nasrallah 2010): 655–6; D. al-Anṭākī 1952, I: 275; Ibn al-Jazzār 2004: 149; al-Tīfāshī 1892: 14 (though elsewhere [31], he claims that it has a diminishing effect because it cuts the flow of sperm); al-Rāzī 1955–69, XXI: 332–5; Ibn al-Bayṭār 1874, IV: 81–2, and 1992: 176, 231–2; Ibn al-Jazzār 2004: 149; Ibn Sīnā 1999, I: 523–4; Ibn al-Quff (H. Kircher 1967): 328–9.

96. *jazar* (also sometimes referred to as *dawqū, aṣṭūfūlin*) – the varieties used included the red (*aḥmar* or *bustānī*), yellow (*aṣfar* or *barrī*) and white (*abyaḍ*). In the medical tradition, carrots (including their seeds) were used against kidney pains, palpitations, cough, and snake blood, and as a diuretic, carminative and emmenagogue. In addition, they were considered a powerful sexual stimulant (especially when picked in vinegar), though al-Kindī prescribed them to cure sexual addiction(!). E. Lev and Z. Amar 2008: 127–8; Ibn Wāfid 2000: 142; Ibn Sīnā 1999, II: 734; al-Kindī (M. Levey 1966): nos 207, 221, 226; al-Rāzī 1955–69, XX: 226–8; Ibn al-Bayṭār 1874, I: 161–3, and 1992: 200, 209; al-Dhahabī 1987: 148; D. al-Anṭākī 1952, I: 105–6; Dietrich 1988, II: 286, 402; al-Warrāq (N. Nasrallah 2010): 786; Issa Bey 1930: 69; Maimonides (F. Rosner and S. Muntner 1970): 21, 80.

97. *maṣṭi/akā* (< Gr. μαστίκη) – dry and hot, mastic (also 'lentisk', which is the aromatic resin of the pistachio tree (*Pistacia lentiscus*), came in a number of varieties (yellow, white – *ᶜilk al-Rūm*, 'Byzantine gum' – and black [Egyptian or Iraqi]), and had a large number of medicinal applications, including to strengthen the stomach, liver and intestines, to improve the appearance of the skin, and to treat ulcers and tumours, as well as being an eructative, expectorant, analgesic (especially for toothache and stomach pains), carminative, breath-sweetener, teeth cleanser and aphrodisiac. E. Lev and Z. Amar 2008: 203–5 ('lentisk'); Ibn al-Bayṭār 1992: 177, 236; Ibn al-Jazzār 2004: 62; Ibn Sīnā 1999, I: 553–4; al-Suyūṭī n.d.: 15; Ibn Wāfid 2000: 154–6; al-Tīfāshī 1892: 14; al-Dhahabī 1987: 261; *Kitāb* (Tunis No

20648[09]): fol. 87a; al-Warrāq (N. Nasrallah 2010): 786; Maimonides (M. Meyerhof 1940): no. 232; Ibn al-Quff (H. Kircher 1967): 340–1.

98. *ʿūd* (also *ʿūd ḥabb, ʿūd bukhūr*) – literally means 'wood', 'rod' or 'stick', and refers to (chips of) agarwood (grown in India, China and Yemen), or its resin extracts. It was variously thought to strengthen the heart and senses, in addition to the uses already mentioned for *ʿūd hindī* (see above). In cooking, it was used for fumigating meat and receptacles to remove unpleasant odours. According to Maimonides, it arouses the lust for coitus, stiffens the penis and increases sexual pleausure, whereas al-Tīfāshī states it arouses women's lust and desire for coitus (*tuhayyij shahwat al-nisāʾ wa tadʿūwhunna ilā ʾl-jimāʿ*). E. Lev and Z. Amar 2008: 97–8; Ibn al-Bayṭār 1992: 182, 224; Ibn al-Jazzār 2004: 65; Ibn Wāfid 1987: 166–7; al-Tīfāshī 1970: 32; Ibn Sahl (O. Kahl 2003): nos 206, 292 ('lignaloes'); A. Dietrich 1988, II: 105; al-Dhahabī 1987: 220; Ibn Sīnā 1999, I: 614–15; al-Warrāq (N. Nasrallah 2010): 676; Issa Bey 1930: 10.

99. 'clove' is omitted in [C].

100. *murr* (lit. 'bitter') – the resin extracted from the bark of trees growing in the south of the Arabian Peninsula (as well as northern Ethiopia and Somalia), myrrh (whose Arabic etymon refers to its taste) was used, for instance, against stomach complaints, coughs and colds, as an anthelmintic, abortifacient, theriac, deodorant, embalming agent and aphrodisiac. Ibn al-Baytār recommended mixing myrrh with olive oil and rubbing the mixture on the big toe of the right foot, which would allow the man to have sex for as long as the substance remained on his toe! E. Lev and Z. Amar 2008: 221–4; al-Rāzī 1955–69, XXI: 500–4; Ibn Sīnā 1999, I: 565; al-Bīrūnī 1973: 345 (transl. 304); al-Kindī (M. Levey 1966): 333–4 (no. 283); Ibn al-Bayṭār 1874, IV: 145–7, and 1992: 237; Ibn al-Jazzār 2004: 85–6; D. Antākī 1952, I: 293–4; A. Dietrich 1988, II: 110; al-Warrāq (N. Nasrallah 2010): 755; Ibn al-Quff (H. Kircher 1967): 338–9. For a detailed discussion of the origins and trade of the substance, see N. Groom 1981.

101. 'Pulverize ...'; [C]: 'and bee honey equalling three times the total amount. Then boil everyting over a fire and turn into an electuary.'

102. 1 *mithqāl* = 4.464 grammes. Hinz 1970: 4.

103. *duyūk* (sg. *dīk*) – in the Arabic tradition, the cock appears often in literature, and was thought to be highly sensual (as well as conceited). The voice of the cock was considered very attractive, and allegedly alleviated pains in those who heard it. According to a hadith, Allah also liked the sound of the cock's voice, while the Prophet used to keep a white cock in his house. In medicine, the bile, brain, comb and blood were used in remedies for colics and fevers, and for those with cold temperaments. According to Maimonides, rooster testicles were very effective in increasing sperm. *EI²*, s.v. 'dīk' (L. Kopf); Ibn Sīnā 1999, I: 436-7; Ibn al-Bayṭār 1992: 184; Ibn al-Jazzār 2004: 209; Maimonides (F. Rosner 1984): 167; al-Ṭabarī 1928: 432–3; al-Kātib 1977: 274.

104. The Arabic *murdāsank* is a (miswritten) calque of the Persian *murdāsang*. In Arabic, it was also known as martak and *mu/ardāsanj*. A by-product of separating silver from lead, litharge (which was considered cold and dry

in the second degree) was used in the treatment of various dermatological conditions (scrofula, vitiligo alba, abscesses, swollen sores), eye diseases and haemorrhoids, and as a deodorant. E. Lev and Z. Amar 2008: 440 ('lead oxide'), 535 ('lead peroxide'); Ibn Sīnā 1999, III: 285, 559–60; W. Lane 1863–74, III: 1,028; Ibn al-Bayṭār 1874, IV: 150; Ibn al-Jazzār 2004: 89; al-Kindī (M. Levey 1966): 334–5; al-Suyūṭī n.d.: 14; Ibn al-Quff (H. Kircher 1967): 336–8; Maimonides (M. Meyerhof 1940): nos 239, 256.

105. [C]: 'sufficient to enable you to knead the collected gall into a fine paste'.

106. This sentence is missing from [C].

107. The reference to the bath is missing from [C], which simply states 'in the morning'.

108. The last two sentences are as follows in [C]: 'Eat the musk electuary after coming out of the bath.'

109. *baṣal* – a number of varieties of onion are mentioned in the literature (red, white, long, and so on). Hot and moist, both the vegetable and its seeds are mentioned as an appetizer and anti-emetic, but most often as a sexual stimulant, to increase sperm (and improve its motility), and as a remedy for impotence. According to Ibn al-Quff, pouring onion juice in the ear was a remedy for tinnitus (*ṭanīn fi 'l-udhun*), while rubbing it in the eyes increased vision. On the other hand, onions could also cause headaches, whereas excessive consumption led to forgetfulness and haemorrhoids. In cooking, it was (and still is) a staple in both North African and Near Eastern dishes (especially meat). D. al-Anṭākī 1952, I: 76; Ibn Sīnā 1999, I: 390–2, and II: 734 ('especially when grilled'); Ibn al-Bayṭār 1874, I: 96, and 1992: 193; Maimonides (F. Rosner 1984): 167; Ibn Lūqā 1974: 13, 16 (transl. 19, 20, 23); *Kitāb* (Tunis No 20648[09]): fol. 87a; *Risāla* (Cairo 362): fol. 3a; Ibn Māssa 1971: 8, 9 (transl. 10, 11); al-Tīfāshī 1892: 13, 14; Ibn Lūqā 1974: 16 (transl. 23); al-Kātib 2002: 36; al-Dhahabī 1987: 129–30; al-Warrāq (N. Nasrallah 2010): 646–7; A. Dietrich 1988, II: 297–8; Ibn al-Quff (H. Kircher 1967): 100–1; E. Lev and Z. Amar 2008: 230–1.

110. *fujl* (also *fajl*) – hot and dry, it had a wide variety of medical applications, ranging from clearing of obstructions in the liver to improving eyesight, combating arthritis, as an emetic, digestive, appetizer, eructative, antidote (against scorpion bites), and to trigger hair-growth. It was also thought to increase sperm and assist in coitus. In cooking, it was eaten both raw and cooked. At the same time, some physicians (including Maimonides) considered it a harmful food. E. Lev and Z. Amar 2008: 257–9; A. Dietrich 1988, II: 260–1; al-Dhahabī 1987: 223–4; al-Rāzī 1955–69, XXI: 218–22; Ibn Sīnā 1999, I: 672–3, and II: 734; Ibn al-Bayṭār 1874, III: 156–8, and 1992: 227; D. al-Anṭākī 1952, I: 248; al-Suyūṭī n.d.: 12; al-Tīfāshī 1892: 14; *Kitāb* (Tunis No 20648[09]): fol. 87a; al-Warrāq (N. Nasrallah 2010): 784; Ibn al-Quff (H. Kircher 1967): 295–6; Maimonides (F. Rosner and S. Muntner 1970): 15:6, 21:80, 22:45.

111. *rashād* (also known as *ḥurf*, *Lepidium sativum*), 'garden cress', sometimes appears under the name *thuffā*. Aside from being an appetizer, anthelmintic, emmenagogue, abortifacient (when the woman inserts the seeds into the vagina) and carminative, the herb (or rather its seeds), was also thought to

increase the lust for coition. There was often terminological confusion between this herb and cardamom because of the similarity in the Greek etyma κάρδαμον and καρδάμωμον, respectively. Cardamom became known as qardamānā, which was used interchangeably with *karawiyā barrī* ('wild caraway'). E. Lev and Z. Amar 2008: 172–4; A. Dietrich 1988, II: 15, 301ff; Ibn al-Jazzār 2004: 206–7; al-Kātib 2002: 36; al-Warrāq (N. Nasrallah 2010): 668–9; Ibn al-Bayṭār 1874, II: 15–17; *Kitāb* (Tunis No. 20648[09]): fol. 86b, *Risāla* (Cairo 362): fol. 3a; al-Shayzarī, *al-Īḍāḥ*: fol. 2b; al-Qazwīnī 1849: 278; Ibn Sīnā 1999, I: 476–7, and II: 734; al-Bīrūnī 1973: 156 (transl. 125); al-Rāzī 1955–69, XX: 319–23; Ibn al-Quff (H. Kircher 1967): 162.

112. [C] has 'ginger' instead of 'turnip seeds'.

113. In the Near and Middle East, *harīsa* usually refers to a dish (stew) of meat and bulghur (cracked wheat). In North Africa – especially Tunisia – it is a hot pepper paste. Ibn al-Bayṭār 1992: 178; Maimonides (F. Rosner 1984): 171 (*harīsiyya*).

114. The rest of the sentence is omitted from [C].

115. *ḥimmiṣ* (also *ḥimmaṣ, ḥummuṣ*), *Cicer arietinum* – the varieties used are white, black and red, all of which were said to cause bloating and had to be soaked and cooked before eating (only during a meal). Medicinally, they were widely known as a diuretic, emmenagogue and aphrodisiac. According to al-Tīfāshī, chickpeas (and eggs) were particularly effective in increasing sexual potency because they combined three basic qualities: to create coarse winds (*muwallid li 'l-riyāḥ al-ghalīẓa*), nutritional (*kathīr al-ghadā*) and moderate in heat (*muʿtadal al-ḥarāra*), balanced to suit the characteristic of the sperm. Because chickpeas allegedly assisted the stiffening and maintenance of the erection, they were fed to male horses. A. Dietrich 1988, II: 253; al-Warrāq (N. Nasrallah 2010): 797; al-Dhahabī 1987: 160; Ibn Sīnā 1999, II: 734; al-Suyūṭī n.d.: 9; al-Ṭabarī 1928: 432–3; Ibn al-Bayṭār 1874, II: 302, and 1992: 205; D. al-Anṭākī 1952, I: 28; al-Tīfāshī 1892: 13, 14; *Risāla* (Cairo 362): fol. 3a; al-Kātib 2002: 36; al-Qazwīnī 1849: 279; al-Bīrūnī 1973: 163 (transl. 129–30); al-Rāzī 1955–69, XX: 356–9.

116. [C]: 'in which it has been cooked.'

117. *ʿaṣāfīr* (sg. *ʿuṣfūr*) – hot and dry, the bird was widely held to increase sperm and potency. According to several hadiths, the Prophet even forbade its killing. al-Tīfāshī 1892: 14; al-Dhahabī 1987: 217; Ibn al-Bayṭār 1992: 185.

118. 'Cook over a low fire ...'; [C]: 'If it starts smelling, remove from the fire and boil with...'

119. '... cinnamon bark...'; [C]: 'six walnuts and ten *dirhams* of cinnamon bark; mix everything together and eat by sprinkling on your food. It is beneficial as we have mentioned.'

120. This is an Egyptian sauce, consisting usually of garlic and (ground) coriander fried in butter, and used as a garnish (especially for stewed vegetables) or to enrich stock or sauce. It is also the main spicing of the famous Egyptian dish *mulūkhiyya* (Jew's mallow [*Corchorus olitorius*], or the soup made with this plant).

121. *shīshak* – the one-year-old lamb is among the meats mentioned by Maimonides (R. Rosner 1984: 171) as being beneficial for coitus.

122. *abāzir* (also *abzār*, *buzūr*, sg. *bizr*), refers to spices and condiments, whether dried or fresh (and may even be extended to include olive oil and vinegar); the other generic for spices, *tawābil* (sg. *tābil*), only denotes dried seasonings; al-Warrāq (N. Nasrallah 2010: 643).
123. *tamr* – considered hot and dry, the fruit of the date palm (*nakhla*, *Phoenix dactylifera*) has been a staple in the Middle Eastern diet for millennia. It is mentioned several times (19 in total) in the Qur'ān, usually as a beneficence granted by Allah to humanity (for example, 6:99; 6:141; 16:11; 16:67; 18:32), and occurs in a large number of hadiths (for example, as one of the fruits of paradise), as well as in poetry and medical treatises. In addition to its flesh (either whole or in a paste), the stones were also used in various applications. Dates were recommended for a variety of illnesses and conditions, such as diarrhoea, colic and poisoning, including to increase sexual lust and potency. E. Lev and Z. Amar 2008: 397–8; E. Lane, 1863–74, I: 316; al-Dhahabī 1987: 138–42; al-Suyūṭī n.d.: 11; *EI*², s.v. 'nakhla' (F. Viré); al-Warrāq (N. Nasrallah 2010): 638–9.
124. 'cow's milk…'; [C]: 'fresh cow's milk.'
125. *thūm* – hot and dry, it came in two varieties: *barrī* ('wild') and *bustānī* ('cultivated). It was used medicinally to relieve flatulence, for various dermatological conditions, and as an emenagogue. Though some authors stated that garlic had a negative effect on coitus (as well as the breath!), others recommended it as a remedy for impotence. E. Lev and Z. Amar 2008: 412–14; Ibn Lūqā 1974: 16 (transl. 23); *Risāla* (Cairo 362): fol. 2a (who claimed it was very effective when drunk with milk and honey); Ibn al-Bayṭār 1874, I: 151–3, and 1992: 199; Ibn al-Jazzār 2004: 202–3; D. al-Anṭākī 1952, I: 101–2; al-Dhahabī 1987: 144–5; al-Suyūṭī n.d.: 13; Ibn Sīnā 1999, I: 695–6; A. Dietrich 1988, II: 298; al-Warrāq (N. Nasrallah 2010): 675; al-Bīrūnī 1973: 125; Ibn al-Quff (H. Kircher 1967): 130–2; Issa Bey 1930: 9 (no. 15).
126. The preceding passage, 'You can also eat *taqliyya*…' is missing from [C], which simply has: 'and cook the carrots with the meat or the chicken and sprinkle on top. The recipe for the broth is as follows.'
127. The ms. has the misspelling *sukūrruja* for *suku/arruja* (< Persian *sukraja*, 'saucer'), which was used 'to put sauces and the like to excite the appetite and to aid digestion' (E. Lane 1863–74). It came in two sizes (six ounces and three ounces, or four *mithqāls*), though as a measure it was often equalled to 125 grammes. Lane 1863–74, IV: 116; W. Hinz 1970; L. Chipman 2009: 91.
128. The preceding five sentences are omitted from [C], which has: 'Throw the grated garlic on, cook over a low fire and sprinkle the above-mentioned spices on top.'
129. 'in a glass vessel' is omitted from [C].
130. This entire sentence and the remainder of the chapter are omitted from [C].
131. *samn* – clarified butter, while *zubd* denotes butter made from churned milk. In medicine, *samn* (often mixed with honey), on its own, was used as an antidote against poisons and snake bites, or (in an unguent) to treat haemorrhoids, for instance. In addition, it figures as an ingredient in many medical preparations for a variety of ills. In cooking, it was particularly used in egg-based dishes. *EI*², s.v. 'samn' (J. Ruska [D. Waines]); Ibn Sahl (O. Kahl

2003); al-Dhahabī 1987: 192–3; al-Suyūṭī n.d.: 9, 13; Ibn Sīnā 1999, I: 602; E. Lev and Z. Amar 2008: 132–4 ('sour cream').

132. *qadīd* – the meat was marinated in sour vinegar mixed with salt and spices (black pepper, coriander, caraway), and then dried in the sun. According to al-Rāzī, it sated what he called the 'false hunger' (*jūᶜ kādhib*) brought about by drinking alcohol, provided the meat was eaten with dry biscuits and *murrī* (liquid fermented sauce); al-Warrāq (N. Nasrallah 2010): 719.

133. *zabīb* – which also denoted currants, have been used extensively in cooking but were also thought to have beneficial medicinal properties (being hot and moist). The seeds and juice, as well as wine based on it (which was said to be lighter than that made from grapes), were all used in remedies. Raisins were recommended, for instance, to strengthen the stomach, and as a remedy for cough, ulcers, and tumours. When eaten to excess, raisins (which are hot and moist in the first degree) were thought to burn the blood, which could be countered by green cucumbers. E. Lev and Z. Amar 2008: 176–80; Ibn Wāfid 2000: 59–62 (especially 61f); *Risāla* (Cairo 362): fol. 3a; al-Warrāq (N. Nasrallah 2010): 642; al-Dhahabī 1987: 282–4; Ibn Sahl (O. Kahl 2003): s.vv. 'raisin', 'raisin-seed', 'raisin water', 'raisin wine'; *EI²*, s.v. 'zabīb' (D. Waines); M. Steinschneider 1900: 74; Ibn al-Quff (H. Kircher 1967): 203–4; al-Suyūṭī n.d.: 11. Also see the note above on '*ᶜinab*'.

134. 'and nature' is omitted from [C].

135. A dessert typically made with wheat flour, rosewater, saffron and cardamom, and garnished with pistachios and almonds.

136. The preceding passage is considerably shorter in [C]: 'Among them Persian halva, which is made from fine flour, cow ghee and bee honey, and eaten with dry bread and...'

137. *ḥamām* – like other poultry, it was said to be very moist. Pigeon blood was used to stop nasal bleeding and in remedies for paralysis. Ibn Sīnā 1999, I: 492; Ibn al-Bayṭār 1992: 184–5, 207.

138. *afrākh* (sg. *firākh*) – their medicinal properties were similar to those of chickens (*dajāj*); see note below.

139. *iwazz* (sg. *wazz*) – goose blood and fat were used in electuaries for the treatment of ear diseases, as an emmenagogue or to stem excessive menstrual bleeding. Al-Ṭabarī 1928: 433.

140. *dajāj* – considered cold and moist, its properties were praised in a number of hadiths, as it was thought to be beneficial to the mind, to relieve stomach inflammation and increase sperm. Ibn Sīnā 1999, I: 436–7; al-Dhahabī 1987: 184–5; Ibn al-Bayṭār 1992: 184; Ibn al-Jazzār 2004: 209.

141. *farārīj* (sg. *farrūj*) – their medicinal uses were thought to be identical to those of chickens (*dajāj*), including benefits for coition and as a sperm booster; al-Tīfāshī 1892: 14; Ibn Sīnā 1999, II: 734; Ibn al-Bayṭār 1992: 184; al-Warrāq (N. Nasrallah 2010): 724.

142. *samak* (pl. *asmāk*) – generally considered cold and moist, fish were recommended in the treatment of, for instance, arthritis, whereas a number of them (such as the eel) were aphrodisiacs; Ibn Sīnā 1999, I: 605–7, and II: 734; Ibn al-Bayṭār 1992: 218.

143. *birisht*, which is a term used in ECA. It is borrowed from Persian, *nīm birisht*,

'poached egg (half-boiled)' (F. Steingass 1892: 1,445). Hard-boiled eggs were said to be harmful, as they are difficult to digest and cause colic and stones (both in kidney and bladder); Ibn al-Quff (H. Kircher 1967): 97–8.

144. This is a rather strange comment, as eggs (considered cold and moist) from most poultry were generally held to be beneficial. Their ability to increase potency (and sperm) is often mentioned in the literature. According to Ibn al-Quff, the best eggs were those from young, black hens. Ibn al-Bayṭār 1992: 182; Ibn Sīnā 1999, II: 734; Maimonides (F. Rosner 1984): 167; al-Tīfāshī 1892: 14; M. al-Fallātī [BN 5662]: fol. 83a; al-Dhahabī 1987: 135; Ibn al-Quff (H. Kircher 1967): 97–9; al-Suyūṭī n.d.: 11.

145. The reference to soft-boiled eggs and the harmfulness of other types of eggs is omitted from [C].

146. [A]: *(al-ᶜaṣāfīr) al-darwiyya* (for *al-dūriyya*).

147. *admigha* (sg. *dimāgh*) – various animal brains, such as those of bulls, veal, camel and sheep, were used medicinally in the treatment, for instance, of ulcers, tumours, sciatica and colic, as well as being endowed with aphrodisiacal qualities. According to Ibn al-Bayṭār (1992: 209), the best brains were those of birds and quadrupeds (chiefly the camel). Sparrows' brains are also mentioned by al-Kātib (2002: 36), who recommends using the brains of birds when they are sexually excited (1977: 280), and by Ibn Sīnā (1999, II: 734), alongside those of pullets, ducks and squabs, to enhance coitus. Also see Ibn al-Quff (H. Kircher 1967): 347–8; Ibn Sīnā 1999, I: 573, 635.

148. *laban* (also *ḥalab*) – milk was considered particularly useful for hot and cold temperaments, and had a number of medicinal applications – such as to treat stomach complaints, ulcers and cough (especially donkey and goat's milk), and as an emmenagogue. Physicians warned, however, of the fact that milk was difficult to digest, causing flatulence and colic. It was considered a potent aphrodisiac (even the sour variety), fresh milk and butter being prescribed to strengthen the erection. Some (such as al-Kindī) recommended breastmilk in medical treatments. Al-Kindī (M. Levey 1966): nos 9–11, 28, 37, 40, 46, 96, 127, 140, 142, 166, 170, 178, 180, 258; Ibn Sīnā 1999, II: 546–50, and II: 732; E. Lev and Z. Amar 2008: 132–4; Ibn al-Bayṭār 1874, I: 157–9, and IV, 93–100, 132–4; al-Kātib 2002: 36; D. al-Anṭākī 1952, I: 103.

149. *lift* – also commonly known in Arabic as *s[h]aljam* (< Persian *shalgham*), a number of varieties being mentioned in the literature (*barrī*, 'wild'; *bustānī*, 'garden'; *ṣaghīr*, 'small'). The seeds and root of the plant were used in medicine – for instance, to improve the eyesight. It was also thought to increase sperm and heighten sexual appetite. A. Dietrich 1988 II: 257–9, 621–2; Maimonides (F. Rosner 1984): 167; al-Warrāq (N. Nasrallah 2010): 794; Ibn al-Bayṭār 1874, III: 67–8, and IV, 110; D. al-Anṭākī 1952, I: 198, 283; al-Dhahabī 1987: 199–200; Ibn al-Quff (H. Kircher 1967): 230–1; Ibn Sīnā 1999, I: 679–80.

150. *kurrāt* (for *kurrāth*) – in addition to commonly used *kurrāth shāmī* ('Syrian') and *nabatī* ('Nabataean', also known as *kurrāth al-baql and k. al-mā'ida*), the leek varieties mentioned include *kurrāth Fārisī* ('Persian l.'),

k. Rūmī ('Byzantine l.'), *k. al-karm* ('vine l.', also known as *k. barrī,* 'wild l.') and *k. jabalī* ('mountain l.'). The term *kurrāth al-ḥayya* ('snake leek') refers, however, not to a leek but to a type of garlic (*thūm ḥayya*), which occasionally is even equated (wrongly) with gentian. Medically, leeks were used as a diuretic and antihelmintic, in the treatment of ulcers, swellings, colic, haemorrhoids and headaches, and as an aphrodisiac. Maimonides recommended them to prevent the growth of pubic and armpit hair. According to Ibn Lūqā (1974: 14), Syrian leek was one of the substances that could 'loosen the sperm if it was solid, make it more fluid, soluble and eager to be expelled' (*tuḥallil al-minā idhā kāna jāmidan wa yaṣīru fihi ilā 'l-dhawbān wa 'l-sayalān wa ṭalab al-khurūj*). Al-Tīfāshī stated the benefit of leek for increasing female sperm and coital vigour (1970: 22). E. Lev and Z. Amar 2008: 433–4; A. Dietrich 1988, II: 296–7, 299; Ibn al-Bayṭār 1874, IV: 61–3, and 1992: 233; Ibn Sīnā 1999, I: 532–3; D. al-Anṭākī 1952, I: 271; al-Rāzī 1955–69, XXI: 383–8; al-Kindī (M. Levey 1966): nos 29, 148; al-Bīrūnī 1973: 315; Maimonides (M. Meyerhof 1940): No 198; al-Kindī (M. Levey 1966): nos 29, 148; al-Warrāq (N. Nasrallah 2010): 660–2.

151. 'cow ghee' is omitted from [C].

152. *lawz* (*Prunus amygdalus*) – considered moderately hot, it usually refers to the 'sweet' almond (*lawz hulw*), in addition to which the literature mentions bitter (*murr*), 'fresh' (*ṭarī*) and 'salted' (*mamlūḥ*). In the medical tradition, almonds were recommended against coughs and skin diseases, to purify the blood and increase the sperm (especially when eaten with sugar), and as an analgesic and aphrodisiac. The bitter variety was used to relieve blockages (especially in the liver) and cure uteral pains and renal calculus. E. Lev and Z. Amar 2008: 91–4; A. Dietrich 1988, II: 187–8; Maimonides (F. Rosner 1984): 167 ('peeled dried almonds'); Ibn Wāfid 2000: 92–3; Ibn al-Bayṭār 1874, IV: 111–2, III: 86, and 1992: 175, 235; Ibn al-Jazzār 2004: 118–19; Ibn Sīnā 1999, I: 544–5; D. al-Anṭākī 1952, I: 284; al-Dhahabī 1987: 252–3; al-Suyūṭī n.d.: 9; al-Bīrūnī 1973: 334–5; al-Warrāq (N. Nasrallah 2010): 633.

153. *bunduq* (> Gr. Ποντικόν) – also known as *jillawz* (< Persian *j/galūz*), they originally hailed from Turkey and were considered hot and dry. In medicine, hazelnuts were used, for instance, to cleanse and strengthen the intestines, improve memory, and treat palpitations, urinary infections and epilepsy. They were sometimes subdivided into 'Indian' and 'non-Indian' hazelnuts. Both were generally thought to have a number of negative properties: they were difficult to digest, generate bile, and cause vomiting and headaches. As a result, they were often not administered on their own but as part of a syrup or preserve – added with honey, for instance. But non-Indian hazelnuts were said to strengthen the brain and serve as an antidote, as well as being a sexual stimulant. The Indian variety was an emmenagogue and relieved asthma symptoms, whereas roasted hazelnuts mixed with olive oil could cure alopecia when the mixture was rubbed into the scalp. A. Dietrich 1988, II: 189–90; E. Lev and Z. Amar 2008: 416–17; al-Dhahabī 1987: 134; al-Tīfāshī 1892: 14; Maimonides (F. Rosner 1984): 167; Ibn Sīnā 1999: 734; Ibn al-Bayṭār 1874, I: 119; Ibn Sīnā 1999, I: 406–8; Ibn Wāfid 2000: 140–

1; D. al-Anṭākī 1952, I: 85; al-Rāzī 1955–69, XXI: 383–8; al-Bīrūnī 1973: 101–2; Maimonides (M. Meyerhof 1940): no. 43; al-Warrāq (N. Nasrallah 2010): 627; Ibn al-Quff (H. Kircher 1967): 114–16; Maimonides (M. Meyerhof 1940): no. 335.

154. *fustuq* (also *fustaq* < Gr. Πιστάκια) – hot and dry (more so than walnuts and almonds), it was used to unblock obstructions (especially in the liver) and thought to be beneficial for chest and lung ailments, as a purgative, and to invigorate coitus. A. Dietrich 1988, II: 188; E. Lev and Z. Amar 2008: 468–70; Maimonides (F. Rosner 1984): 167, (M. Meyerhof 1940): no. 301; al-Dhahabī 1987: 224; al-Tīfāshī 1892: 14; Ibn Sīnā 1999: 734; Ibn al-Bayṭār 1874, III: 163, and 1992: 227–8; Ibn Wāfid 2000: 80; D. al-Anṭākī 1952, I: 249–50; al-Rāzī 1955–69, XXI: 214; al-Bīrūnī 1973: 289; al-Warrāq (N. Nasrallah 2010): 628.

155. *ruṭab*, hot and moist, comes in two varieties – 'one that cannot be dried and spoils soon if not eaten; one that dries, and is made into *ᶜajwa*' (E. Lane 1863–74, III: 1,101). This type of date was believed to heat and increase thickness of the blood, but was discouraged for those with a hot temperament or prone to headaches. Ibn Wāfid 2000: 84–5; al-Dhahabī 1987: 179; al-Warrāq (N. Nasrallah 2010): 638. Also see note on '*tamr*', above.

156. *tīn* – figs came in many varieties, but the fresh, peeled white (or yellow) type was thought to be the best, while generally being the most nutritious of all fruit. Unripe figs were known as *al-tīn al-fijj/barrī* ('winter, unripe figs'). Both the fruit and the leaves were used in medicine. Its applications included as a diuretic, appetizer, antidote against poisons, laxative, anti-cough treatment, and to relieve obstructions. Figs (especially fresh ones) were also thought to increase sperm and fecundity, and were thus often considered an aphrodisiac; fig was also a key ingredient in electuaries for vaginal treatments. It was also thought to attract lice to the body. The fruit appears in the title of a Qur'ānic *sūra* (95) as well as in a large number of hadiths, the most famous of which states that the Prophet considered it descended from paradise. Ibn al-Bayṭār 1874, I: 146–8, and 1992: 167, 197; al-Tīfāshī 1892: 14, and 1970: 31 (transl. 46), 35 (transl. 51); D. al-Anṭākī 1952, I: 99–100; al-Warrāq (N. Nasrallah 2010): 639–40; Ibn Wāfid 2000: 176–9; al-Dhahabī 1987: 143; al-Ṭabarī 1928: 381; al-Qazwīnī 1849: 251–2; Ibn al-Quff (H. Kircher 1967): 122–3; A. Dietrich 1988, II: 192–3.

157. *ᶜinab* – hot and moist, the white variety was considered the best and more easily digestible than the red, and highly nourishing (often invoking comparisons to figs). Sour unripe grapes were known as *ḥisrim*. The fruit is given great prominence in Islam (on a par with the date); it occurs a number of times in the Qur'ān, where it is listed as one of the fruits of paradise (2:266, 6:99, 16:67, 17:91, 23:19; 36:34; 80:28). Even wine made from it (and from dates) is said to be good nourishment (Qur'ān 16:69), though the relevant verse was later superseded by others prohibiting intoxicating substances (4:46; 5:92). In Arabic literature, too, there are numerous references to the grape, particularly in relation to wine of course, which is the object of a genre in poetry known as *khamriyyāt*. Grapes were used in a

variety of ways (fresh, dried, vinegar, its lees as fertilizer). In pharmacology and medicine, the fruit, leaves, juice and wine of grapes were used for the stomach, as a diuretic, against vaginal ulcers and eye ailments, as an anti-emetic for pregnant women, and as an aphrodisiac. Old wine was used in the treatment of impotence. *EI*², s.vv. 'khamr' (A. J. Wensinck-J. Sadan), 'karm' (L. Bolens and Cl. Cahen); E. Lev and Z. Amar 2008: 176–80; Maimonides (F. Rosner 1984): 167; al-Tīfāshī 1892: 14; Ibn al-Bayṭār 1874, IV: 56–7, and 1992: 225; Ibn Wāfid 2000: 59–61; D. al-Anṭākī 1952, I: 270; Ibn Sīnā 1999, I: 615–6, 622–3; al-Rāzī 1955–69, XXI: 318–22; al-Qazwīnī 1849: 263–5; al-Kindī (M. Levey 1966): no. 121; al-Warrāq (N. Nasrallah 2010): 630; al-Dhahabī 1987: 219; al-Suyūṭī n.d.: 11; P. Heine 1982: 111–12.

158. *rummān* (*Punica granatum*) – the sweet variety (*ḥulw*) of the fruit is mentioned several times in the Qur'ān, including as one of the fruits of paradise (6:99; 6:144; 55:68). In cooking, the sour variety (*ḥāmiḍ*) was used as an aromatic, whereas it was also said to be an appetizer. In medicine, both the fruit and peel were used in the treatment of diarrhoea (especially the juice), fevers, cough, stomach and liver ailments, to curb yellow bile, and as a diuretic and anaphrodisiac (because of its acidity). The sour variety was considered cold and dry, whereas the sweet one was hot and dry. E. Lev and Z. Amar 2008: 248–50; Ibn Wāfid 2000: 119–20; Ibn al-Bayṭār 1874, II: 142–4, and 1992: 167, 169; al-Tīfāshī 1892: 31; D. al-Anṭākī 1952, I: 169–70; al-Dhahabī 1987: 179–80; Ibn Sīnā 1999, I: 666–7; al-Suyūṭī n.d.: 12; al-Qazwīnī 1849: 290–1; al-Rāzī 1955–69, LXX, 512–19; al-Warrāq (N. Nasrallah 2010): 637; A. Dietrich 1988, II: 170–1; al-Kindī (M. Levey 1966): nos 36, 38, 42, 55, 59, 77, 86, 91; Ibn al-Quff (H. Kircher 1967): 187–8. See also the note on *jullanār*, below.

159. [A]: *bāliᶜ* (for *bāligh*).

160. *safarjal* – considered cold and dry, both the sour and sweet varieties of the quince were used in medicine, mainly to strengthen the stomach, as a digestive, appetizer and anti-emetic, against headaches, and to prevent hangovers. Syria was renowned for quince (though its original birthplace was Babylon), with the best variety being allegedly found around Aleppo (Ibn al-Bayṭār). Ibn Wāfid 2000: 123–4; al-Rāzī 1955–69, XXI: 10–13; Ibn al-Bayṭār 1874, III: 17, and 1992: 217; al-Kindī (Levey 1966): nos 166, 173; al-Bīrūnī 1973: 357; al-Warrāq (N. Nasrallah 2010): 637–8; D. al-Anṭākī 1952, I: 189–90; al-Dhahabī 1987: 189–91; Ibn Sīnā 1999, I: 607–8; A. Dietrich 1988, II: 176–7; E. Lev and Z. Amar 2008: 255–7; R. Degen 1978; Issa Bey 1930: 64.

161. 'which do not contain any trace of bitterness any more. All of the things that we have mentioned strengthen sexual potency, the brain and organs. There are many others but this selection is sufficient'; [C]: 'All of these are beneficial to strengthen the brain and organs.'

162. This entire chapter is omitted from the Cairo ms., whereas the content of Chapter 4 in [A] corresponds to Chapter 3 in [C], which thus lacks a Chapter 4.

163. *ᶜanbar* – the term denotes grey amber (or ambergris, the secretion of the sperm whale's gall bladder), so named to distinguish it from yellow amber (fossilized tree resin). Both have been used in perfumes (Ibn al-Bayṭār called

it 'the king of scents') and medicines, but only the latter was (and still is) prized as a gemstone. The ancient Greeks knew it as *elektron*, which gave the word 'electricity', initially denoting static electricity because of (yellow) amber's capacity to attract other materials after friction. Islamic scholars were unsure about its origins, but distinguished between the types; Ibn al-Quff stated that the best amber was fatty and grey, whereas the black one was of the lowest quality. In the medical tradition, amber(gris), which was said to be hot and dry, was used to strengthen the brain and senses. It was especially beneficial for old men and those with a cold disposition. E. Lev and Z. Amar 2008: 331–3; Ibn Wāfid 2000: 164–5; *EI*², s.v. 'ᶜanbar' (J. Ruska/M. Plessner); Ibn al-Bayṭār 1874, III: 134–6, and 1992: 182, 223; Ibn al-Jazzār 2004: 73–4; Ibn Sīnā 1999, I: 613–14; al-Qazwīnī 1849: 245; al-Yaᶜqūbī 1892: 366ff; Ibn al-Quff (H. Kircher 1967): 276–7.

164. *shaqāqul* (*Pastinaca schekakuli*), also appears under the following names in the literature: *shaqāqīl, jamjam, shaḥmīla, filla, ḥashqāl, ḥurṣ al-Nīl.* This vegetable was thought to be highly beneficial for coitus, increasing lust and potency, and helping erection, especially when used in a preserve mixed with honey. E. Lev and Z. Amar 2008: 462; Ibn Wāfid 2000: 96; Ibn al-Bayṭār 1992: 219; Ibn al-Jazzār 2004: 31–2; Ibn Sīnā 1999, I: 675–6, II: 734; Maimonides (F. Rosner 1973: 21, 72, and (F. Rosner 1984): 176; al-Tīfāshī 1892: 13, 14; *Kitāb* (Tunis No. 20648[09]): fol. 86b; al-Shayzarī, *al-Īḍāḥ*, fol. 2a; R. Muschler 1912: 468; M. Steinschneider 1900: 91.

165. *qanṭāriyūn* (also *qanṭūr[i]yūn*). This genus contains some 600 species; the ones that are most commonly referred to in Arabic pharmacology are the 'small' (*ṣaghīr, daqīq*) and 'great' (*tūmāghā, kabīr, jalīl, ghalīẓ*) centaury (*Centaurium minus/maximus*), the former of which was also known as *ᶜarbaz* (< Syriac *ᶜarbzaz*). Medicinally, it was used in the treatment of cramps, sciatica, backache, liver and spleen obstructions, and as an emmenagogue. Dietrich 1988, II: 348ff, and 1991: 152ff (note 9); E. Lev and Z. Amar 2008: 377–8; Ibn al-Jazzār (G. Bos 1997): 140, 204; Ibn Sīnā 1999, I: 645–6; D. Antākī 1952, I: 263; Ibn Sahl (O. Kahl 2003): nos 38, 45; al-Kindī (M. Levey 1966): no. 241; Ibn al-Bayṭār 1874, IV: 33–4; Maimonides (M. Meyerhof 1940): no. 333; Ibn al-Quff (H. Kircher 1967): 310.

166. *kabāba* (also *kubāba, kabbāba*; *Piper cubeba*), also known as 'Java pepper'. Hot and dry (in the second degree), it comes in two main varieties – big (*ḥabb al-ᶜarūs*, 'seed of the bride') and smaller (*falanja*). In addition to its aromatic qualities, it was used in the treatment of septic ulcers and gum disease, whereas the saliva of a man chewing cubeb was believed to be pleasurable for the woman during intercourse. E. Lev and Z. Amar 2008: 393; Ibn al-Bayṭār 1874, IV: 48–9; Ibn al-Jazzār 2004: 30–1; Ibn Sīnā 1999, I: 519–20, and II: 746; al-Kindī (M. Levey 1966): nos 69, 77, 91, 102, 106; al-Rāzī 1955–69, XXI: 391; al-Warrāq (N. Nasrallah 2010): 654; D. Antākī 1952, I: 255.

167. *Abū Zaydān* – this was also used by al-Tīfāshī (1970: 33/ transl. 48) in a recipe aimed at arousing the lust for coitus in women to such a degree that they would go out on the street to look for it (*yakhrujna ilā al-ṭuruq min buyūtihinna fī ṭalab al-jimāᶜ*)!

168. *lakk* – considered hot and dry (in the second degree), this resinous excretion

of a number of insects left on trees was also used in the treatment of palpitations, jaundice, dropsy and liver aches, to release obstructions (in the stomach and liver), and as an emmenagogue (especially when prepared in a honey syrup). In addition, it was thought to cause weight loss, and was used in red dye and ink. E. Lev and Z. Amar 2008: 193; Ibn al-Quff (H. Kircher 1967): 330–1; Ibn Sīnā 1999, I: 539; Ibn al-Bayṭār 1874, IV: 110, and 1992: 234; Ibn Wāfid 2000: 153–4.

169. *lisān ʿuṣfūr* (also *lisān al-ʿuṣfūr, lisān al-ʿaṣāfīr*) – the fruit of the *dardār* tree was said to be very potent, and was recommended for the treatment of ulcers and palpitations, as a diuretic, carminative, theriac and purgative, but especially to increase sexual potency (stiffness of erection) and invigorate coition. E. Lev and Z. Amar 2008: 340–1; Ibn al-Bayṭār 1874, IV: 108–9, and 1992: 234; Ibn Sīnā 1999, I: 541, and II: 734, 735; *Kitāb* (Tunis No. 20648[09]): fol. 86b; *Risāla* (Cairo 362): fol. 3b; al-Kātib 2002: 36; Ibn al-Jazzār 2004: 40; Issa Bey 1930: 84, 184; Ibn Wāfid 2000: 181–2; al-Warrāq (N. Nasrallah 2010): 662; Maimonides (M. Meyerhof 1940): No 212; al-Bīrūnī 1973: 157.

170. *qishr al-utrunj* – the uses of lemons (also *utrujj, turunj, tuffāḥ māʾī,* 'water apple') in both cooking and medicine are legion, the peel, in particular, being used in preserves, stews soured with citron pulp (*hummāḍiyyāt*), sniffed, as a breath sweetener, and so on. In medicine, it was used to strengthen the stomach, against poisonous bites and stings, jaundice and haemorrhoids, and as a digestive, anti-diarrhoeal, and anti-emetic. In erotological literature, lemons (both the fruit and peel) were considered aphrodisiacs, and are ingredients in a number of remedies. Somewhat confusingly, it was also recommended as an anaphrodisiac for women. Palestine was particularly renowned for its high-quality lemons. A. Dietrich 1988, II: 178; E. Lev and Z. Amar 2008: 147–9; al-Tīfāshī 1892: 14; Ibn Lūqā 17 (transl. 31); *Kitāb* (Tunis No. 20648[09]): fol. 86b; al-Shayzarī, *al-Īḍāḥ*: fol. 2a; Ibn al-Bayṭār 1874, I: 10–11, and 1992: 169, 189; Ibn Wāfid 2000: 34; D. Antākī 1952, I: 37; al-Dhahabī 1987: 114–15; al-Ṭabarī 1928: 302–3; al-Bīrūnī 1973: 21–3; al-Warrāq (N. Nasrallah 2010): 278–82, 641–2; al-Masʿūdī 1960–79, II: 438–9; al-Qazwīnī 1849: 216–17.

171. *anīsūn* (< Gr. ἄνησσον) – in addition to the variant *yānīsūn*, it was confusingly also known as *rāzyānāj*, which actually denotes fennel. Anise, which is native to Asia Minor, was said to be hot and dry. In medicine, mainly the seeds were used as a carminative, diuretic and emmenagogue, to strengthen the stomach, and to treat colds and inflammations. It was also recommended as an aphrodisiac and, for women, to tighten the vagina and heal the womb. Ibn al-Bayṭār 1874, I: 59–60, and 1992: 187, 215; Ibn al-Jazzār 2004: 164–5; al-Tīfāshī 1892: 14, and 1970: 21 (transl. 35); *Kitāb* (Tunis No. 20648[09]): fol. 86b; *Risāla* (Cairo 362): fol. 3a; al-Shayzarī, *al-Īḍāḥ*: fol. 2a; al-Kindī (M. Levey 1966): nos 114, 162, 225; al-Kātib 2002: 36; D. Antākī 1952, I: 59; Maimonides (F. Rosner and S. Muntner 1970): 20, 86; al-Warrāq (N. Nasrallah 2010): 645, 668; al-Ghassānī 1990: 12; A. Dietrich 1988, II: 406; E. Lev and Z. Amar 2011: 102–4; al-Dhahabī 1987: 124.

172. *khiyār* (*Cucumis sativis*), also known as *qiththāʾ* (also *quththāʾ*), which is the

word that appears in the Qur'ān (2:61); even though the two are sometimes used interchangeably, the latter is actually the vegetable melon (*Cucumis melo*), with *qiththā' shāmī/al-Shām* ('Syrian cucumber') denoting *khiyār*. Another variety of cucumber, *faqqūṣ* (small sour Egyptian melon) is also often mentioned. Other names for *khiyār* are *jalmatha* and *qathadh* (also known as *khiyār badharanq*). In the medical tradition, the cucumber's cold and moist properties caused it to be prescribed for a hot liver (*kibd ḥārra*), and as a diuretic and antipyretic. It was also used to sweeten the breath. In erotological literature, it was considered an anaphrodisiac; Maimonides, for instance, claimed it was extremely harmful for coitus (as were melons and other 'sour substances'). Al-Rāzī 1982: 229–30, and 1955–69, XX: 389; Ḍ. al-Anṭākī 1952, I: 148; al-Bīrūnī 1973: 173 (*khiyār*), 300 (*qiththā'*); al-Suyūṭī n.d.: 12; Maimonides (F. Rosner 1984), (F. Rosner 1995): 307–8, 170, and (M. Meyerhof 1940): nos 343 (*qiththā'*), 388 (*khiyār*); al-Warrāq (N. Nasrallah 2010): 627, 788–9, 792–3; Ibn Butlān (H. Elkhadem 1990): 168–71; Ibn al-Bayṭār 1874, II: 80–1 (*khiyār*), IV: 4 (*qiththā'*), and 1992: 175, 176; Ibn Sīnā 1999, I: 656–7; al-Isrā'ilī 1992: 355–8; al-Ṭabarī 1928: 380; H. S. Paris et al. 2011: 121–4; Issa Bey 1930: 61–2; E. Lev and Z. Amar 2011: 394; Ibn al-Quff (H. Kircher 1967): 170–1; A. Dietrich 1988, II: 283, 656, 692 (note 14).

173. *dār fulful* (*Piper longum*) also appears in the literature as *fulful ṭawīl* and *falfūlaniyya*; it involves the dried fruit catkins of this vine, which is closely related to the standard pepper (*Piper nigrum*), and often confused with it. It is endowed with the qualities attributed to pepper and is also considered a sexual stimulant. Ibn Sīnā 1999, I: 438–9, and II: 734; Ibn al-Bayṭār 1874, II: 86, and III: 166–7; Ibn al-Bayṭār 1992: 210; Ibn al-Jazzār 2004: 130; al-Kindī (M. Levey 1966): nos 108, 111, 151, 178, 216, 217, 225; al-Tīfāshī 1892: 13, 14; al-Kātib 2002: 36; Ibn Lūqā 1974: 16 (transl. 23); *Kitāb* (Tunis No. 20648[09]): fol. 86b; al-Shayzarī, *al-Īḍāḥ*: fol. 2a; Risāla (Cairo 362): fol. 3b; D. al-Anṭākī 1952, I: 150; al-Bīrūnī 1973: 188; E. Lev and Z. Amar 2011: 208–9; al-Warrāq (N. Nasrallah 2010): 648; Issa Bey 1930: 141 (nos 2–4); Maimonides (F. Rosner and S. Muntner 1970): 21, 38.

174. *qusṭ* (< Gr. κόστος). Hot and dry, this plant was known as an aromatic and aphrodisiac by Greek and Arab physicians and pharmacologists. There were said to be three varieties: white (Arab), Indian (black) and 'clove-like' (*qaranfulī*). In addition, it was also said to be beneficial for the liver, back, spleen and womb, to remove tumours, and as a theriac (especially for snake bites). According to Ibn al-Jazzār (2004), it should be drunk with wine and honey in order for it to act as a sexual stimulant, whereas al-Rāzī and al-Dimashqī claimed it prevented palpitations resulting from (excessive) intercourse. See A. Dietrich 1988, II: 99–100; E. Lev and Z. Amar 2011: 157–8; Ibn al-Jazzār 2004: 125–6; Ibn Sīnā 1999, I: 648, and II: 734; al-Tīfāshī 1892: 14, 18; *Kitāb* (Tunis No. 20648[09]): fol. 86b; al-Bīrūnī 1973: 307; al-Rāzī 1955–69, XXI: 262–4; al-Dhahabī 1987: 227–9; Ibn al-Jazzār (G. Bos 1997): 83–4; al-Kātib 1977: 283; D. al-Anṭākī 1952, I: 259; R. Dozy 1877–81, II: 344; al-Warrāq (N. Nasrallah 2010): 774; Dioscorides 2000: 21; Ibn al-Quff (H. Kircher 1967): 311–12.

175. *khaṭmiyat al-thaʿlab* (*Althaea officinalis*) – also known as *kha/iṭmi*, it was used to prevent tumours in various parts of the body, and as a painkiller, diuretic and antidote against poisons. Ibn Sīnā 1999, I: 701–2; Ibn al-Bayṭār 1992: 207; Ibn al-Jazzār 2004: 113–14; Ibn Wāfid 2000: 88–9; al-Warrāq (N. Nasrallah 2010): 788; Ibn Sahl (O. Kahl 1900): 134 (no. 267), 140 (no. 290), 141–2 (no. 296), 173 (no. 390); Ibn al-Quff (H. Kircher 1967): 165–6.

176. [A]: *baḍḍ*; [B]: *hinā*. It is clear that this is a misprint in [A], as *baḍḍ* is not a botanical term (Lane 1863–74, I: 213).

177. *khūlinjān* (also *khūlanj*) – hot and dry (in the third degree), it is a variety of the cyperus (see note on *suʿd*, above). Its aromatic dried root is used in cooking and in medicine against colic, as a digestive, carminative and aphrodisiac, whether drunk with milk or by chewing it. If it was chewed together with a bit of musk, it caused a powerful erection (Ibn al-Jazzār). Ibn al-Jazzār 2004: 147–8; Ibn Sīnā 1999, I: 709, and II: 734; Ibn Lūqā 1974: 16 (transl. 23); al-Kātib 2002: 36; al-Tīfāshī 1892: 14; al-Shayzarī, *al-Īḍāḥ*: fol. 2a; *Risāla* (Cairo 362): fol. 3a; al-Warrāq (N. Nasrallah 2010): 660.

178. *ʿāqir qarḥ* (for *ʿāqir qarḥā*, which is also how it appears in Chapter 16) was used as a digestive and to control saliva flow, as well as being an aphrodisiac. According to Ibn al-Bayṭār it was a remedy for impotence when boiled down in water and then cooked in olive oil. A. Dietrich 1988, II: 422–3; al-Tīfāshī 1892: 14; al-Shayzarī, *al-Īḍāḥ*: fol. 3b; *Risāla* (Cairo 362): 5; al-Kātib 2002: 36; al-Bīrūnī 1973: 261; Ibn Sīnā 1999, II: 734; al-Rāzī 1955–69, XXI: 191; Ibn al-Bayṭār 1874, III: 115–16, and 1992: 223; Ibn al-Jazzār 2004: 190; D. al-Anṭākī 1952, I: 235; Ibn al-Quff (H. Kircher 1967): 272.

179. *shaḥm al-asad* – all fats were hot and moist in the first degree and were used, among other things, to ripen wounds. Among the most effective fats were those of lions, wolves and bear – lion's fat, in particular, being an effective aphrodisiac. Ibn al-Quff (H. Kircher 1967): 240; al-Ṭabarī 1928: 428; al-Tīfāshī 1892: 14; *Kitāb* (Tunis No. 20648[09]): fol. 86b; *Risāla* (Cairo 362): fol. 3a; al-Kātib 2002: 36.

180. *liḥyat tays* (*Tragopogon pratensis or Tragopogon porrifolius*) is also known as 'salsify', and appears more commonly as *liḥyat al-tays*; it was used to treat ulcers, diarrhoea and uteral discharge. Ibn al-Bayṭār 1874, IV: 104–5; Ibn Wāfid 2000: 113–14; al-Rāzī 1955–69, XXI: 479–81; Maimonides (M. Meyerhof 1940): nos 37, 174; D. al-Anṭākī 1952, I: 281; A. Dietrich 1988, II: 292.

181. *zift rūmī* – sometimes used interchangeably with *qaṭrān* or *qīr*, it is a residue of tar production, pitch tended to be harvested from pine trees (*zift raṭb*, 'liquid pitch'), which was also cooked and dried (*zift yābis*). Medicinally, it was primarily used as an antiseptic. Dietrich 1988, II: 118–20; Ibn al-Bayṭār 1874, II: 164–5; D. al-Anṭākī 1952, I: 140; Ibn Sīnā 1999, I: 463; Ibn al-Quff (H. Kircher 1967): 199–200; al-Warrāq (N. Nasrallah 2010): 759–60. See also note on *qaṭrān*, below.

182. *khashkhāsh*, 'black Egyptian poppy'. Medicinally, it was thought to be beneficial as a soporific, and to treat ailments as varied as corneal ulcers and cough. In erotological literature it is mentioned as an aphrodisiac. A. Dietrich

1988, II: 568–9; Ibn al-Bayṭār 1992: 177, 207, and 1874, II: 59–60; Ibn al-Jazzār 2004: 199; Ibn Sīnā 1999, I: 699–701; D. al-Anṭākī 1952, I: 140; al-Ishbīlī 1995, I: 237 (*al-khashkhās al-aswad*); al-Tīfāshī 1892: 14; *Kitāb* (Tunis No. 20648[09]): fol. 86b; al-Shayzarī, *al-Īḍāḥ*: fol. 3a; E. Lane 1863–74, I: 70; al-Ṭabarī 1928: 376; M. Steinschneider 1900: 62 (no. 749).

183. *jawz* – hot and dry, the leaves, shells, nut (both cooked and dried) and oil from the pit were used in cooking and medicine. In the medical tradition, walnuts were known to be difficult to digest (the dried ones more than the fresh green ones, *jawz raṭb*), harmful to the stomach (cf. hazelnuts) and to cause pustules in the mouth. As a result, they should be mixed with honey (*ᶜasal*), combined with other substances such as rue (*sadhāb*) or onions (*baṣal*). Nuts were recommended, for instance, to treat throat aches (when taken in a honey syrup), tumours and ulcers. Roasted walnut shells were also used to dye the hair black. Ibn al-Bayṭār 1874, II: 173–5, and 1992: 201; al-Warrāq (N. Nasrallah 2010): 592, 630–1; Ibn Wāfid 2000: 140ff; al-Rāzī 1955–69, XX: 267–71; Ibn Sīnā 1999, I: 415–17; Maimonides (M. Meyerhof 1940): no. 82; al-Dhahabī 1987: 149; al-Suyūṭī n.d.: 9; D. al-Anṭākī 1952, I: 109–10; A. Dietrich 1988, II: 188–9; al-Tīfāshī 1892: 14; al-Bīrūnī 1973: 144; Ibn al-Quff (H. Kircher 1967): 135–8.

184. *basbāsa* – the covering of the seed of the *jawz bawwā* nutmeg tree (*Myristica fragrans*), the spice was reported to come from India. Its other names include *darkīsa* (< Persian) and *ṭālīsfar* (< Sanskrit). In the medical tradition, it was used against stomach ulcers, whereas some authors attributred aphrodisiacal qualities to it. Ibn Wāfid 2000: 34–5; al-Tīfāshī 1892: 14; *Kitāb* (Tunis No. 20648[09]): fol. 86b; al-Shayzarī, *al-Īḍāḥ*: fol. 2b; A. Dietrich 1988, II: 134; D. al-Anṭākī 1952, I: 74–5, 229; Ibn Sīnā 1999, II: 734; al-Warrāq (N. Nasrallah 2010): 648; al-Bīrūnī 1973: 191; Ibn al-Bayṭār 1874, I: 93, and 1992: 193; Ibn al-Jazzār 2004: 67; Maimonides (M. Meyerhof 1940): no. 38.

185. *bawraq* (sodium borate) – hot and dry (in the second degree), borax, which consists of salt and soda mined in the Egyptian desert (especially Wādi Naṭrūn), came in two varieties, African (*Ifrīqī* or red) and Armenian (*Armanī*). It was also known as *naṭrūn* (natron), though some authors reserved this term for Armenian borax. In cooking, it was used in bread-baking, whereas the medical authorities recommend it as a remedy for a large number of conditions (70, according to al-Qazwīnī), including eye diseases, constipation and impotence (especially when borax is mixed with honey and rubbed on the genitals). Others, including al- Bīrūnī, warned about the toxicity of the borax when taken internally. Ibn Lūqā 1974: 21 (transl. 28); Ibn al-Bayṭār 1874, IV: 166, and 1992: 195–6; Ibn al-Jazzār 2004: 216–17; al-Dhahabī 1987: 134; Ibn Sīnā 1999, I: 389–90, 580 (*naṭrūn*); al-Warrāq (N. Nasrallah 2010): 760–1; Ibn al-Quff (H. Kircher 1967): 106–7, 351–2; E. Lev and Z. Amar 2008: 118–20; al-Bīrūnī 1973: 80; Maimonides (M. Meyerhof 1940): no. 51.

186. *zurunbād*, or *zurunbādh* – considered to be hot in the second degree and moderately dry, it was recommended for reptile bites, to mask the smell of garlic and alcohol on the breath, and as a carminative, anti-emetic and

antidpressant. In cooking, it was used as an aromatic. Ibn al-Jazzār 2004: 155; Ibn Sīnā 1999, II: 734; Ibn Wāfid 2000: 146; M. Steinschneider 1900: 90 (no. 937); Ibn al-Bayṭār 2001, II: 157–8; Ibn al-Jazzār 2004: 155; Ibn Sahl (Kahl 1900): nos 8, 25, 31, 41, 8, 49, 50, 57, 66, 232, 312, 371; al-Ishbīlī 1995, I: 273; al-Warrāq (N. Nasrallah 2010): 679 ('zurnubād').

187. *halīlaj* – considered cold and dry, it was thought to be beneficial for, among other things, strengthening the stomach, removing black bile, relieving haemorrhoids, aiding digestion, dispelling winds, sharpening the senses, and increasing memory, as well as being a remedy for leprosy, colic, headaches, vomiting and fever. Together with the other myrobalans, it was often used in electuary recipes to cure impotence. Ibn Sīnā 1999, I: 447–8; Ibn Lūqā 1974: 19 (transl. 27); Ibn Wāfid 2000: 107–11; Ibn Sahl (O. Kahl 2003): 119 (note 145); Ibn al-Bayṭār 1992: 188; Ibn al-Jazzār 2004: 13–14.

188. *balīlaj* was thought to be particularly effective in strengthening the body, improving the complexion, and even preventing black hair from turning grey; Ibn Wāfid 2000: 100; Ibn Lūqā 1974: 19 (transl. 27).

189. *amlaj*, the fruit of *Phyllanthus emblica* ('Indian gooseberry'). The last three items, which are often discussed together because of their similarities, are all myrobalans (*ahlīlaj*). For a discussion and overview, see E. Lev and Z. Amar 2008: 218ff (Chapter 6); Ibn al-Quff (H. Kircher 1967): 83–6. *Amlaj* was said to strengthen the stomach, as well as serving as an anti-emetic and sexual stimulant; Ibn Wāfid 2000: 100–1; Ibn Lūqā 1974: 19 (transl. 27); Ibn al-Jazzār 2004: 14.

190. *ḥabba sawdā'* ('black grain'), *Nigella sativa* – hot and dry in the second or third degree, depending on the author, the spice, which is also referred to as *kammūn aswad* ('black cumin'), *k. hindī* ('Indian c.'), *k. ḥabashī* ('Ethiopian c.'), *ḥabb al-baraka* ('the seed of blessing') or by its Persian name *shōnīz*, was considered a remedy for a variety of ailments, including leprosy, and also a diuretic, appetizer, emmenagogue, anthelmintic and carminative. Dietrich 1988, II: 429-30; al-Dhahabī 1987: 150–2; al-Suyūṭī n.d.: 13; E. Lev and Z. Amar 2008: 362–4; Ibn al-Bayṭār 1874, III: 72–3; Ibn al-Bayṭār 1992: 176, 220; al-Warrāq (N. Nasrallah 2010): 651, 656, 672; Dioscorides 2000: 45 (*Melanthelaion*); al-Rāzī 1955069, XXI: 123; al-Bīrūnī 1973: 21–3; D. al-Anṭākī 1952, I: 219–20; Ibn al-Quff (H. Kircher 1967): 238; Ibn Sīnā 1999, I: 677–8.

191. [A]: *ḥawz* (for *jawz*) *hindī* (also *al-Hind*) – the coconut was said to be very effective as an aphrodisiac and to strengthen the erection (*in*ᶜ*āz*). It was also used as an anthelmintic, and against haemorrhoids, backache and throatache. Ibn al-Quff (H. Kircher 1967): 135–8; al-Warrāq (N. Nasrallah 2010): 631; al-Dhahabī 1987: 148.

192. *su*ᶜ*d* – also known as *su*ᶜ*dā*, the plant (especially its root) was used as an aromatic in cooking, with the one from Kufa being considered the best. Medicinally, it was thought to have warming and drying properties, and was recommended against oral ulcers, and as as a diuretic, anthelmentic and emmenagoue. It was also chewed to sweeten the breath. According to Ibn al-Quff, excessive use of the plant leads to leprosy. Ibn Wāfid 2000: 162–3; Ibn al-Bayṭār 1874, III: 15–16, and 1992: 217; Ibn al-Jazzār 2004: 102; al-

Kātib 1977: 257 (who recommends that it be eaten together with saltwort and claims it strengthens the gums); al-Bīrūnī 1973: 220; D. al-Anṭākī 1952, I: 188; al-Shayzarī, *al-Īḍāḥ*: fol. 2b; al-Rāzī 1955–69, XXI: 1–3; al-Warrāq (N. Nasrallah 2010): 776; A. Dietrich 1988, II: 89; Ibn al-Quff (H. Kircher 1967): 223–4.

193. cf. Ibn Sīnā 1999, II: 734.

194. *zayt*, as its name indicates, is the juice extracted from olives (*zaytūn*, *Olea europaea*). Oil obtained from plants is referred to as duhn (though, for an opposite view, see Ibn al-Quff). Cold and dry, olives were thought to have a large number of benefits, including as an aphrodisiac. See *EI*[2], s.v. 'zayt' (D. Waines); al-Dhahabī 1987: 186–8; Ibn al-Quff (H. Kircher 1967): 182–3; Ibn al-Bayṭār 1992: 211–12, 216.

195. *milḥ andarānī* ([C]) – the adjective is a corruption of *dhar'ānī*, which is related to the noun *dhur'a*, meaning 'excessive whiteness'. It also appears as *milḥ macdanī* ('mineral salt') or *tabarzad*. The salt was used to extract phlegm and sharpen the mind, and as an emetic; Ibn Sīnā 1999, I: 571–2; Ibn Warrāq (N. Nasrallah 2010): 579. Al-Tīfāshī uses it in a recipe (boiled with alum) to warm the vagina and reduce its moistness (1970: 30, transl.: 45).

196. *ᶜūd ṣalīb* – the medicinal uses of the plant were known in Indian, Chinese and Arab medicine, where it was primarily recommended as an emmenagogue and to treat heartburn, and pains in the womb, liver and bladder. It was also known as *ward al-ḥamīr* ('donkeys' rose'); Ibn Sīnā 1999, I: 623; F. Corriente 1997: 309; A. Dietrich 1988, II: 496–7.

197. '... that have been cooked in oil and fry everything until it is mixed well. Take a *dirham* each of cinnamon bark, galingale and peony. Pound all of these spices and sprinkle them on top of the cooked onions' [C]: 'boil until everything is mixed. Take a *dirham* each of cinnamon bark, galangale and peony and sprinkle on the dish'.

198. This sentence is omitted from [C].

199. 'Pulverize these ingredients' is missing from [C].

200. The variant in [C] of this passage ('stir until everything is mixed ...') is considerably shorter: 'stir until everything is mixed, remove from the fire and drink. It is beneficial, as we have mentioned, Allah willing.'

201. This is a correction from [B], as the verb is missing from [A].

202. The entire previous recipe up until this point is abridged in [C] to: 'cook and throw on five *dirhams* of common ash, a *dirham* of coconut and clove, and heat up until it becomes mixed with the rest. Remove from the fire and eat in the evening. It is beneficial, as we have mentioned. The following are some of the sweets that restore the temperament, strengthen the principal organs, cure impotence and increase innate heat: ...'

203. 'heat', [B]: 'boil'.

204. 'Add some olive oil ...'; [C]: 'Thicken the honey and sprinkle on it cinnamon bark and lemon peel (five *dirhams* each).'

205. 'half a *dirham* of saffron ...'; [C]: 'one *dirham* of saffron, remove from the fire, pour into a glass jar and eat the mixture every evening before going to sleep. You will see (it works wonders).'

206. *ṣanawbar* – considered hot and moist, it increases sperm, potency and lust

for coition, as well being used to treat burns, and liver and toothaches. Ibn al-Bayṭār 1874, III: 87–9, and 1992: 206; al-Dhahabī 1987: 202; al-Tīfāshī 1892: 14; *Risāla* (Cairo 362): fol. 3b; al-Kātib 2002: 36; D. al-Anṭākī 1952, I: 224; Ibn Sīnā 1999, I: 490–1, 640, and II: 734; Ibn Wāfid 2000: 81–2; al-Bīrūnī 1973: 249; Ibn Warrāq (N. Nasrallah 2010): 628–9; Ibn al-Quff (H. Kircher 1967): 253; al-Ṭabarī 1928: 383; Maimonides (M. Meyerhof 1940): no. 317.

207. *dār ṣīnī* (< Persian *dār chīnī*, 'Chinese wood'), *Cinnamomum* cassia, also known as 'Chinese cassia', was said to be hot and dry in the third degree. In medicine, it was used, among other things, to strengthen the stomach, liver and spleen, and as a diuretic, emmenagogue and antidote against scorpion poison. In erotological literature, it is often credited with aphrodisiacal properties. A. Dietrich 1988, II: 97–8; *EI*[2], *Sup.*, s.v. (A. Dietrich); al-Tīfāshī 1892: 13, 14; *Kitāb* (Tunis No. 20648[09]): fol. 86b; Ibn Sahl (O. Kahl 2003); E. Lev and Z. Amar 2008: 143–4; al-Dhahabī : 173; al-Rāzī 1955–69: XXI: 490–6; Ibn al-Bayṭār 1874, II: 83–5, and 1992: 208; Ibn al-Jazzār 2004: 130–1; D. al-Anṭākī 1952, I: 149; Ibn Sīnā 1999, I: 431–3, II: 734; al-Bīrūnī 1973: 189; Ibn Warrāq (N. Nasrallah 2010): 648; Ibn al-Quff (H. Kircher 1967): 183–5; M. Steinschneider 1900: 65 (no. 792). For an overview of the variation in terms for various types of cinnamon, see J. Leibowitz and S. Marcus 1974: 233.

208. 'mix with white skimmed bee honey...'; [C]: 'pour on it the same measure of skimmed honey until everything is mixed. Sprinkle on top five *dirhams* of lemon peel, half a *dirham* of saffron, stir and use one *mithqāl* daily before going to sleep. You will see the wonders it works, as has been mentioned.'

209. A reference to the Iranian city of Yazd, which has been a centre of Zoroastrian culture for many centuries.

210. 'invigorate coitus ...'; [C]: 'and which is known as the 'threefold syrup'. Take grape water and add three times the quantity of freshwater. Boil until a third remains and take a measure of three *dirhams* from it and fifty *dirhams* of the bee honey.'

211. 'or white sugar, and cook until the froth apears. Then take ...'; [C]: 'Then add to it ...'

212. The passage 'Crush all of these into dust ...' is as follows in [C]: 'until everything is mixed. Then remove and decant into a glass vessel. If you want to use it, take a measure of forty *dirhams* of the mixture, mix with the same amount of freshwater and drink it. It is beneficial, as we have mentioned, Allah willing.'

213. [B] adds 'yellow bile'.

214. 'cure headache, catarrh and innate heat' is omitted from [C].

215. The passage 'to such a great extent that ...' is missing from [C], which simply has 'The recipe for the cardamom electuary is ...'

216. *ḥaṣā lubān; lūbān* (< Gr. λίβανος; Lat. *Olibanum*), also known by its Persian name *kundur* (< Gr. χόνδρος, 'grain'), is a resin (*ṣamgh*) harvested from the olibanum tree. It was thought to have originated in the Shiḥr region of Oman (i.e. the coastal area stretching all the way to Aden). In addition to its being burned for the smell, *lūbān* was recommended for a large number of

ailments, such as bronchitis, stomach ulcers, diarrhoea, skin conditions and dysentery, as a digestive, and to prevent the spread of tumours. But it was also said to be highly dangerous as it could cause madness and, when taken with wine, even death. The term *ḥaṣā* (or *ḥass*) *lūbān* was a synonym of *iklīl al-jabal*, 'rosemary', which was traditionally used to treat jaundice, as a diuretic and emmenagogue, to improve body odour, relieve obstructions in the liver and spleen, to treat headaches, and to preserve meat. *EI*[2], s.v. 'lūbān' (A. Dietrich); E. Lev and Z. Amar 2008: 266–8; Ibn al-Bayṭār 1874, I: 51, IV: 83–6, 116-7, and 1992: 231; Ibn al-Jazzār 2004: 165; Ibn Warrāq (N. Nasrallah 2010): 662–3; Ibn al-Quff (H. Kircher 1967): 157–60; A. Dietrich 1988, II: 113–14; al-Suyūṭī n.d.: 15; Ibn Sīnā 1999, I: 515–17, and II: 734; al-Rāzī 1955–69, XXI: 313–18; D. al-Anṭākī 1952, I: 275–6; al-Bīrūnī 1973: 324.

217. *kuḥl* (also known as *ithmid* and *surma*) was initially antimony sulphide (stibnite), which was pulverized and used as a cosmetic (especially applied to eyebrows, lashes and edges of the eyelids). More often, *kuhl* denoted any eye cosmetic made from a wide variety of substances and, in some cases, a particular lead mineral, whose exact identity remains to be ascertained. The primary source of kuḥl was Iran. *EI*[2], s.v. 'al-kuḥl' (E. Wiedemann [J.W. Allan]); al-Suyūṭī n.d.: 52–4.

218. According to [C], one should take one *mithqāl* after the evening meal.

219. [A]: *ḥawz* (for *jawz*).

220. *simsim* (also known as *juljulān*, *Sesamum indicum*) – used both hulled (*abyaḍ*, 'white') and unhulled (*aḥmar*, 'red'). In cooking, it appears in a paste, the famous tahina (*ṭaḥīn simsim*, *rahshī*), whereas its oil (*shayraj*, *shayraq*) was used for deep-frying. It was considered bad for the stomach and to cause vomiting. It was also thought to increase sperm and sexual potency (according to Ibn Sīnā, especially when eaten with flax and cotton seeds). Ibn Lūqā 1974: 17 (transl. 24); al-Tīfāshī 1892: 14; Ibn Wāfid 2000: 94–5; Ibn al-Bayṭār 1874, III: 30–1, and 1992: 177, 219; Ibn Sīnā 1999, I: 604–5, II: 734; al-Rāzī 1955–69, XXI: 36–9; al-Bīrūnī 1973: 233; Ibn Warrāq (N. Nasrallah 2010): 621–2, 672–3; A. Dietrich 1988, II: 249–60.

221. This sentence is missing from [C].

222. *ḥasak* – sometimes known as *ḥimmaṣ al-amīr* ('the Prince's chickpeas'), it was said to come in wild (*barrī*) and cultivated (*bustānī*) varieties. It was used (both dried and fresh) in the treatment of tumours and kidney stones. Ibn al-Bayṭār 1874, II: 20–1; Ibn Sīnā 1999, I: 478, and II: 734; Ibn Lūqā 1974: 21 (trans.: 28); *Kitāb* (Tunis No. 20648[09]): fol. 86b; *Risāla* (Cairo 362): fol. 5a; al-Kātib 2002: 36; al-Rāzī 1955–69, XX: 327; Ibn Wāfid 2000: 112; al-Bīrūnī 1973: 158; Dietrich 1988, II: 528–9.

223. [C]: 'one *dirham*'.

224. [A]: *(al-ʿaṣāfīr) al-darūriyya* (for *al-dūriyya*).

225. 'half a *dirham* of ginger'; [C]: 'and ginger, two *dirhams* of each; sparrow brains, ten *dirhams*. Vigorously pound everything and thicken with bee honey.'

226. 'When you wish to engage in coitus ...'; [C]: 'When needed, drink from the threefold syrup that is mentioned here and it will achieve its aim, and Allah knows best.'

227. This refers to compounds based on a number of myrobalans (*amlaj*, *balīlaj*, *halīlaj*) which come in a 'smaller' (*al-aṣghar*) and 'greater' (*al-akbar*) variety. The mixture referred to here would appear to be the 'larger', as mentioned by Sābūr Ibn Sahl, who recommends it as a treatment for a cold stomach and haemorrhoidal pains, whereas Ibn al-Jazzār records it as an established therapy for hernias. According to Maimonides, it strengthens the limbs, delays aging and aids coitus. This compound is distinct from *iṭrīful*, 'bitumen trefoil' (*Bituminaria bituminosa*), whose identity is obscure. Both terms would seem to go back to the Greek τρίφυλλον ('three-leaved'). A similar recipe appears in the Trotula as *trifera saracenica* ('the Saracen trifera'), alongside a *trifera magna* ('greater trifera'). See Ibn al-Jazzār (G. Bos 1997): 122; Ibn Lūqā 1974: 15 (transl. 22); Ibn Sahl (O. Kahl 2003): 119, 120; al-Ṭabarī 1928: 480; E. Lev and Z. Amar 2008: 209, 219, 341, 362 (with the vowelling *iṭrīful* for the myrobalan-based compounds); al-Rāzī 2007: 310. and 1955–69, XXI: 159ff; A. Dietrich 1988, II: 461ff; M. Ullmann 1970: 295–6, 349; W. Schmucker 1969: 48; Ibn al-Bayṭār 2001, II: 131 and 1874, III: 101–2; al-Bīrūnī 1973: 255; Maimonides (M. Levey 1966): 21, 38; M. Green 2002: 134.

228. The following is ommited in [C]: 'has great benefits and innumerable advantages. It strengthens the intellect.'

229. [A]: *al-nazalā* (for *al-nazalāt*).

230. 'its brightness opens blockages in the head and eyes'; [C]: 'intellect'.

231. 'strengthens the principal organs and innate heat; strengthens potency; tautens the nerves'; [B]: 'strengthens the organs'.

232. For a similar recipe, see al-Tīfāshī 1892: 15; Ibn Lūqā 1974: 19 (transl. 27).

233. 'strengthens potency ...'; [C]: 'tautens the nerves and the penis; heats the kidneys, bladder and sperm; and greatly strengthens coitus. The recipe is made up of myrobalan, emblic myrobalan and belleric myrobalan.'

234. *shaʿīr* – considered (moderately) cold and dry, this cereal (or one of its derivates like meal or water), was used in a number of remedies, ranging from skin blemishes to fever and bowel infections, as a diuretic, and as a cure for impotence. *EI*², s.v. '*shaʿīr*' (D. Waines); Ibn Sahl (O. Kahl 2003): e.g. nos 20, 23, 195, 285, 290, 296351, 353, 354, 407; Ibn al-Bayṭār 1874, III: 62–3; al-Bīrūnī 1973: 401; Ibn al-Jazzār (G. Bos 1997): 94, 167, 170, 173, 174, 190; D. al-Anṭākī 1952, I: 215–16; A. Dietrich 1988, II: 242; al-Warrāq (N. Nasrallah 2010): 574; Ibn al-Quff (H. Kircher 1967): 233; al-Suyūṭī n.d.: 9.

235. The same recipe is also included in the anonymous medical text that follows [A] in the binding (fol. 104).

236. [C]: 'It is beneficial, as we have mentioned, Allah willing.'

237. 'remove coldness from the back and hip' is omitted from [C].

238. 'finely pound everything so that it becomes like kohl dust'; [C]: 'pulverize'.

239. 'Pound the two...'; [B]: 'Pulverize, strain through a fine cloth and mix with the ingredients. Add the same amount of bee honey and use before going to sleep.'; [C]: 'and cinnamon bark, clove and ginger, one *dirham* of each. Pulverize and mix with the honey. Use before going to sleep. It is very beneficial.'

240. *ḥabb al-quṭn* – in the Islamic medical tradition, cotton (especially tree cotton, *Gossypium arboreum*, and Levant cotton, *Gossypium herbaceum*)

was recommended for coughs, whereas the oil derived from it was used for sunspots and freckles. Cotton was also said to increase the lust for coitus, and appears as a regular ingredient in a number of aphrodisiacs. *EI*[2], s.v. 'ḳuṭn' (H. Inalcik); A. Dietrich 1988, II: 159 (note 11); Ibn al-Bayṭār 1874, IV: 24–9, and 1992: 229; Ibn al-Jazzār 2004: 193; al-Kātib 2002: 36; al-Dhahabī 1987: 230; D. al-Anṭākī 1952, I: 260; Ibn Wāfid 2000: 84; al-Ṭabarī 1928: 282; *Risāla* (Cairo 362): 5; al-Shayzarī, *al-Īḍāḥ*: fol. 2b; al-Rāzī 1955–69, XXI: 307; Maimonides (M. Meyerhof 1940): no. 349.

241. *sūra/injān* (also known as 'meadow saffron'). The red and black were thought to be harmful and only the white was used in medicine. It was recommended as a laxative, and antiseptic, to cure gout and pain in the joints, and as an aphrodisiac. Ibn al-Bayṭār 1874, III: 41–2; Ibn al-Jazzār 2004: 176; al-Ṭabarī 1928: 302; D. al-Anṭākī 1952, I: 204; al-Rāzī 1955–69: XXI: 39; Ibn Wāfid 2000: 163–4; Ibn Sīnā 1999, I: 589–90 (who recommends taking it with ginger, pennyroyal and cumin to increase its aphrodisiacal potency); al-Bīrūnī 1973: 240; A. Dietrich 1988, II: 589–90; Ibn al-Quff (H. Kircher 1967): 221–2; al-Ṭabarī 1928: 402.

242. Animal testicles (and penises, especially of bulls and wolves) were often thought to be effective as a sexual stimulant, as they increased the sperm; in addition to those of lambs, the testicles of donkeys, wild asses and cocks were also often used. The 'fox testicles' (*khaṣiy al-thaᶜlab*) often cited in erotological works as an aphrodisiac should not be taken literally; rather, this refers to orchids, whose Greek name (οόρχις, 'testicle') also denotes their shape, as does the archaic English word 'ballockwort'. Their aphrodisiacal quality was already referred to in ancient Greece, as the plant was commonly associated with the priapic satyrs, after whom it was even named ('satyrion'). Ibn al-Bayṭār 1992: 182; Ibn Sīnā 1999, II: 734; *Kitāb* (Tunis No. 20648[09]): fol. 86b; M. al-Fallātī (BN 5662): fol. 80a; al-Shayzarī, *al-Īḍāḥ*: fol. 2b; *Risāla* (Cairo 362): folios 4b, 5a–b; al-Kātib 2002: 64.

243. *furn*, brick oven – al-Warrāq (N. Nasrallah 2010): 681–2.

244. [A]: *marr* (for *marra*).

245. *qarᶜa*, *dubbā'* and, more commonly, *yaqṭīn* (compare Qur'ān 37:146) – cold and moist, it was thought to be beneficial for cough and headaches, and as a soporific for people with a fever (especitally the seeds and oil). There are a number of hadiths praising the gourd, for instance because it increases the intellect and mind; indeed, the Prophet himself was very partial to it. When eaten with lentils, it acts as a sexual stimulant; with sour pomegranat and sumac, it is beneficial for yellow bile. A. Dietrich 1988, II: 282; Ibn al-Quff (H. Kircher 1967): 298–9; Maimonides (M. Meyerhof 1940): no. 332; Ibn al-Bayṭār 1874, II: 87, and 1992: 172, 230; D. al-Anṭākī 1952, I: 256; al-Rāzī 1955–69: XXI: 284–7; Ibn Sīnā 1999, I: 656; al-Ṭabarī 1928: 380; al-Warrāq (N. Nasrallah 2010): 791–2, 796; al-Dhahabī 1987: 2267.

246. *shibitt* ([C]) – in medicine, it was used as a carminative and soporific, as a remedy against kidney and bladder stones, and in the treatment of wounds. Ibn al-Quff (H. Kircher 1967): 236–7; A. Dietrich 1988, II: 407–8; Ibn al-Bayṭār 1874, III: 50–1; Ibn al-Jazzār 2004: 108; al-Rāzī 1955–69: XXI: 121–3; al-Ṭabarī 1928: 380; Maimonides (M. Meyerhof 1940): no. 363; al-

Bīrūnī 1973: 391–3; al-Warrāq (N. Nasrallah 2010): 671 (‘*shabat*’).

247. ‘pepper’ is omitted from [B].

248. A cylindrical dome-shaped oven used mainly for baking bread, cakes and pies. *EI*², s.v. ‘maṭbakh’ (J. Burton-Page); al-Warrāq (N. Nasrallah 2010): 88–9, 820.

249. ‘the fat and testicles…’; [C]: ‘a small amount of lamb fat and a thin piece of lamb meat; place in a pot and cover with water. Put the lid on the top and place in the oven overnight until everything is cooked thoroughly. Then, administer an enema with it, which is called “the aperient one”.’

250. The present translation is based on [B], which has *al-ṣūf wa ’l-mansūj wa’l-tafkīk*, as the text in [A], *al-ṣūf al-mansūj min al-tankīk*, is clearly a misprint. The version in [C] is, simply, ‘woven wool’ (*al-ṣūf al-mansūj*).

251. Tu. *kemer* (‘waistband’) *qashāghi* (‘currycomb’); J. Redhouse 1880: 722, 754 (1890: 1,415).

252. This chapter is considerably shorter in [C]: ‘So, you have to wear the clothes that are appropriate for the season in order to tighten and strengthen the organs. In spring the appropriate attire is made out of cotton so that the organs remain temperate and the temperament does not become foul. In summer, only flax is appropriate, whereas in autumn woven wool should be worn. As for fur, this should be sabre, ermine, squirrel, and white or black sheep. It is beneficial against the weakening of the organs and preserves the temperament.’

253. ‘coitus and how to conduct it so as to as to avoid weakness, harm, premature old age and grey hair’; [C]: ‘conditions and manner of coitus’.

254. The rest of this paragraph is missing from [C].

255. This position was discouraged by most authors and physicians, including Ibn Sīnā, through whom it entered the Christian European medical tradtion – for example, Ibn Lūqā 1973: 33; al-Nafzāwī n.d.: 30; al-Kātib 2002: 103–4 (transl. 1977: 305); al-Tīfāshī 1892: 66–7; D. Jacquart and C. Thomasset 1988: 132.

256. cf. al-Kātib 1977: 305 (‘The side position is harmful to a man who has weakness in one of his organs [and] also makes difficult the ejaculation of the seminal fluid and causes kidney pain and a swelling in the penis’).

257. The entire passage from ‘These are all dangerous diseases …’ onwards, is missing from [C].

258. The passage starting here and ending in the next chapter (‘… narcissus bulbs’) is considerably shorter in [C]: ‘a burning sensation when urinating, urinary stammer, blood in urine. A wise man should be wary of engaging in coitus in the aforementioned positions. The best position is when the woman is lying flat on her back. Put a cushion underneath her hips, with the woman lifting her thighs. The man then goes on all fours until he is close to ejaculating, at which point he lies down on the woman, who puts her arms around him until the ejaculation has been completed. The advantage of this [position] is that it provides protection against the above-mentioned ailments, Allah the Almighty willing. Chapter Twelve. Description of medicines to strengthen and thicken the penis. Take narcissus bulbs….’

259. *ᶜinab al-dhi’b* (literally, ‘wolf grapes’), which is also known as *ᶜinab al-thaclab*

('fox grapes'). Its medicinal use was often linked to the curing of tumours in various parts of the body. When used with wine, it acts as a soporific. In erotological literature, it is considered one of the anaphrodisiacs. A. Dietrich 1988, II: 573–7; Ibn al-Bayṭār 1992: 225, and 1874, III: 135–7; Ibn al-Jazzār 2004: 115–16; Ibn Sīnā 1999, III: 297, 612–13; al-Shayzarī, *al-Īḍāḥ*, fol. 2b; al-Bīrūnī 1973: 274–6; al-Rāzī 1955–69: XXI: 195–7; R. P. Dozy 1877–81, II: 179; D. al-Anṭākī 1952, I: 240–1; Ibn al-Quff (H. Kircher 1967): 267–8; al-Ṭabarī 1928: 381, 401; Maimonides (M. Meyerhof 1940): no. 297.

260. The author uses the Persian word *ardij* (Ar. *ʿarʿar, abhal*). The type of juniper meant here is probably *Juniperus savina* (savin), which was known to have a number of medicinal purposes and often occurs in Arab pharmacology, for instance, as a purgative, diuretic, carminative, anthelminic, emmenagogue and abortifacient. In cooking, juniper berries were added to stews as an aromatic, as well as being used for juniper brandy. A. Dietrich 1988, II: 125–6; al-Warrāq (N. Nasrallah 2010): 645; Ibn al-Bayṭār 1874, III: 120–1; Ibn al-Jazzār 2004: 126–7; D. al-Anṭākī 1952, I: 236; al-Rāzī 1955–69, XXI: 179; Maimonides (M. Meyerhof 1940): no. 22.

261. *sukkar al-qand* – the latter word denotes crystallized cane sugar, resulting from straining and boiling cane juice. Sugar was used to remedy catarrh, cough and fever, while it invigorated coitus (when taken with milk). Ibn al-Bayṭār 1992: 218; al-Warrāq (N. Nasrallah 2010): 599–600, 601; A. Dietrich 1988, II: 238.

262. cf. al-Kātib 1977: 305.

263. *baṣal al-narjis* (< Gr. νάρκισσος); hot and cold (in the second degree), it was said that the mere fragrance of the narcissus could relieve obstructions in the brain. It was also used as an emetic (especially its boiled root), to cleanse wounds and cure chronic joint aches. The oil was thought to be good for the nerves. Ibn al-Bayṭār 1874, IV: 179, and 1992: 238; Ibn al-Jazzār 2004: 80–1; Ibn Sīnā 1999, I: 575; D. al-Anṭākī 1952, I: 330; Ibn Wāfid 2000: 158; al-Rāzī 1955–69, XXI: 590–2; al-Bīrūnī 1973: 362; al-Dhahabī 1987: 267; Maimonides (M. Meyerhof 1940): no. 254; al-Ṭabarī 1928: 396; al-Warrāq (N. Nasrallah 2010): 774.

264. This refers to an area in Yemen that allegedly produced the best variety of grapes, both in terms of appearance and taste. al-Warrāq (N. Nasrallah 2010): 630.

265. The passage 'pulverize them ... This is treated by', is as follows in [C]: 'Pulverize, throw into grape water and oil, then boil over a fire, remove and rub onto the penis.'

266. *jullanār* (< Persian *gul-i anār*, 'granate rose/blossom'), which is also sometimes referred to as 'a small seedless pomegranate', was thought to be useful against ulcers and bleeding, as well as being an aphrodisiac. It came in wild (*barrī*) and cultivated (*bustānī, janbad al-rummān*) varieties. Ibn Wāfid 2000: 184–5; Ibn al-Jazzār 2004: 117–18; Dietrich 1988, II: 150, 171–2; al-Tīfāshī 1892: 14; Ibn al-Bayṭār 1874, I: 164, and 1992: 202; Ibn al-Jazzār 2004: 117–18; D. al-Anṭākī 1952, I: 106; Ibn al-Quff (H. Kircher 1967): 133. See also note on *rummān*, above.

267. 'Take a white copper plate and place it on live embers'; [C]: 'Take live embers'.
268. 'and beat the grounds on the plate. Turn over and roll until all the oil has been extracted. Proceed in this fashion for all cores'; [C]: 'Knead the aforementioned core until the oil is released. Continue in the same manner with all cores.'
269. It has not been possible to ascertain who is referred to here.
270. This is a reference to the famous physician. See Introduction.
271. The passage starting from the second sentence until this point is missing from [C].
272. *afrībūn*, which is a rare variant of the more common *ū/afarbiyūn* (< Gr. εὐφόρβιον), *Euphorbia resinifera* – a resin from a tree mainly found in the Atlas mountains. It was used for those with cold temperaments and in the treatment of rabies, sciatica and colic. D. al-Anṭākī 1952, I: 53 (*afarbiyūn*); al-Tīfāshī 1892: 14, 18 (*farbiyūn*); Ibn al-Quff (H. Kircher 1967): 290–2; Ibn al-Bayṭār 1874, III: 158–9, and 1992: 227 (*fārbiyūn*); Ibn al-Jazzār 2004: 192 (*afarbiyūn*); Ibn Sīnā 1999, I: 268–9 (*farbiyūn*); al-Rāzī 1955–69, XXI: 229–31; Maimonides (M. Meyerhof 1940): no. 25; A. Dietrich 1988, II: 433–4.
273. The information in this and the next chapter may be compared with the information provided in al-Kātib 1977: 284–5; Ibn Sīnā 1999, II: 747.
274. *marsīn* (< Gr. Μυρσίνη), which is the word commonly used in Egyptian Arabic, as well as being the term in Ottoman Turkish (J. Redhouse 1880: 802). In Arabic botany, it is usually referred to as ās (also *marsīm*). Both the leaves and (black) berries of this evergreen shrub, which came in wild (*barrī*) and cultivated (*bustānī*) varieties, were used for medicinal purposes (often boiled down to a syrup or in a poultice): as a diuretic and against ulcers, bleeding haemorrhoids (especially the leaves), headaches, spider bites, diarrhoea, tumours (especially hot ones, as in the testicles), hair loss and dandruff. The fruits were used to clean the teeth. According to Maimonides, myrtle oil constricted the glans of the penis, whereas al-Tīfāshī (1970: 28) recommended green myrtle leaves mixed with rosewater to make the vagina narrower and sweet smelling. Ibn Wāfid 2000: 98–9; D. al-Anṭākī 1952, I: 43–4; Ibn al-Bayṭār 1874, I: 27–30; al-Rāzī 1955–69, XX: 14–9; al-Qazwīnī 1849: 216; Maimonides (M. Meyerhof 1940): no. 10; Ibn al-Quff (H. Kircher 1967): 74–6; E. Lev and and Z. Amar 2008: 223–5; A. Dietrich 1988, II: 172–3; al-Warrāq (N. Nasrallah 2010): 748, 765.
275. *sharāb* (pl. *ashriba*) – usually denotes a syrup (which is how it is used elsewhere in the text), made from a wide range of sweetened fruits and vegetables. According to Ibn al-Quff, the term is synonymous with *khamr* in the medical literature. Ibn Sīnā, for his part, equates it with *qahwa* (coffee). E. Lev and Z. Amar 2008: 567; Ibn Sīnā 1999, I: 685; Ibn Māssa 1971: 9; Ibn al-Quff (H. Kircher 1967): 234; al-Warrāq (N. Nasrallah 2010): 748; al-Ṭabarī 1928: 391 (*ra's al-ashriba al-khamr*).
276. The last two sentences are missing from [C].
277. *ballūṭ*, referring to both the tree and the fruit – cold and dry, it was recommended (often cooked) against diarrhoea and stomach ulcers, and was thought to counter bedwetting. The term *shāhballūṭ* denoted the chestnut,

which was also known as *k/qastāna* (< Gr. καστανία) or *qas/ṣṭal*. Ibn Wāfid 2000: 102-3; Ibn al-Bayṭār 1874: I, 110-11; Ibn al-Jazzār 2004: 101; Ibn Sīnā 1999: I, 408-9; D. al-Anṭākī 1952, I: 83; al-Dhahabī 1987: 133; al-Ṭabarī 1928: 383; A. Dietrich 1988, II: 166–7; al-Warrāq (N. Nasrallah 2010): 638.

278. *kalīl*, which is a corruption of *iklīl*, as it appears in [C], can refer to either *iklīl al-jabal* (also known as *ḥass lubān*), 'rosemary' (*Rosmarinus officinalis*), or *iklīl al-malik*, 'sweet clover' (white melilot, *Melilotus albus*). One may speculate it is the former, which was used as a diuretic and emmenagogue, to relieve obstructions, and to cure cough. According to Ibn al-Bayṭār, there was consensus on the medicinal uses of the latter; Ibn al-Quff recommended it against joint aches and to purify the body. Al-Kātib (1977: 272) recommends it to strengthen erection. E. Lev and Z. Amar 2008: 266–8 (*iklīl al-jabal*), 492–4 (*iklīl al-malik*); Ibn al-Bayṭār 1874, I: 50–1 (*iklīl al-malik*); Ibn al-Quff (H. Kircher 1967): 57–8 (*iklīl al-malik*); Maimonides (M. Meyerhof 1940): no. 7.

279. *ḥayy ᶜālam* (for *ḥayy al-ᶜālam*) – cold in the third degree and dry in the first, used mainly against headaches. Ibn al-Quff (H. Kircher 1967): 144–5; Ibn al-Bayṭār 1874, II: 43; D. al-Anṭākī 1952, I: 134–5; Maimonides (M. Meyerhof 1940): no. 162; A. Dietrich 1988, II: 595–6.

280. *qaṭrān*. In Arabic pharmacological and botanical literature, *qa/iṭrān* refers to the substance extracted from conifers, especially cedarwood (*Cedrus libani*), i.e. cedar oil. The medicinal use of tar goes back to Antiquity, when its beneficial properties were first reported, and to this day it is used to treat dermatological conditions (especially psoriasis). See A. Dietrich 1988, II: 118–19; *EI*[2], s.v. 'ḳaṭrān' (A. Dietrich); M. Ullman 1970: 217; H. Kichner 1967: no. 206; Ibn al-Bayṭār 1874, IV: 25, and 1992: 230; Ibn Sīnā 1999, I: 647; D. al-Anṭākī 1952, I: 261; al-Bīrūnī 1973: 310–12; Ibn al-Quff (H. Kircher 1967): 306–8; al-Warrāq (N. Nasrallah 2010): 756–7.

281. 'will experience…'; [C]: 'will prevent conception and provide pleasure to the man. Another recipe: [take] acacia and acorn, ten *dirhams* of each; gallnuts and dried aubergine, fifteen *dirhams* of each. Pulverize and strain. Then, vigorously pound in a pestle. The woman inserts a piece [of cloth] soaked in it [into her vagina] for three days. You will see the wondrous result in terms of her tightness and hotness.' See also al-Kātib 1977: 311–12.

282. *ᶜafṣ*, also known as 'oak apples' – they were recommended as a 'tightening' tonic and a remedy against ulcers and festering wounds. They have also been used as a black hair-dye and to make ink. Ibn al-Quff (H. Kircher 1967): 269–70; al-Tīfāshī 1970: 27, 28, 29, 30 (various electuaries used to improve the vagina); Ibn al-Bayṭār 1874, III: 127–8, and 1992: 224; Ibn al-Jazzār 2004: 67–9; Ibn Wāfid 2000: 187–8; D. al-Anṭākī 1952, I: 238; al-Bīrūnī 1973: 270; al-Ṭabarī 1928: 404; A. Dietrich 1988, II: 167–8; M. Hinds and E. Badawi 1986: 586.

283. The manuscript spelling *idkhir* reflects the colloqual pronunciation of *idhkhir*. This herb was recommended as a diuretic and emmenagogue, to treat swellings, as well as kidney and gall stones, and for toothache. A. Dietrich 1988, II: 100–1; al-Dhahabi 1987: 118; Ibn al-Quff (H. Kircher 1967): 70–1; D. al-Anṭākī 1952, I: 39; Ibn al-Jazzār 2004: 148; Ibn Wāfid 2000:

47–8; al-Shayzarī, *al-Īḍāḥ*: fol. 2b; Ibn al-Bayṭār 1874, I: 15–16; al-Ṭabarī 1928: 400; al-Rāzī 1955–69, XX: 6–9; al-Bīrūnī 1973: 27.

284. *balaḥ*, date 'while continuing green and small'; within the growth cycle of the fruit, it comes after *ṭala*ᶜ and *khilāl* and before *busr*, *ruṭab* and *tamr*. E. Lane 1863–74, I: 246; Ibn Sīnā 1999, I: 393–4. See the note on *tamr*, above, for medical applications.

285. *shabb* (also *shabba*), potassium (*potash*) alum. In Islamic medicine, the mineral was used in the treatment of leprosy and ulcers, or as an astringent and coagulant. It has also been used as a dye and in cosmetics (for example, mixed with henna, as an axillary deodorant or depilator). Contrary to European usage, alum did not have any culinary applications in the Middle East. In erotological literature, it is an ingredient in recipes to invigorate the vagina. Ibn al-Bayṭār 1992: 220; Ibn al-Jazzār 2004: 217–18; Ibn Sahl (O. Kahl 2003): nos 209, 389, 391; al-Tīfāshī 1970: 27, 30.

286. *ṣamgh* ᶜ*arabī* – considered warm and dry, it was used in remedies for cough, lung ulcers, pharyngitis and eye inflammation. Ibn Wāfid 2000: 190; Ibn al-Jazzār 2004: 93; Ibn Sīnā 1999, I: 639–40, II: 734; Ibn al-Bayṭār 1992: 30, 220; Ibn al-Quff (H. Kircher 1967): 256–7; al-Warrāq (N. Nasrallah 2010): 670; al-Kātib 1977: 282.

287. [A]: (*ḥabba*) *sawdah* (for *sawdā*').

288. [C]: 'bitter orange peel, one *dirham*. Pound and boil in fine old wine. The woman puts some of it on a woollen cloth before coitus and she will become like a virgin and become pregnant with the help of Allah. This ends the Book, with the assistance of the beneficent King, on the 18th day of Rabīᶜ I of the year 1224 [= 3 May 1809]'.

289. 'and grant them salvation until the Day of Judgement, He is the Lord of the Worlds. In the Name of Allah, the Merciful, the Compassionate', [B]: 'There is no strength and no power save in Allah, the Supreme. [The book] has been completed with the grace and help of Allah.'

290. 3 August 1793–27 July 1794 AD.

APPENDIX

List of Erotological Works

AUTHOR ([C] = Christian; [J] = Jewish)	WORKS ([*] = lost; [M] = mss only)
[ANON]	[*Untitled*] (On aphrodisiacal electuaries and pills)[1] [M]
[ANON]	[*Untitled*] (On aphrodisiacal electuaries and talismans)[2] [M]
[ANON]	[*Untitled*] (Recipes for cosmetics,charms, aphrodisiacs)[3] [M]
[ANON]	*Jāmiᶜ al-masarrāt fīmā li 'l-nafs min al-mufriḥāt* ('Compendium of Pleasures as Regards Things that Gladden the Soul')[4] [M]
[ANON]	*Nubdha min kitāb fī 'l-bāh* ('Excerpt from the Book on Coitus')[5] [M]
[ANON]	*Irtiyāḥ al-arwāḥ fī ᶜādāt al-nikāḥ* ('The Delight of the Souls Regarding the Customs of Lawful Intercourse')[6] [M]
[ANON]	*Miṣbāḥ fī asrār al-nikāḥ* ('Light on the Secrets of Lawful Intercourse')[7] [M]
[ANON]	*Risāla fī 'l-jimāᶜ* ('Treatise on Lawful Intercourse')[8] [M]
[ANON]	*Ḍuᶜf al-intishār* ('On Impotence')[9] [M]
[ANON]	*Risāla fī 'l-jimāᶜ* ('Treatise on Lawful Intercourse')[10] [M]
[ANON]	*Tuḥfat al-aṣḥāb fī muᶜāsharat al-aḥbāb* ('Gift of the Friends in Relations with Lovers')[11] [M]
[ANON]	*Qiṣṣat Lūṭ* ('The Story of Lot')[12] [M]
[ANON]	*Risāla fī dhikr adwiyat al-bāh* ('Treatise on Aphrodisiacs'[13] [M]
[ANON]	*Kitāb al-ḥayk fī ᶜilm al-nayk* ('The Book of Weaving in the Science of Fucking')[14] [M]
[ANON]	*Kitāb fī ᶜilm al-bāh* ('Book on the Science of Coitus')[15] [M]

AUTHOR ([C] = Christian; [J] = Jewish)	WORKS ([*] = lost; [M] = mss only)
[ANON]	*al-Rawḍa al-bahiyya fī 'l-ladhdha al-bāhiyya* ('The Brilliant Garden of Coital Pleasure')[16]
[ANON]	*Risāla fī aᶜḍā' al-tanāsul* ('Treatise on the Sexual Organs')[17] [M]
[ANON]	*Kitāb fī ᶜilm al-bāh wa adwiyatihi* ('Book on the Science of Coitus and Its Medicines')[18] [M]
[ANON]	*al-Risāla al-jāmi'a*[19] ('Treatise on Intercourse') [M]
[ANON]	*Risāla fī waṣf al-nisā' wa ādāb al-jimāᶜ* ('Treatise on the Description of Women and the Rules of Conduct for Coitus')[20] [M]
[ANON]	*Kitāb al-īḍāḥ fī ᶜilm al-nikāḥ* ('Book of Elucidation on the Science of Lawful Intercourse')[21]
al-Aqfahsī, Shihāb al-Dīn [d. 1406, Egypt]	*Rafᶜ al-janāḥ ᶜammā huwa min al-mar'a al-mubāḥ* ('The Raising of the Wings as Regards the Lawful Woman')[22]
al-Baghdādī, Abū 'Abd al-Raḥmān [14th century, Egypt]	*Kitāb al-zahr al-anīq fī 'l-lubūs wa 'l-taᶜnīq* ('The Book of Delicate Flowers Regarding the Kiss and the Embrace')[23] [M]
al-Fallātī, Muḥammad Ibn Muḥammad Tuqur [d. 1741, Sudan]	*Muᶜāwanat al-ikhwān fī muᶜāsharat al-niswān* ('Assistance of the Brothers Regarding the Association with Women')[24] [M]
al-Ghazlāwī, Muḥammad Ibn ᶜUmar [17th century]	*Yāsamīn al-rawḍ al-ᶜāṭir fī nuzhat al-khāṭir* ('Jasmine of the Scented Garden in the Excursion of Desire')[25] [M]
al-Ḥawrānī, ᶜAbd al-Raḥīm [14th century – Bilād al-Shām]	*Kashf asrār al-muḥtalīn wa nawāmīs al-ḥayyālīn* ('Uncovering the Secrets of Swindlers and the Laws of Tricksters')[26] [M]

AUTHOR ([C] = Christian; [J] = Jewish)	WORKS ([*] = lost; [M] = mss only)
al-Ḥimṣī, al-Muẓaffar Bin Nāṣir Bin ᶜAlī al-Qurayshī [d. 1215 – Bilād al-Shām]	*Maqāla fī 'l-bāh* ('Treatise on Coitus')[27] [M]
Ḥunayn Ibn Isḥāq [C] [809–73, Iraq]	*Kitāb asrār al-falāsifa fī 'l-bāh* ('Book on the Secrets of the Philosophy of Coitus')[28] [M]
Ibn ᶜĀdī, Yaḥyā [d. 974]	*Kitāb fī manāfiᶜ al-bāh wa maḍārrihi wa jihāt istiᶜmālihi* ('Book on the Benefits and Disadvantages of Coitus and the Ways of Practising it')[29] [M]
Ibn Bukhtīshūᶜ, Jibrā'īl Ibn Jūrjiūs [C] [d. 827, Persia]	*Kitāb fī 'l-Bāh* ('The Book on Coitus')[30] [*]
Ibn Falīta al-Yamanī, Aḥmad Ibn Muḥammad Ibn ᶜAlī Abū al-ᶜAbbās [d. 1331, Yemen]	*Rushd al-labīb ilā muᶜāsharat al-ḥabīb* ('An Intelligent Man's Guide to Intercourse with a Loved One')[31]
Ibn Ḥājib al-Nuᶜmān, Muḥammad Ibn ᶜAbd al-Azīz [d. 1031]	*Kitāb al-qiyān* ('The Book of Dancing Girls')[32] [M]
Ibn Hishām, Abū Ahmad [13th century]	*Maḥāsin al-nisā'* ('The Beauties of Women')[33]
Ibn Ishāq, ᶜAlī [mid-14th century]	*Kitāb fī ᶜilm al-bāh* ('Book on The Science of Coitus')[34]
Ibn Kannān, Muḥammad Ibn ᶜĪsā al-Khalūtī [1663–1740, Bilād al-Shām]	*Nuzhat al-nufūs wa daftar al-ᶜilm wa rawḍat al-ᶜarūs fī 'umūr al-nikāḥ wa ghayrihi* ('Excursion of the Souls, the Book of Science and the Garden of the Bride in Matters of Lawful Sexual Intercourse, etc.')[35] [M]
Qusṭā Ibn Lūqā [C] [820–912, Bilād al-Shām]	*Kitāb fī 'l-bāh wa mā yuḥtāju ilayhi min tadbīr al-badan fī istiᶜmālihi* ('The Book on Coitus and what Regimen is Required to Practise It')[36]

AUTHOR ([C] = Christian; [J] = Jewish)	WORKS ([*] = lost; [M] = mss only)
Qusṭā Ibn Lūqā [C] [820–912, Bilād al-Shām] *(Cont.)*	*Kitāb fi 'l-bāh wa mā yuḥtāju ilayhi min tadbīr al-badan fi istiᶜmālihi* ('The Book on Coitus and what Regimen is Required to Practise It')[36] *Kitāb fi 'l-Bāh* ('The Book on Coitus')[37]
Ibn Mandawayh, Abū ᶜAlī [d. 1019, Persia]	*Risāla fi asbāb al-bāh* ('Treatise on the Reasons for Coitus')[38] [M]
Ibn Marzūq, Shams al-Dīn Abu ᶜAbd Allāh [d. 472/1080, Tunis]	*al-Intibāh li-muᶜālajat al-bāh* ('Vigilance Regarding the Treatment of Coitus')[39] [M]
Ibn Māssa, ᶜĪsā [C] [9th century, Persia]	*Masā'il fi 'l-nasl wa 'l-dhurriyya wa 'l-jimāᶜ* ('Questions about Progeny, Offspring and Coitus')[40]
Ibn Maymūn (Maimonides) [J] [1135–1204, al-Andalus]	*Fi 'l-jimāᶜ* ('On Coitus')[41]
Ibn al-Qaṭṭāᶜ [1041–1121, Sicily]	*Kitāb al-nikāḥ fi 'l-lugha* ('The Book on the Language of Lawful Intercourse')[42]
Ibn Raḥmūn, Sallāma [J] [d. 1136, Egypt], doctor	*Maqāla fi khiṣb abdān al-nisā' bi-Miṣr ᶜinda tanāhī al-shabāb* ('Treatise on the Fertility of Egyptian Women's Bodies upon the Expiration of Youth')[43] [*]
Ibn Raqīqa, Maḥmūd Ibn ᶜUmar al-Shaybānī [1169–1238, Turkey]	*Kitāb muwaḍḍaḥat al-ishtibāh fi adwiyat al-bāh* ('The Revelation of Doubts about Aphrodisiacs')[44] [M]
Ibn Sīnā [d. 1037, Persia]	*Urjūza fi'l-bāh* ('*Urjuza* on Coitus')[45] [M] *Asrār al-jimāᶜ* ('The Secrets of Lawful Intercourse')[46] [M]
Ibn Sulaymān, Aḥmad	*Zahr al-bustān fi maᶜrifat aḥwāl al-bāh fi 'l-insān* ('Garden Flowers in the Knowledge of the Situations in which People Engage in Coitus')[47] [M]

AUTHOR ([C] = Christian; [J] = Jewish)	WORKS ([*] = lost; [M] = mss only)
Ibn al-Takrītī, Yaḥyā Ibn Jarīr [second half of 11th century, Iraq]	*Kitāb fī 'l-bāh wa manāfiᶜ al-jimāᶜ wa maḍarrihi* ('The Book on Coitus, the Benefits of Intercourse and Its Harmful Effects')[48] [M]
al-Isrā'ilī, Samaw'āl Ibn Yaḥyā Ibn ᶜAbbās al-Maghribī [J] [d. 1180]	*Nuzhat al-aṣḥāb fī muᶜāshirat al-aḥbāb* ('The Friends' Jaunt in Coitus Between Lovers')[49] *Kitāb fī 'l-Bāh* ('The Book on Coitus')[50] [*]
al-Jāḥiẓ, Abū ᶜUthmān [781–868, Iraq]	*Mufākharāt al-jawārī wa 'l-ghulmān* ('Boasts of Girl and Boy Slaves')[51] *Kitāb al-ᶜurs wa 'l-ᶜarā'is* ('The Book of Marriage and Brides')[52] [M]
al-Jildakī, Īdmar Ibn ᶜAlī ᶜIzz al-Dīn [d. 1342, Egypt]	*Kitāb durrat al-ghawāṣṣ wa kanz al-ikhtiṣāṣ fī ᶜilm al-khawāṣṣ* ('The Diver's Pearls and the Specialist Treasure regarding the Science of Characteristics')[53] [M]
al-Kātib, Abū 'l-Hasan ᶜAli Ibn Nasr al-Samnānī (active 10th century, Bagdad)	*Jawamiᶜ al-ladhdha* ('The Encyclopaedia of Pleasure')[54] *Kitāb kīmiyā' al-bāh* ('Book on The Chemistry of Coitus')[55] [*]
Khān, Muḥammad al-Ṣādiq Ḥassan [d. 1878]	*Nashwat al-sakrān min ṣahbā' tidhkār al-ghizlān* ('The Intoxication of the Drunkard on the Wine of the Commemoration of Youths')[56]
al-Khaṭīb, Abū Naṣr	*Kitāb akhbār al-nisā'* ('Book on the News of Women')[57] [M]
al-Khuwārizmī, Abū Bakr [d. 993, Persia]	*Kitāb fī 'l-Bāh* ('The Book on Coitus')[58] [M]
al-Kindī [d. 873, Iraq]	*Kitāb al-Bāh* ('The Book on Coitus')[59]
al-Maghribī, Ibrāhīm [first half 17th century, Morocco]	*Ṣanf fī 'l-bāh* ('Categories of Coitus')[60] [M]

AUTHOR ([C] = Christian; [J] = Jewish)	WORKS ([*] = lost; [M] = mss only)
al-Masīhī, ᶜIzz al-Dīn [C]	*al-Munākaḥa wa 'l-mufātaḥa fī aṣnāf al-jimāᶜ wa ālātihi* ('Coitus and Preamble to the Categories of Coitus and Its Tools')[61] [*]
al-Mufaḍḍal, Ibn ᶜUmar	*Kitāb al-haft wa 'l-azilla* ('The Book of Nonsense and Slips of the Tongue')[62]
al-Mughalṭāy, al-Ḥāfiẓ [13th century]	*al-Wāḍiḥ al-mubīn fī dhikr man ustushhida min al-muḥibbīn* ('Clarity Regarding the Memory of Those Who Were Martyred Because of the Loved Ones')[63]
al-Nafzāwī, Muḥammad Ibn Muḥammad [16th century, Tunis]	*al-Rawḍ al-ᶜāṭir fī nuzhat al-khāṭir* ('The Scented Garden in the Excursion of Desire')[64] *Tanwīr al-wiqāᶜ fī asrār al-jimāᶜ* ('Illumination of Coition in the Secrets of Intercourse')[65] [*]
al-Nam(a)lī, Hassān Ibn Muḥammad [9th century, Iraq]	*Kitāb Burjān wa Ḥubāḥib* ('The Book of Burjan and Hubahib')[66] [*] *Kitāb khiṭāb al-makārī li-jāriyat al-Baqqāl* ('Address of the Muleteer to the Greengrocer's Slave Girl')[67] [*] *Kitāb Bighā'* ('The Book of Prostitution')[68] [*] *Kitāb al-saḥq* ('The Book of Lesbianism')[69] [*]
al-Nawājī, Shams al-Dīn Muḥammad Ibn Ḥasan [1386–1455, Egypt]	*Marātiᶜ al-ghizlān fī waṣf al-ḥisān min al-ghilmān* ('The Gazelles' Pasture Regarding the Description of the Beautiful among Boys')[70] [M]
al-Niḥillī	*Kitāb al-bāh* ('The Book on Coitus')[71] [*]

AUTHOR ([C] = Christian; [J] = Jewish)	WORKS ([*] = lost; [M] = mss only)
al-Qusṭanṭīnī, Maḥmūd Ibn Muḥammad [d. 1568, Tunis]	*Kitāb adwiyat al-Bāh* ('The Book of Medicines for Coitus')[72] [M]
al-Rāzī, Muḥammad Ibn Zakariyyā' [865–925, Persia]	*Kitāb al-Bāh wa manāfiᶜihi wa maḍārrihi wa mudawātihi* ('The Book on Coitus, Its Benefits, Harmful Effects and Treatments')[73] *Maqāla fīmā su'ila ᶜanhu fī annahu bimā ṣāra man qalla jimāᶜuhu min al-insān ṭāla 'umruhu* ('Treatise on Whether Engaging in Coitus with Low Frequency Increases Lifespan')[74] [M] *Risāla fī 'l-ubna* ('Treatise on Passive Sodomy')[75] [M]
al-Sāᶜātī, Muḥammad Rājī al-Ḥalabī	*Rashf al-ruḍāb wa fākihat al-aḥbāb* ('The Sipping of Saliva and the Fruit of Lovers')[76]
al-Ṣaymarī, Muḥammad Ibn Isḥāq Abū al-ᶜAnbas [827–88, Iraq]	*Kitāb al-saḥḥāqāt wa 'l-baghghā'īn* ('The Book of Lesbians and Homosexual Prostitutes')[77] [*] *Kitāb al-khaḍkhaḍa fī jald ᶜUmayra* ('The Book of Masturbation')[78] [*] *al-ᶜĀshiq wa 'l-maᶜshūq* ('The Lover and the Loved One')[79] [*] *Kitāb nawādir al-khaṣī* ('The Book of Rare Anecdotes on Eunuchs')[80] [*] *Kitāb nawādir al-quwwād* ('The Book of Rare Anecdotes on Pimps')[81] [*] *Kitāb faḍl al-surm ᶜalā 'l-fam* ('The Book on the Superiority of the Rectum over the Mouth')[82] [*]

AUTHOR ([C] = Christian; [J] = Jewish)	WORKS ([*] = lost; [M] = mss only)
al-Shādhilī, ᶜAbd al-Qādir Ibn Aḥmad Ibn Muḥammad al-Māliki [d. 1529, Tunis]	*Tashnīf al-asmāᶜ bi-fawāʾid al-tasmiya ᶜinda ʿl-jimāᶜ* ('Delighting the Ears by the Benefits of Hearing the Formula "In The Name of God" during Coitus')[83] [M]
al-Shāfiᶜī, ᶜAlā ʿl-Dīn	*al-Nikāḥ* ('On Lawful Intercourse')[84] [M]
al-Shayzarī al-Ṭabarī, ᶜAbd al-Raḥmān Ibn Naṣr [d. 1193, Egypt]	*al-Īḍāḥ fī asrār il-nikāḥ* ('Elucidation of the Secrets of Lawful Intercourse')[85]
al-Suyūṭī, Jalāl al-Dīn [1445–1505, Egypt]	*al-Wishāḥ fī fawāʾid al-nikāḥ* ('The Sash in the Benefits of Lawful Intercourse')[86] *Rashf al-zulāl min al-siḥr al-ḥalāl* ('The Sipping of the Pure Water of Lawful Charm')[87] *Nawāḍir al-ayk fī nawādir al-nayk* ('The Blooming of the Jungle in the Rareties of Fucking')[88] *al-ayk fī maᶜrifat al-nayk* ('Jungle in the Knowledge of Fucking')[89] *Fi ʾl-jimāᶜ wa ālātuhu* ('On Coitus and Its Tools')[90] *Shaqāʾiq al-utrunj fī daqāʾiq al-ghunj* ('Halves of the Lemon Regarding the Intricacies of Coquetry')[91] *Nuzhat al-ᶜumr fī ʿl-tafḍīl bayn al-bīḍ wa ʿl-sūd wa ʿl-sumr* ('Jaunt in Preferences in Terms of the White, Black and Brown')[92] *Ghāyat al-iḥsān fī khalq al-insān* ('The Height of Charity in the Creation of Human Beings')[93] [M]?

AUTHOR ([C] = Christian; [J] = Jewish)	WORKS ([*] = lost; [M] = mss only)
	Ādāb *al-nikāḥ wa kasr al-shahwatayni* ('The Rules of Conduct for Lawful Intercourse and the Breaking of the Two Passions')[94]
	Nuzhat al-julasā' fī ishʿār al-nisā' ('Jaunt of the Table Companions in the Notification of Women')[95]
	Mu'akkad al-maḥabba bayn al-muḥibb wa man aḥabba ('The Certainty of the Attachment Between the Lover and the One He Loves')[96] [M]
	al-Uss fīman ra'asa bi 'l-kuss ('The Foundation in He Who Is in Charge of the Cunt')[97] [*]
al-Suyūṭī, Jalāl al-Dīn [1445–1505, Egypt] *(cont.)*	*al-Ifṣāḥ fī asmā' al-nikāḥ* ('Declaration regarding the Names for Lawful Intercourse')[98] [M]
	al-Yawāqīt al-thamīna fī ṣifāt al-samīna ('Precious Stones in the Description of the Fat Woman')[99]
	Wuḍū' al-ṣabāḥ fī lughāt al-nikāḥ ('Morning Ablutions in the Language of Lawful Intercourse')[100] [M]
	al-Mustaẓrafa fī aḥkām dukhūl al-ḥashafa ('The Elegant Woman as regards Provisions for the Entry of the Glans Penis')[101] [*]
	al-Mustaẓraf fī akhbār al-jawārī ('The Elegant Man regarding News of Slave Girls')[102]

AUTHOR ([C] = Christian; [J] = Jewish)	WORKS ([*] = lost; [M] = mss only)
al-Suyūṭī, Jalāl al-Dīn [1445–1505, Egypt] *(cont.)*	*Nuzhat al-Nadīm* ('Excursion of the Boon Companion')[103] *Nuzhat al-muta'ahhil wa murshid al-muta'ahhal fī faḍā'il al-nikāḥ* ('Excursion of the Spouse and the Guide to His Wife Regarding the Virtues of Lawful Intercourse')[104] *Mabāsim al-milāḥ wa manāsim al-ṣabāḥ fī mawāsim al-nikāḥ* ('The Mouths of Wittiness and the Foot Soles of the Morning in the Seasons of Lawful Intercourse')[105] [*] *al-Zanjabīl al-qāṭiᶜ fī waṭ' dhāt al-barāqiᶜ* ('Cut Ginger in Coitus with Face-Veiled Women')[106] [*] *al-Īḍāḥ fī asrār al-nikāḥ* ('Elucidation of the Secrets of Lawful Intercourse')[107] *al-Kanz al-madfūn wa 'l-falak al-mashḥūn* ('The Hidden Treasure and the Loaded Star')[108]
al-Ṭabarī, ᶜAlī Abū 'l-Ḥasan Ibn Rabban [C] [active mid-9th century, Persia]	*Kitāb al-īḍāḥ min al-simān wa 'l-huzāl wa tahayyuj al-bāh wa 'ibṭālihi* ('The Book of Elucidation Regarding the Fat and the Skinny, Stimulation of Coitus and Its Thwarting')[109] [*]
al-Tadaghī, Abū Ṣāliḥ A. Ibn Ṣāliḥ	*Tuḥfat al-falāḥ fī ᶜilm al-nikāḥ, Manẓūma* ('Gift of the Peasant regarding the Science of Lawful Intercourse')[110] [M]

AUTHOR ([C] = Christian; [J] = Jewish)	WORKS ([*] = lost; [M] = mss only)
al-Ṭāhirī, Ibn al-Shāh (9th century?)	Kitāb akhbār al-ghilmān ('The Book of News on Catamites')[111] [*]
	Kitāb akhbār al-nisā' ('The Book of News on Women')[112] [*]
	Kitāb al-bighā' wa ladhdhatihi ('The Book of Prostitution and Its Pleasures')[113] [*]
	Kitāb al-khaḍkhaḍa ('The Book of Masturbation')[114] [*]
al-Tamakrūtī, Muḥammad ʿAbd Allāh Ibn Muḥammad Ibn Masʿūd al-Darʿī al-Tafjarūtī [10th–11th centuries]	al-Rawḍ al-yāniʿ fī aḥkām al-tazwīj wa-ādāb al-majāmiʿ ('The Ripe Gardens in the Rules for Marrying off a Woman and Etiquette for Congregation')[115] [M]
Ṭayfūr, Aḥmad Ibn Abī Ṭāhir [819–93, Iraq]	Balāghāt al-nisā' ('Information about Women')[116]
al-Tīfāshī, Shihāb al-Dīn Aḥmad Ibn Yūsuf [1184–1253, Tunis]	Nuzhat al-albāb fīmā lā yūjad fī 'l-kitāb ('Delights of Hearts in Things that Cannot Be Found in Any Book')[117]
	Rujūʿ al-shaykh ilā ṣibāhi fī 'l-quwwa wa 'l-bāh ('Returning the Old Man to His Youthful Sexual Potency')[118]
	Risāla fīmā yaḥtajī ilayhi al-rijāl wa 'l-nisā' fī istiʿmāl al-bāh mimmā yaḍurr wa yanfaʿ ('Treatise on What Men and Women Need during Coitus and Its Harms and Benefits')[119]
al-Tījānī, Muḥammad Ibn Aḥmad [13th to early 14th centuries, Tunis]	Tuḥfat al-ʿarūs wa nuzhat al-nufūs ('The Bride's Gift and the Delight of the Souls')[120]

AUTHOR ([C] = Christian; [J] = Jewish)	WORKS ([*] = lost; [M] = mss only)
al-Ṭūsī, Naṣīr al-Dīn	*Kitāb albāb al-bāhiyya wa 'l-tarākīb al-sulṭāniyya*
al-Ẓāhirī, ʿAlī Ibn Muḥammad [d. 963, Iraq]	*Akhbār al-Ghilmān* ('News about Boys')[121] [*] *Akhbār al-Nisā'* ('News about Women') [*] *al-Bighā' wa Ladhdhātuhu* ('Prostitution and Its Pleasures') [*]
Zarrūq, Aḥmad [1442–93, Morocco]	*al-Nikāḥ* ('Lawful Intercourse')[122] [M]

Notes

1. BN 3039.5, fols. 61–82 (copy dated 1075/1664–65).
2. BN 3039.13, fols. 125–7 (copy dated 1075/1664–65).
3. BN 3039.14, fols. 127–38 (copy dated 1075/1664–65).
4. BN 3039.15, 138ff (copy dated 1075/1664–65).
5. Damascus, al-Ẓāhiriyya, No. 7524.
6. BN 3039.11, fols. 109–10 (copy dated 1075/1664–65).
7. BN 3039.4, fols. 36-61 (copy dated 1075/1664–65).
8. BN 3039.3, fols. 30 (copy dated 1075/1664–65).
9. BN 3039.1, fols. 28–30 (copy dated 1075/1664–65).
10. BN 3039.12, fols. 111–25 (copy dated 1075/1664–65).
11. BN 3039, fols. 151–259 [3039.17], 267–8 [3039.20] (copy dated 1075/1664–65).
12. BN 1932, fols. 105–15.
13. Cairo, Dār al-Kutub, Ṭ Taymūr 362.
14. Berlin, 6385 Spr. 1920.
15. A. Ihsanoglu 1984: 449; Shahid Ali library, No 2145.
16. ᶜA. Hishām and ᶜĀ. ᶜAbd al-Hamīd 1999: 177–215.
17. Tunisian National Library 18248.
18. Tunisian National Library 20648 (09).
19. Aya Sofya 2938.
20. Tunisian National Library 18228 (2).
21. al-Nafzāwī n.d.: 64–84.
22. Aḥmad Farīd al-Mazīdī, ed., Cairo: Dār al-Āfāq al-ᶜArabiyya, 2007, pp. 371–402. ᶜU. al-Kaḥḥāla n.d.: I, 214.
23. R. Irwin, 'ᶜAlī al-Baghdādī and the Joy of Mamluk Sex', in H. Kennedy. ed., *The Historiography of Islamic Egypt* (c. 950–1800), Leiden: Brill, 2000, pp. 45–57; L. Lopez-Baralt 1992: 258–60 – translated into French by R. Khawam as *Les Fleurs éclatantes dans les baisers et l'accolement*, Paris: Albin Michel, 1973 (revised translation, Paris: Phébus, 1989).
24. BN 5622, ff 78b–90a. See ᶜU. Kaḥḥāla n.d. XI: 132.
25. BN 3069, 3070.1 (128ff; in this ms, the author's name is erroneously given as Muḥammad al-Nafzāwī, presumably because of the similarity in title between the two works).
26. BN 2042, 3564–6, 3612, 6146. French translation, R. Khawam, *Les ruses des femmes*, Paris: Phébus, 1994.

27. ᶜU. Kaḥḥāla n.d. XII: 12; mss Aleppo.
28. *GAS* III: 254 (No. 25); P. Sbath 1938–40, I: 43 (No. 312); mss Aleppo. The book is quoted in al-Rāzī's *Kitāb al-Ḥāwī fi 'l-ṭibb* as *al-Bāh or al-Kunnāsh fi 'l-bāh* (1955–69, X: 263–295–7).
29. *GAS* III: 304; P. Sbath 1938–40, I: 69, No. 562.
30. ᶜU. Kaḥḥāla n.d., III: 113; *GAS* III: 243; L. Shaykhū 1924: 224.
31. Aḥmad Ibn Muḥammad al-Yamanī, ed., *Rushd al-labīb ilā maᶜāshirat al-ḥabīb*, Beirut: Tāla li 'l-Ṭibāᶜa wa 'l-Nashr, 2002. Partial editions: Ghadhban Al-Bayati (Chapters 1–3), unpublished PhD dissertation, Friedrich-Alexander University Erlangen-Nürnberg, 1976; Adnan Husni-Pascha (Chapter 4), unpublished PhD dissertation, Friedrich-Alexander University Erlangen-Nürnberg, 1975; Jalal Elias Yousif (Chapter 5), unpublished PhD dissertation, Friedrich-Alexander University Erlangen-Nürnberg, 1977; Boulus Al-Khouri (Chapter 6, Part 1), unpublished PhD dissertation, Friedrich-Alexander University Erlangen-Nürnberg, 1975; Abdul Hassan Abdul Khador (Chapter 6, Part 2), unpublished PhD dissertation, Friedrich-Alexander University Erlangen-Nürnberg, 1983; Adnan Zeni (Chapter 6, Part 3), unpublished PhD dissertation, Friedrich-Alexander University Erlangen-Nürnberg, 1978; Mohamed Zouher Djabri (Chapters 9–11), unpublished PhD dissertation, Friedrich-Alexander University Erlangen-Nürnberg, 1968; Elian Sabbagh (Chapters 12–14), unpublished PhD dissertation, Friedrich-Alexander University Erlangen-Nürnberg, 1973. Translated into English by A. Jarkas and S. Khawwam as *An Intelligent Man's Guide to the Art of Coition by Ibn Falita Ahmad Ibn Muhammad*, Toronto: Aleppo, 1977. See S. Habib 2007: 25–31; D. Jacquart and C. Thomasset 1988: 126; *GAL* I: 232, *GALS* I: 415; ᶜU. Kaḥḥāla n.d., II: 20, 136; A. Ihsanoglu 1984: 82.
32. al-Tīfāshī 1892: 2 (this is probably a reference to al-Jāḥiẓ's work); R. Burton 1885, X: 175. ᶜU. Kaḥḥāla n.d.: X, 173.
33. H. ᶜAbd al-ᶜAziz and ᶜAbd al-Ḥamīd 1999: 37–148.
34. A. Ihsanoglu 1984: 299, Tera No. 3/259 (165pp), copy dating to 1136 AH/1723AD.
35. Damascus, Ẓāhiriyya. ᶜU. Kaḥḥāla n.d., XI: 108; *GAL* II: 299–300; *GALS*: 410–1; Ṣ. al-Munajjid 1975: 24.
36. G. Haydar 1973; *GAS* III: 272, No 14; D. Jacquart and C. Thomasset 1988: 123.
37. N.A. Barhoum 1974; H. Fähndrich, *Abhandlung über die Ansteckung*, Berlin: Deutsche Morgenländische Gesellschaft, 1987; *GAS* III: 272, No. 15; M. Ullmann 1970: 194. A. Ihsanoglu 1984: 314; *Aya Sophia* No. 10/3729; University of Istanbul, Arabic Section No. 2/242.
38. *GAS* III: 328; ᶜU. Kaḥḥāla n.d., I: 269; XIII: 261.
39. Tunis National Library, No. 17970; ᶜA. Manṣūr 1975: 408; M. Maḥfūẓ 1992, IV: 302–3.
40. Mohamed Walid Anbari, ed., *Masā'il fi 'l-nasl wa 'l-dhurriyya wa 'l-jimāᶜ*, 1971. This book is also known as *Maqāla fi 'l-jimāᶜ wa mā yataᶜalliqu bihi* ('Treatise on Coitus and Related Matters'). See M. Ullmann 1970: 122f, 194; A. Ihsanoglu 1984: 87 (*Kitāb al-jimāᶜ aw masā'il fi 'l-nasl wa l-dhurriyya wa*

*'l-jimā*ᶜ); *GAL* I (*Kitāb al-Jimā*ᶜ), 232, 267; *GALS* I: 417; *GAS* III: 257; ᶜU. Kaḥḥāla n.d., VIII: 31.

41. This is the name of two works attributed to Maimonides. However, it is now generally accepted that only the shorter of the two (consisting of ten chapters) was written by Maimonides himself. For a brief discussion, see F. Rosner, *The Medical Legacy of Moses Maimonides*, New York: Ktav Publishing House, 1997, pp. 10–11; M. L. Wilensky, 'Health Conduct in Intercourse Taken from Rabbi Moshe Maimon', *Proceedings of the American Academy for Jewish Research* 56 (1990), pp. 101–10, at pp. 103–4. The Hebrew translations of both texts were edited and rendered into German by Hermann Kroner (*Ein Beitrag zur Geschichte der Medizin des XII. Jahrhunderts: an der Hand zweier medizinischer Abhandlungen des Miamonides auf Grund von 6 uneditierten Handschriften*, Oberdorf-Bopfingen, 1906), who concurred with M. Steinschneider (1902: 213) that both works were composed by Maimonides. The Arabic manuscript of the shorter version was later also edited by Kroner ('Eine medizinische Maimonides-Handschrift aus Granada. Ein Beitrag zur Stilistik des Maimonides und zur Charakteristik der hebraischen Übersetzungsliteratur. Im Urtexts herausgegeben, übersetzt und kritisch erlautert', *Janus* 21 [1916], pp. 203–47). It was subsequently translated into Italian by U. De Martini as *Maimonides. Segreto dei segreti*, Rome: Istituto di storia della Medicina dell'Universita di Roma, 1960, into Spanish by E. Chelminiski as 'Notas introductorias al "Guia sobre el contacto sexual de Maimonides"', *An de ars medica-Mexico*, 1961, 5, pp. 240–8, and into English M. Gorlin as *Maimonides' On Sexual Intercourse* (*Fi'l-Jima*), New York: Rambash Publishing, 1961. See also F. Rosner, Sex Ethics in the Writings of Moses Maimonides, New York: Bloch Publishing Company, 1974; F. Rosner 1984: 162–82. The Hebrew translations were critically re-edited by Susman Muntner as *Pseudo-Maimonides and Sexual Life: Collection of Medieval Treatises*, Jerusalem: Geniza, 1965.

42. *EI*², s.v. 'Ibn al-Qaṭṭaᶜ' (U. Rizzitano); *GAL* I: 308; *GALS* I: 540; Ṣ. al-Munajjid 1975: 142; al-Suyūṭī 2001: 125.

43. ᶜU. Kaḥḥāla n.d., IV: 237.

44. ᶜU. Kaḥḥāla n.d., XII: 185–6.

45. M. Ullmann 1970: 195; *GALS* I: 827; British Library 1349. This work is also known as *Risāla fī 'l-bāh* ('Treatise on Coitus').

46. Cairo: Dār al-Kutub, *Ṭ-ṭibb* No. 509.

47. Damascus: Ẓāhiriyya, No. 8315.

48. ᶜU. Kaḥḥāla n.d., XIII; L. Shaykhū 1924: 75–6; *GALS* I: 862.

49. Aḥmad Farīd al-Mazīdī, Cairo: Dār al-Āfāq al-ᶜArabiyya, 2007, pp. 7–288; Partial editions: F. Mansour (Part 2, Sections 1–5), unpublished PhD dissertation, Universität Erlangen-Nürnberg, 1975; K. Hallak (Part 2, Section 6), unpublished PhD dissertation, Universität Erlangen-Nürnberg, 1973; T. Haddad (Part 1, Sections 6–8), unpublished PhD dissertation, Universität Erlangen-Nürnberg, 1976. Translated into English by A. Jarkas and S. Khawwam as *A Jaunt in the Art of Coition*, Toronto: Aleppo Publishing, 1978. See A. Ihsanoglu 1984: 251; D. Jacquart and F. Thomasset 1988: 124; *GAL* I: 488; *GALS* I: 892; F. Rosenthal, 'Die arabische

Autobiographie', in F. Rosenthal, G. von Grünebaum and W. J. Fischel, eds, *Studia Arabica* I (Analecta Orientalia 14), Rome: Pontificum Institutum Biblicum, 1937; A. Ambouba, 'As-Samaw'al Ibn Yahya al-Magribī (570 H.)', *al-Machriq* 55 (1961), pp. 89–112; L. Leclerq 1877 II: 14–17.

50. M. Steinschneider 1902: 189; *GAL* II: 643.
51. Charles Pellat, ed., Beirut: 1957.
52. A. Ihsanoglu 1984: 158–9; *Ahmad* III, No 2538.
53. Berlin 4186. ᶜU. al-Kaḥḥāla n.d., III: 28.
54. Mss, Aya Sofia 3836 (dated 533/1139), Aya Sofia 3837 (dated 634/1236), Fatih 3729 (dated 582/1186): al-Kātib 1977: 41 (where a ms held by the Alexandria municipal library is also mentioned); A. Ihsanoglu 1984: 52. Partial ed., 2002; Beirut: Tāla li 'l-Tibāᶜa wa 'l-Nashr, 2006 (under al-Qazwīnī, ᶜAlī al-Kātibī), translated into English by A. Jarkas and S. Khawwam 1977. *GALS* I: 945 (No. 339); Ṣ. al-Munajjid 1975: 156–8; Burton 1885, X: 175. This work is listed as a source by al-Tīfāshī (1892: 2).
55. Al-Kātib 1977: 108. According to the author, the book dealt with masturbation.
56. Constantinople: al-Jawā'ib, n.d.; Beirut: Arab Diffusion Company, 2007.
57. Ahmad III: 259 (A. Ihsanoglu 1984).
58. Istanbul University Library No 242, Folio 63–117.
59. A. Ihsanoglu 1984: 314, Aya Sophia 4832 (written 568 AH); Ullmann 1970: 194; *GALS* I: 374; *GAS* III: 245 (No. 2). Giuseppe Celentano, ed., *Due scritti medici di al-Kindī*, Napoli: Istituto Orientale di Napoli, 1979.
60. ᶜU. Kaḥḥāla n.d., I: 107; *GAL* II: 465.
61. Al-Tīfāshī 1892: 2; R. Burton 1885: X, 175.
62. ᶜA. Tāmir and I. Khalifa (eds), Beirut, 1960.
63. Beirut: Mu'assasat al-Intishār al-ᶜArabī, 1997.
64. L. A. Giffen, in J. Lowry and D. Stewart 2009: 309–21. Tunis: Maktabat al-Manār, n.d., pp. 1–64; Jamāl Jumᶜa, ed., London/Beirut: Riyad El-Rayess, 1993; al-Jins ᶜinda 'l-ᶜArab, Vol. 1, Cologne, Al-Kamel Verlag, 1997, pp. 35–120. Translated into English by R. Burton 1886 and J. Colville 1999. Translated into French by le Baron R... as *Le Jardin parfumé*, Paris: Isidore Liseux, 1886 (1906; Paris, Leopold Blondeau, 1960), new edition, Mohamed Lasly, ed., Paris: Philippe Picquier, 1999 (2002); R. Khawam, *La Prairie parfumée ou s'ébattent les plaisirs*, Paris: Phébus, 1976 (Paris: Pocket, 1993); K. Holmes, *La Prairie parfumée ou s'ébattent les plaisirs*, Paris: Phébus, 2003; M. Maḥfūẓ 1992, V: 39–43.
65. This work formed the nucleus of al-Rawḍ al-ᶜāṭir.
66. Yāqūt 1936–38, II: 1,474; Ibn al-Nadīm 1871–72, I: 152 (trans. B. Dodge 1970, I: 334); R. Burton 1885, X: 175; ᶜU. Kaḥḥāla n.d., IX (which states that it involves Horan-born Muḥammad Ibn Ḥasan al-Namīlī). A similar sounding *Burjān wa Janāhib* is mentioned by al-Tifāshī (1892: 2), without the name of an author. A fuller title of the work, *Burjān wa Habāhib fī akhbār al-bāh*, appears in al-Kātib's *Jawāmiᶜ al-ladhdha*, with a number of quotations from it (al-Kātib 1977: 37, 219, 231ff, 246, 275, 376).
67. Ibn al-Nadīm 1871–72, I: 152 (trans. B. Dodge 1970, I: 334).
68. Ibid.

69. Ibid.
70. Translated into French by R. Khawam as *La Prairie des gazelles: éloge des beaux adolescents*, Paris: Phébus, 1989. On the author, see *EI*[1], s.v. 'al-Nawādjī' (I. Krachkovskij); T. Bauer, in J. Lowry and D. Stewart 2009: 321–31.
71. al-Tīfāshī 1892: 2; R. Burton 1885, X: 175 ('al-Nahli').
72. Tunis National Library 18556. ᶜA.; Mansūr 1975: 407.
73. Hishām ᶜAbd al-ᶜAzīz and ᶜĀdil ᶜAbd al-Ḥamīd 1999: 149–76; Aḥmad Farīd al-Mazīdī, ed., Cairo: Dār al-Āfāq al-ᶜArabiyya, 2007, pp. 291–370; *GAL* I: 270; *GALS* I: 420, No. 10; *GAS* III: 285, No. 9. Mss: Ihsanoglu 1984: 110 (Aya Sofia 1/3725, University of Istanbul, Arabic Section, No 1/242).
74. *GAS* III: 294. In al-Rāzī's *al-Ḥāwī* (1955–69, X: 263–4, 267, 298, 303, 308), there is also a reference to *Masā'il Arisṭāṭālīs fi'l-bāh* (Ibn Abī Uṣaybi'a 184: I, 69), though this is actually Aristotle's *Problemata Physica*. *GAS* III: 51; R. Kruk 1976: 255.
75. For a discussion of the various manuscripts, as well as an English translation of one of them, entitled, 'Treatise on the Hidden Disease', see F. Rosenthal 1978.
76. ed. Jurj Kadr, Beirut: Aṭlas li 'l-Nashr wa 'l-Intāj al-Thaqāfī, 2013.
77. Ibn al-Nadīm 1871–72, I: 152 (trans. B. Dodge 1970: I, 333). This work was one of the sources for al-Kātib's *Jawāmiᶜ al-ladhdha*. On the author, see *EI*[2], s.v. 'al-Ṣaymarī' (C. Pellat); ᶜU. Kaḥḥāla n.d., IX: 38; C. Pellat, '*Un curieux amuseur bagdādien: Abu 'l-ᶜAnbas as-Ṣaymarī*', *Studia Orientalia in Memoriam C. Brockelmann*, Halle: Universität Halle-Wittenberg, 1968, pp. 133–7; M. B. ᶜAlwān, 'Abū 'l-ᶜAnbas Muḥammad Ibn Isḥāq al-Ṣaymarī', *al-Abḥāth* XXVI: 1973–77, pp. 35–50.
78. Ibn al-Nadīm 1871–72, I: 152 (trans. B. Dodge 1970, I: 333).
79. Ibid. (trans. B. Dodge 1970, I: 332).
80. Ibid. (trans. B. Dodge 1970, I: 333).
81. Ibid.
82. Ibid.
83. Tunisian National Library 19904.
84. BN 3039, fol. 111.
85. Beirut, Dār al-Bayān al-ᶜArabī, 2002. Mss., BN 2776, fol. I–72; Berlin 6389; Gotha 2033, 2, 2,040–44; National Library of Medicine (Washington, DC) MS A89.2; A. Ihsanoglu 1984: 270–1; Aya Sofa 3573, Fatih 5317, I, 3,687–90; Karatay Topkapi Saray No 7296; Rabat, Maktabat Zāwiyyat al-Ḥamzāwī; Casablanca, Maktabat Mu'assassat al-Malik ᶜAbd al-ᶜAzīz. *GAL* I, 461, 488, *GALS* I, 832ff.; ᶜU. Kaḥḥāla n.d., V: 197; M. de Slane 1883–95: 427, 542.
86. Ḥ. Jughām 2001: 193–228; Beirut, Tāla li 'l-Ṭibāᶜa wa 'l-Nashr, 2002; Damascus, Dār al-Kitāb al-ᶜArabī, 2001. R. Burton 1885, X: 174.
87. Jughām 2001: 129–63; Beirut: Mu'assasat al-Intishār al-ᶜArabī, 1997; Y. Sarkīs (1928) mentions a publication in the nineteenth century. Translated into French by R. Khawam as *Nuits de noces ou comment humer le doux breuvage de la magie licite par 'Abd al-Rahmane al-Souyouti*, Paris: Albin Michel, 1972, pp. 1–94.

88. Ṭalaᶜat Ḥasan ᶜAbd al-Qawī, ed., Damascus: Dār al-Kitāb al-ᶜArabī, n.d. This book is actually the coda (*dhayl*) to *Rashf al-Zulal*. Translated into French by R. Khawam as *Nuits de noces ou comment humer le doux breuvage de la magie licite par 'Abd al-Rahmane al-Souyouti*, Paris: Albin Michel, 1972, pp. 95–234. R. Burton 1885, X: 174.
89. Dār al-Kutub (Cairo), A. Talᶜat 4532; Ḥ. Jughām 2001: 229–39.
90. Faraj al-Ḥiwār, ed., *al-Jins ᶜinda 'l-ᶜArab*, Cologne: Al-Kamel Verlag, 2006, Vol. 4, pp. 35–120.
91. ᶜĀdil al-ᶜĀmil, ed., Damascus: Dār al-Maᶜrifa, 1988, 1994; Muhammad Sayyid al-Rifāᶜī, ed., Damascus: Dār al-Kitāb al-ᶜArabī, (2001?), Ḥ. Jughām 2001: 81–102.
92. Damascus: al-Maktaba al-ᶜArabiyya, 1349/1931; ᶜAbd al-Amīn Mahdī al-Tā'ī, ed., Baghdad: Dār Ibn Nadīm, (1990); Samīr Ḥusayn Ḥalabī, ed., Cairo: Maktabat al-Turāth al-Islāmī 1308/1987; Beirut: Mu'assassat al-Intishār al-ᶜArabī, 2005; Hammam-Sousse: Dār al-Mīzān li 'l-Nashr, 2005; Ḥ. Jughām 2001: 261–6.
93. Ḥ. Jughām 2001: 293–307.
94. Sousse/Tunis: Dār al-Ma'ārif li 'l-Ṭibā'a wa-al-Nashr, 1990.
95. Salāḥ al-Dīn al-Munajjid, ed., Beirut: Dār al-Makshūf, 1958; ᶜAbd al-Latīf ᶜĀshūr, ed., Cairo: Maktabat al-Qur'ān, n.d. Ḥ. Jughām 2001: 243–50.
96. Tunis National Library, 17970 (02; BN 3039, fol. 146 (no author mentioned) – ᶜA. Manṣūr (1975: 421) attributes it to Muḥammad Khalīl al-Ṭawāḥnī al-Tūnisī (d. 1300).
97. *al-Wishāḥ fī fawā'id al-nikāh*, 2001: 198.
98. Ms, Cambridge, No. 2/1008.
99. Faraj al-Ḥawwār, ed., Sousse: Dār al-Mizān li 'l-Nashr, 2003.
100. Ms, Berlin, No 3/7061; Ḥ. Jughām 2001: 352.
101. Ḥ. Jughām 2001.
102. Ṣ. al-Munajjid, ed., Cairo: Dār al-Kitāb al-Jadīdī, 1963; Cairo: Maktabat al-Turāth al-Islāmī, 1998. Ḥ. Jughām 2001: 251–9.
103. Ḥ. Jughām 2001: 103–27; Faraj al-Ḥawwār, ed., Hammam-Sousse: Dār al-Mīzān li 'l-Nashr, 2003.
104. Jūrj Kadr, ed., Beirut: Atlas li 'l-Nashr wa 'l-Intāj al-Thaqāfī, 2013; Ms, Cairo, No. 9424.968; Damascus Ẓāhiriyya No. 1163.
105. Ḥ. Jughām 2001: 352–3. According to al-Suyūṭī, his *al-Wishāḥ* is an abridgement of this work.
106. *Nawādir al-hayk fī nawādir al-nayk*, n.d.: 24.
107. Bibliotheca Alexandrina 7365; Rabat Maktabat Zāwiya Ḥamzāwiyya 127; Ḥ. Jughām 2001: 165–92. This work was mentioned as a source by al-Tīfāshī (1892: 2).
108. Ḥ. Jughām 2001: 323–50.
109. *GAS* III: 239. The work is only referred to in the author's far more famous *Firdaws al-ḥikma* (1928: 113).
110. *GAL* III: 203.
111. Ibn al-Nadīm 1871–72, I: 153 (trans. B. Dodge 1970, I: 335).
112. Ibid.
113. Ibid.

114. Ibid.
115. The author's name is also sometimes written as Tamajrūtī and al-Tamghrūtī. National Library of Medicine (Washington, DC) MS A89.1; Berlin, MS Qu. 1171 (fols 4b–72b); BN, MS ar. 5573, fols 169a–178a; Istanbul, University Library, MS Arab. 3192, fols 1b–70b; G. Vajda 1953, IV: 580; A. Ihsanoglu 1984: 154 (No. 133); *GALS* II: 369: G. Schoeler 1990, II: 152–4.
116. *al-Jins ^{c}inda 'l-^{c}Arab*, Vol. 3, Cologne: Al-Kamel Verlag, 1999 (2nd edn 2006), pp. 6–65. On this author, see Shawkat M. Toorawa, *Ibn Abī Ṭāhir Ṭayfūr and Arabic Writerly Culture: A Ninth-Century Bookman in Baghdad*, Abingdon: Routledge, 2005.
117. Jamāl Jum^{c}a, ed., London: Riyad El-Rayess (Saqi Books), 1994; partial English translation (based on French translation, R. Khawam, *Les Délices des coeurs*, Paris: Jérôme Martineau, 1971 – revised [Phébus] 1981, 1988) by Edward A. Lacey, *The Delight of Hearts: Or What You Will Not Find in Any Book*, Los Angeles: Gay Sunshine Press, 1988. See *EI^2*, s.v. 'al-Tīfāshī' (J. Ruska-[O. Kahl]); *GAL* I: 495; *GALS* I: 904; M. Ullmann 1970: 196–7; M. Maḥfūẓ 1992, I: 205–9; S. Habib 2007: 66–83; F. Malti-Douglas, 'Tribadism/Lesbianism and the Sexualised Body in Medieval Arabo-Islamic Narrative', in F. Canadé Sautman and P. Shengorn, *Same Sex Love and Desire among Women in the Middle Ages*, New York: Palgrave, 2001, pp. 123–41.
118. Cairo: Bulaq, 1309/1892: Muṣṭafā Fahmī, ed. [attributed to Ibn Kamāl Pasha, Aḥmad Ibn Sulaymān]; Beirut, Manshūrāt Samar li 'l-Ṭibā^{c}a wa 'l-Nashr, 1994; Damascus: Dār al-Kitāb al-^{c}Arabī, 2001; in *al-Jins ^{c}inda 'l-^{c}Arab*, Vol 2, Cologne, Al-Kamel Verlag, 2007, pp. 7–182. Translated into English by the anonymous ' English Bohemian', *The Old Man Young Again: Or Age-Rejuvenescence in the Power of Concupiscence*, Paris: Charles Carrington, 1898 (reprinted 2009). R. Burton 1885: X, 175 ('Ahmad bin Sulayman. Surnamed Kamál Pasha').
119. Partial edition Hassan Mohammad El-Haw [al-Tifashi 1970]. *GAL* I: 652; D. Jacquart and C. Thomasset 1988: 125–6.
120. Ed. Jalīl ^{c}Aṭṭiyya, London: Riyad El-Rayess, 1992; Hammamet: Manshūrāt Muḥammad Būdhīnah, 1998; Beirut: Dār al-Jīl, n.d. See *EI^2*, s.v. 'al-Tidjānī' (M. Plessner-[Taïeb El Achèche]); *GAL* II: 334; *GALS* I: 368; Sarkīs 1928: 1,622. Al-Tījānī is also quoted in al-Suyūṭī's work (2001: 193).
121. ^{c}U. Kaḥḥāla n.d., VII: 202–3. None of this author's three works on the subject seems to have survived.
122. Translated into Spanish by L. López-Baralt (1992). See also L. López Baralt, 'El original árabe del "Kama Sutra español" (ms. S-2-BRAH-Madrid)', in Manuel García Martín, ed., *Estado actual de los estudios sobre el Siglo de Oro*, Salamanca: Ediciones Universidad de Salamanca, 1974, pp. 561–8.

Bibliography

Manuscripts

[ANON]: *Risāla fī dhikr adwiyat al-bāh*, Cairo: Dār al-Kutub, Ṭ Taymūr 362.
[ANON]: *Kitāb fī ᶜilm al-bāh wa adwiyatihi*, Tunis: Dār al-Kutub, 20648(09).
al-Fallātī, Muḥammad, *Muᶜāwanat al-ikhwān fī muᶜāsharat al-niswān*, Paris: BN 5662.
al-Ghazlāwī, Muḥammad, *Yāsamīn al-rawḍ al-ᶜāṭir fī nuzhat al-khāṭir*, Paris: BN 3069.
Ibn Sīnā, *Asrār al-jimāᶜ*, Cairo: Dār al-Kutub, No. 509.
al-Shayzarī al-Ṭabarī, ᶜAbd al-Raḥmān, *al-Īḍāḥ fī asrār il-nikāḥ*, Casablanca: Mu'assassat Malik ᶜAbd al-ᶜAzīz.

Printed Works

Arabic

ᶜAbd al-Wāḥid, Muṣṭafā (1961): *al-Islām wa 'l-mushkila al-jinsiyya*, Cairo: Dār al-Iᶜtiṣām li 'l-Ṭibāᶜa wa 'l-Nashr wa 'l-Tawzīᶜ.
Abū Nuwās (1994): *al-Nuṣūṣ al-muḥarrama – The Forbidden Poems*, ed. Jamāl Jumᶜa, Beirut: Riad El-Rayyes [= *al-Fukāha wa ītinās fī mujūn Abī Nuwās*, Cairo, 1898].
al-Anṭākī, Daud (1952): *Tadhkirat ulī 'l-ābāb wa 'l-jāmiᶜ li 'l-ᶜajab al-ᶜujāb*, 2 vols, Cairo.
——(1999): *al-Nuzha al-mubhaja fī tashḥīdh al-adhhān wa taᶜdīl al-amzija*, Beirut: Mu'assassat al-Balāgh.

al-Bīrūnī (1973): *al-Ṣaydana fī 'l-ṭibb. al-Bīrūnī's book on pharmacy and materia medica*, ed. H. M. Said and R. E. Elahie, Karachi: Hamdard National Foundation.

al-Dhahabī, Shams al-Dīn (1987): *al-Ṭibb al-nabawī*, ed. ᶜĀdil Abū al-Maᶜātī, Cairo: Dār al-Bashīr.

al-Dimashqī, Shams al-Dīn (1866): [*Nukhbat al-dahr fī ᶜajā'ib al-barr wa 'l-baḥr*] *Cosmographie de Chems-ed-Din Abou Abdallah Mohammed ed- Dimichqui. Texte arabe, publié d'après l'édition commencé par M. Fraehn d'après les manuscrits de St-Pétersbourg, de Paris, de Leyde et de Copenhague*, ed. A. F. Mehren, Saint Petersburg/Copenhagen: C. A. Reitzel.

al-Ghassānī, Abū 'l-Qāsim (1990): *Ḥadīqat al-azhār fī māhiyat al-ᶜushb wa-l-ᶜaqqār*, ed. Muḥammad al-ᶜArbī al-Khaṭṭābī, Beirut: Dār al-Gharb al-Islāmī.

Ḥajjī Khalīfa (1835–84): *Kashf al-zunūn ᶜan ᶜasāmi 'l-kutub wa 'l-funūn*, 7 vols, ed. G. Flügel, Leipzig/London: F. C. W. Vogel.

Hishām, ᶜAbd al-ᶜAziz and ᶜĀdil ᶜAbd al-Ḥamīd (1999): *al-Nisā': Thalāth makhṭūṭāt nādira fī 'l-jins, Cairo: Dār al-Khayyāl.*

Ibn Abī Uṣaybiᶜa (1882): *ᶜUyūn al-anbā' fī ṭabaqāt al-aṭibbā'*, 2 vols, Cairo: al- Maṭbaᶜa al-Wahbiyya.

Ibn al-Bayṭār, Abū Muhammad (1291/1874): *al-Jāmiᶜ li-mufradāt al-adwiya wa 'l-aghdhiya*, 2 vols, Būlāq, Cairo: Dār al-Kutub al-ᶜIlmiyya, 2001; French translation, Lucien Leclerq, 'Traité des simples par Ibn el-Beïthar', in *Notices et extraits des manuscrits de la Bibliothèque nationale et autres bibliothèques*, 23: 1 (1877), 25: 1 (1881), 26: 1 (1883), Paris: Imprimerie Nationale.

——(1992): *Tuḥfat Ibn al-Bayṭār fī 'l-ᶜilāj bi 'l-aᶜshāb wa'l-nabātāt*, ed. Abū Musᶜib al-Badrī, Cairo: Dār al-Faḍīla.

Ibn al-Jawzī, ᶜAbd al-Raḥmān (1319/1902): *Akhbār al-nisā'*, Cairo, n.p.

Ibn al-Jazzār, Abū Jaᶜfar (2004): *al-Iᶜtimād fī 'l-adwiya al-mufrada*, ed. Idwār al-Qishsh, Beirut: Sharikat al-Maṭbūᶜāt li 'l-Tawzīᶜ wa 'l-Nashr.

Ibn Lūqā, Qusṭā (1974): *Das Buch über die Geschlechtichkeit (Kitāb fī 'l-Bāh) von Qusṭā Ibn Lūqā. Edition und Übertragung des arabischen Textes nach der Handschrift Nr. 242 der Universitätsbibliothek Istanbul*, ed. Najdat Ali Barhoum, Universität Erlangen-Nürnberg.

——(1973): Kitāb fī 'l-Bāh wa mā yuḥtāju ilayhi min tadbīr al-badan fī istiᶜmālihi des Qusṭā Ibn Luqā. 1. Abhanduling. (Das Buch über die Kohabitation und die für ihre Ausübung notwendigen

korperlichen Voraussetzungen) Edition, Übertragung und Bearbeitung des arabischen Textes auf der Grundlage der Handschrift der Universitätsbibliothek Istanbul Nr.243, ed. Gauss Haydar, Universität Erlangen-Nürnberg.

——(1992): *Qusṭā Ibn Lūqā's Medical Regime for the Pilgrims to Mecca: The Risāla Fī Tadbīr Safar al-Hajj*, ed. Gerrit Bos, Leiden: Brill.

Ibn Manẓūr, Jamāl al-Dīn (1299/1881–1308/1890–91): *Lisān al-ᶜArab*, 20 vols, Būlāq.

Ibn Māssa, ᶜĪsa (1971): [*Masā'il fī 'l-nasl wa al-dhurriyya wa 'l-jimāᶜ*] Streitfragen über die Zeugung, Nachkommenschaft und über den Geschlechtsverkehr. Verfaßt von Isa ibn Massah. Edition, Übersetzung und Bearbeitung des arabischen Textes auf der Grundlage der Handschrift Ayasofya 3724, ed. Mohamed Walid Anbari, Universität Erlangen-Nürnberg.

Ibn al-Nadīm (1871–72): *Kitāb al-fihrist*, 2 vols, ed. Gustav Flügel, Leipzig: F. C. W. Vogel; English translation, Bayard Dodge, *The Fihrist of al-Nadim*, 2 vols, New York: Columbia University Press, 1970.

Ibn Qutayba, Muḥammad (1343–48/1925–30): *ᶜUyūn al-akhbār*, ed. Aḥmad Zakī al-ᶜAdawī, Cairo.

Ibn Sīnā (1999): *al-Qānūn fī 'l-ṭibb*, 3 vols, ed. Muḥammad Amīn al-Ḍannāwī, Beirut: Dār al-Kutub al-ᶜIlmiyya.

Ibn Wāfid al-Andalusī, al-Wazīr Abū 'l-Muṭarraf (2000): *Kitāb al-adwiya al-mufrada*, ed. Aḥmad Ḥasan Basaj, Beirut: Dār al-Kutub al-ᶜIlmiyya.

Ihsanoglu, Akmāl al-Dīn (1984): *Fihris makhṭūṭāt al-ṭibb al-Islāmī bi 'l-lughāt al-ᶜArabiya wa 'l-Turkiyya wa 'l-Fārisiyya fī maktabāt Turkiyā*, Istanbul: Markaz al-Abḥāth li 'l- Tārīkh wa 'l-Funūn wa 'l-Thaqāfa al-Islāmīyya.

al-Ishbīlī, Abū 'l-Khayr (1995): *ᶜUmdat al-ṭabīb fī maᶜrifat al-nabāt*, ed. Muḥammad al-ᶜArbī al-Khattābī, 2 vols, Beirut: Dār al-Gharb al-Islāmī.

al-Isrā'ilī, Isḥāq Ibn Sulaymān (1992): *Kitāb al-aghdhiya wa 'l-adwiya*, ed. M. Ṣabbāh, Beirut.

al-Jāḥiẓ, Abū ᶜUthmān (1938): *Kitāb al-ḥayawān*, 7 vols, Cairo: al-Maṭbaᶜa al-Bābī al-Ḥalabī.

Jughām, Ḥasan Aḥmad (2001): *al-Jins fī aᶜmāl al-imām Jamāl al-Dīn al-Suyūṭī*, Tunis: Dār al-Maᶜārif li 'l-Ṭibāᶜa wa 'l-Nashr.

Kaḥḥāla, ᶜUmar Riḍā (n.d.): *Muᶜjam al-mu'allifīn. Tarājim muṣannifīn al-kutub al-ᶜArabiyya*, 15 vols, Beirut: Dār al-Aḥyā' al-Turāth al-ᶜArabī.
al-Kātib, Abū 'l-Hasan (2002): *Jawāmiᶜ al-ladhdha*, Beirut: Ṭāla li 'l-Ṭibāᶜa wa 'l- Nashr; English translation, Adnan Jarkas and Salah Addin Khawwam, *Encyclopedia of Pleasure by Abul Hasan 'Ali Ibn Naser al Katib*, Toronto: Aleppo, 1977.
Maḥfūẓ, Muḥammad (1992): *Tarājim al-mu'allifīn al-Tūnisiyyīn*, 5 vols, Beirut: Dār al-Gharb al-Islāmī.
Maḥmūd Ibrāhīm (2000): *al-Mutᶜa al-maḥẓūra: al-shudhūdh al-jinsī fī tārīkh al-ᶜArab*, Beirut: Riyāḍ al-Rayyis li 'l-Kutub wa 'l-Nashr.
Manṣūr, ᶜAbd al-ᶜAzīz (1975): *Tūnis. Dār al-Kutub. Al-fihris al-ᶜāmm li 'l-makhṭūṭāt*, Tunis.
al-Masᶜūdī, ᶜAlī Ibn Ḥusayn (1960–79): *Murūj al-dhahab wa maᶜādin al-jawhar*, Barbier de Meynard and Pavet de Courteille (rev. C. Pellat), 7 vols, Beirut: Université Libanaise de Beirut; French translation, C. Pellat: Les Prairies d'Or, 5 vols, Paris: Paul Geuthner (1962–97).
al-Munajjid, Ṣalāḥ al-Dīn (1957, 1969): *Jamāl al-mar'a ᶜinda 'l-ᶜArab*, Beirut: Dār al-Kitāb al-Jadīd.
——(1975): *al-Ḥayāt al-jinsiyya ᶜinda 'l-ᶜArab*, 2nd rev. edn, Beirut: Dār al-Kitāb al-Jadīd.
al-Muqaddasī (1906): *Aḥsan al-taqāsīm fī maᶜrifat al-aqālīm*, ed. M. J. de Goeje, Leiden: Brill.
al-Nafzāwī, Muḥammad Ibn ᶜUmar (n.d.): *al-Rawḍ al-ᶜāṭir fī nuzhat al-khāṭir*, Tunis: Maktabat al-Manār; English translations: R. Burton, *The Perfumed Garden of the Cheikh Nefzoui: A Manual of Arabian Erotology (XVI Century)*, Cosmopoli: Kama Shastra Society of London and Benares, 1886; J. Colville, *The Perfumed Garden of Sensual Delight*, London: Kegan Paul International, 1999.
al-Qazwīnī, Zakariyyā' Ibn Muhammad (1849): [*ᶜAjā'ib al-makhlūqāt wa āthār al- bilād*], ed. Ferdinand Wüstenfeld, *Zakarija Ben Muhammed Ben Mahmud el- Cazwini's Kosmographie. Erster Theil. ᶜAjā'ib al-makhlūqāt. Die Wunder der Schöpfung. Aus den Handschriften der Bibliotheken zu Berlin, Gotha, Dresden und Hamburg*, Göttingen: Dieterischen Buchhandlung.
al-Rāzī, Abū Bakr Muḥammad b. Zakariyyā (1955–69): *al-Ḥāwī fī 'l-tibb*, 23 vols, Hyderabad.
——(1982): *Manāfiᶜ al-aghdhiya wa-dafᶜ maḍarrihā*, Beirut: Dār Iḥyā' al- ᶜUlūm.

——(2007): *Kitāb al-bāh wa manāfiᶜihi wa maḍārrihi wa mudawātihi*, ed. Aḥmad Farīd al-Mazīdī, Cairo: Dār al-Āfāq al-ᶜArabiyya, pp. 291–370.

al-Saffārīnī, Ibn Aḥmad, Rashīd Ibn ᶜĀmir Ghufaylī (1412/1991–92): *Qarᶜ al-siyāṭ fī qamᶜ ahl al-Liwāṭ*, Riyadh: Dār al-Ṭaḥawi.

Sarkīs, Yūsuf Ilyās (1928): *Muᶜjam al-maṭbūᶜ*āt al-*ᶜArabiyya wa 'l-muᶜarabba*, 2 vols, Cairo: Maktabat al-Thaqāfa al-Dīniyya.

al-Sharīf, ᶜAdnān (1990): *Min ᶜilm al-ṭibb al-Qur'ānī: al-thawābit al-ᶜilmiyya fī 'l-Qur'ān al-karīm*, Beirut: Dār al-ᶜIlm li 'l-Malāyīn.

Shaykhū, Luwīs (1924): *Kitāb al-makhṭūṭāt al-ᶜArabiyya li 'l-katabat al-Naṣrāniyya. Catalogue des manuscrits des auteurs arabes chrétiens depuis l'Islam*, Beirut: Maṭba'at al-Ābā' al-Yasū'iyyīn.

al-Suyūṭī, Jalāl al-Dīn (2001): *al-Wishāḥ fī fawā'id al-nikāḥ*, ed. Ṭalaᶜat Ḥasan ᶜAbd al- Qawī, Damascus: Dār al-Kitāb al-ᶜArabī.

——(n.d.): *al-Raḥma fī 'l-ṭibb wa 'l-ḥikma*, Cairo: Dār al-Kutub al-ᶜArabiyya al-Kubrā.

al-Ṭabarī, Abū 'l-Ḥasan (1928): *Firdaws al-ḥikma*, M. Z. al-Ṣiddīqī, Berlin: Sonne.

al-Tīfāshī, Shihāb al-Dīn (1892): *Rujūᶜ al-shaykh ilā ṣibāh fī 'l-quwwa wa 'l-bāh*, Būlāq.

——(1970): *Risāla fīmā yaḥtajī ilayhi al-rijāl wa 'l-nisā' fī istiᶜmāl al-bāh mimmā yaḍurr wa yanfaᶜ. Abhandlung darüber, was Männer und Frauen zur Ausübung des Geschlechtsverkehrs brauchen, was dabei nützt und schadet. Die Edition des arabischen Textes auf der Grundlage der Handschrift Al-Azhar Halim 34687 und der Handschrift Dar al-Kutub Kairo Mim Tibb unter Hinzuziehung der Handschrift Paris 3056*, ed. Hassan Mohammad El-Haw (partial edn), Universität Erlangen-Nürnberg.

——(1992): *Nuzhat al-albāb fīmā lā yūjad fī 'l-kitāb*, ed. Jamāl Jumᶜa, London/Cyprus: Riad El-Rayess.

al-Wāsiṭī, Shams al-Dīn Muḥammad Ibn ᶜUmar Ghamrī (1988): *al-Ḥukm al-maḍbūṭ fī taḥrīm fi'l qawm Lūṭ*, Tanta: Dār al-Ṣaḥābah li 'l-Turāth.

al-Yaᶜqūbī, Aḥmad Ibn ᶜAbd Yaᶜqūb (1892): [*Kitāb al-buldān*] *Kitāb al-boldān auctore Ahmed ibn abî Jakûb ibn Wādhih al-Kātib al-Jakûbî*, (Bibliotheca Geographorum Arabicorum, VII: 1), 2nd edn, ed. M. J. de Goeje, Leiden: Brill.

Yāqūt al-Ḥamawī (1866–73): *Muᶜjam al-buldān*, 6 vols, ed. Ferdinand

Wüstenfeld, Leipzig: F.A. Brockhaus.
——(1936–38): *Muʿjam al-udabāʾ: irshād al-arīb ilā maʿrifat al-adīb*, ed. A. F. Rifāʿī, Cairo: Matbaʿat al-Maʾmūn.

European languages

Abu Khalil, As'ad (1993): 'A Note on the Study of Homosexuality in the Arab/Islamic Civilization', *Arab Studies Journal* 1: 2, pp. 32–4.
Ali, Kecia (2006): *Sexual Ethics and Islam: Feminist Reflections on Qur'an, Hadith and Jurisprudence*, New York: Oneworld.
Al-Sammani, Hanadi (2008): 'Out of the Closet: Representation of Homosexuals and Lesbians in Modern Arabic Literature', *Journal of Arabic Literature* 39: 2, pp. 270–310.
Al-Sayyid-Marsot, Afaf Lutfi, ed. (1979): *Society and the Sexes in Medieval Islam*, Malibu, CA: Undena Publications.
Amar, Zev, and Ephraim Lev (2011): 'Watermelon, Chate Melon, and Cucumber: New Light on Traditional and Innovative Field Crops in the Middle Ages', *Journal Asiatique* 299, pp. 193–204.
Amer, Sahar (2009): 'Medieval Arab Lesbians and Lesbian-Like Women', *Journal of the History of Sexuality* 18: 2, pp. 215–36.
Ashtiany, Julia, T. M. Johnstone, J. D. Latham, R. B. Serjeant and G. Rex Smith, eds (1990): *The Cambridge History of Arabic Literature: ʿAbbasid belles-lettres*, Cambridge: Cambridge University Press.
Babayan, Kathryn and Afsaneh Najmabadi (2008): *Islamicate Sexualities: Translations across Temporal Geographies of Desire*, New Haven, MA: Harvard University Press.
Benton, John F. (1985): 'Trotula, Women's Problems, and the Professionalization of Medicine in the Middle Ages', *Bulletin of the History of Medicine* 59: 1, pp. 30–53.
Bos, Gerrit (1997): *Ibn al-Jazzār on Sexual Diseases and their Treatment: A Critical Edition of* Zād al-musāfir wa qūt al-hādir, *Provisions for the Traveller and Nourishment for the Sedentary, Book 6*, London/New York: Kegan Paul International.
Bouhdiba, Abdelwahab (1975): *La sexualite en Islam*, Paris: PUF.
Bousquet, G. H. (1966): *L'ethique sexuelle en Islam*, Paris: Desclée de Brouwer.
Brockelmann, Carl (1937–49): *Geschichte der arabischen Literatur*, 2 vols, 3 supplementary vols, Leiden: Brill.
Bummel, Julia (1999): *Zeugung und pränatale Entwicklung des Menschen*

nach Schriften mittelalterlicher muslimischer Religionsgelehrter über die 'Medizin des Propheten', unpublished PhD dissertation, University of Hamburg.

Burnett, Charles S. F. (2001): 'The Coherence of the Arabic–Latin Translation Program in Toledo in the Twelfth Century', *Science in Context* 14: 1–2, pp. 249–88.

Burnett, C. S. F., and Danielle Jacquart, eds (1994): *Constantine the African and ʿAlī Ibn Al-ʿAbbās Al-Mağūsī: The Pantegni and Related Texts*, Leiden: Brill.

Burton, Richard (1885–89): *A Plain and Literal Translation of the Arabian Nights' Entertainments, Now Entitled The Book of the Thousand Nights and a Night; with Introduction Explanatory Notes on the Manners and Customs of Moslem Men and a Terminal Essay upon the History of the Nights*, 10 vols, 7 supplementary vols, Benares: Kamashastra Society.

Cadden, Joan (1993): *Meanings of Sex Difference in the Middle Ages: Medicine, Science, and Culture*, Cambridge: Cambridge University Press.

Cervulle, Maxime (2008): 'French Homonormativity and the Commodification of the Arab Body', *Radical History Review* 100, pp. 171–9.

Cervulle, M. and Nick Rees-Roberts (2009): 'Queering the Orientalist Porn Package: Arab Men in French Gay Pornography', *New Cinemas: Journal of Contemporary Film* 6: 3, pp. 197–208.

Chebel, Malek (1984): *Le corps en Islam*, Paris: PUF (2nd edn 1999, 3rd edn 2004).

——(1986): *Le livre des séductions suivi de Dix Aphorismes sur l'amour*, Paris: Payot (2nd edn 1997).

——(1988): *L'Esprit de sérail, mythes et pratiques sexuelles au Maghreb*, Paris: Payot (2nd edn 1997).

——(1995): *Encyclopédie de l'amour en Islam. Érotisme, beauté et sexualité dans le monde arabe, en Perse et en Turquie*, Paris: Payot (2nd edn 2003).

——(2004): *Dictionnaire amoureux de l'islam*, Paris: Plon.

——(2006): *Le Kama sutra arabe, 2000 ans de littérature érotique en Orient*, Paris: Pauvert.

Chipman, Leigh (2009): *The World of Pharmacy and Pharmacists in Mamluk Cairo*, Leiden: Brill.

Colligan, Colette (2003): '"A Race of Born Pederasts": Sir Richard Burton, Homosexuality, and the Arabs', *Nineteenth-Century Contexts* 25: 1, pp. 1–20.

Compier, Abdul Haq (2012): 'Rhazes in the Renaissance of Andreas Vesalius', *Medical History* 56: 1, pp. 3–25.

Conrad, Lawrence I., Michael Neve, Vivian Nutton, Roy Porter and Andrew Weart (1995): *The Western Medical Tradition, 800BC to 1800AD*, Cambridge: Cambridge University Press.

Correinte, Federico (1997): *A Dictionary of Andalusi Arabic*, Leiden: Brill.

Dakhlia, Jocelyne (2007): 'Homoérotismes et trames historiographiques du monde islamique', *Annales. Histoire, Sciences Sociales* 5, pp. 1,097–120.

Degen, R. (1978): 'Al-Safarjal: A Marginal Note to Ibn al-Bayṭār: *Kitāb al-Jāmi' li-mufradāt al-adwiya wal-aghdhiya*', *Journal of the History of Arabic Science* 2, pp. 143–8.

De Slane, William Mac Guckin (1883–95): *Catalogue des manuscrits arabes*, 2 vols, Paris: Imprimerie nationale.

Devereux, Robert (1966): 'XIth Century Muslim Views on Women, Marriage, Love and Sex', *Central Asiatic Journal* 11, pp. 134–40.

Dietrich, Albert (1988): *Dioscurides triumphans. Ein Anonymer Arabischer Kommentar (Ende 12. Jahrh. N. Chr.) Zur Materia Medica*, 2 vols, Göttingen: Vandenhoeck and Ruprecht.

——(1991): *Die Dioscurides-Erklärung des Ibn al-Baitār. Ein Beitrag zur arabischen Pflanzensynonymik des Mittlealters*, Göttingen: Akademie der Wissenschaften in Göttingen, Philologisch-Historische Klasse.

Dioscorides, Pedanios (2000): *De Materia Medica: Being an Herbal with Many Other Medicinal Materials*, trans. Tess Anne Osbaldeston, Johannesburg: Ibidis Press.

Dols, Michael (1984): *Medieval Islamic Medicine. Ibn Riḍwān's Treatise 'On the Prevention of Bodily Ills in Egypt'*, Berkeley, CA: University of California Press.

Dover, Kenneth Richard (1984): *Greek Homosexuality*, Cambridge, MA: Harvard University Press.

Dozy, Pieter Reinhart (1877–81): *Supplément aux dictionnaires arabes*, 2 vols, Leiden: Brill.

Dunne, Bruce (1990): 'Homosexuality in the Middle East: An Agenda for Historical Research', *Arab Studies Quarterly* 12: 3–4, pp. 55–82.

——(1998): 'Power and Sexuality in the Middle East', *Middle East Report* 206, 28: 1, pp. 8–12.

Duran, Khalid (1993): 'Homosexuality in Islam', in *Homosexuality and World Religions*, Valley Forge, PA: Trinity P. International, pp. 181–97.

Edwardes, Allen (1963): *The Jewel in the Lotus: A Historical Survey of the Sexual Culture of the East*, London: Tandem Books.

El Feki, Shereen (2013): *Sex and the Citadel: Intimate Life in a Changing Arab World*, London: Chatto and Windus.

Elkhadem, Hossam (1990): *Le Taqwim al Sihha (Tacuini Sanitatis) d'Ibn Butlan: Un traité médical du XIe Siècle*, Louvain: Peeters.

El-Masri, Y. (1962): *Le drame sexuel de la femme dans l'Orient arabe*, Paris: Lafont.

El Menyawi, Hassan (2012): 'Same-Sex Marriage in Islamic Law', *Wake Forest Journal of Law and Police* 2: 2, pp. 375–531.

El Rouayheb, Khaled (2005): *Before Homosexuality in the Arab-Islamic World, 1500–1800*, Chicago, IL: University of Chicago Press.

Farah, Madelaine (1984), *Marriage and Sexuality in Islam: A Translation of al Ghazzali's Book on the Etiquette of Marriage*, Salt Lake City, UT: University of Utah Press.

Foucault, Michel (1978–90): *The History of Sexuality*, 3 vols, trans. Robert Hurley, New York: Pantheon Books.

Gadelrab, Sherry Sayed (2010): 'Discourses on Sex Differences in Medieval Scholarly Islamic Thought', *Journal of the History of Medicine and Allied Sciences*, pp. 1–42.

Ghoussoub, Mai, and Emma Sinclair-Webb, eds (2000): *Imagined Masculinities: Male Identity and Culture in the Modern Middle East*, London: Saqi.

Giffen, Lois Anita (1971): *Theory of Profane Love among the Arabs: The Development of the Genre*, New York: New York University Press.

Goitien, S. D. (1967–88): *A Mediterranean Society: The Jewish Communities of the Arab World as Portrayed in the Documents of the Cairo Geniza*, Berkeley, CA: University of California Press.

Green, Monica Helen (1985): *The Transmission of Ancient Theories of Female Physiology and Disease through the Early Middle Ages*, unpublished PhD dissertation, Princeton, NJ: Princeton University Press.

——(2002): *The Trotula: An English Translation of the Medieval*

Compendium of Women's Medicine, Philadelphia, PA: University of Pennsylvania Press.

Groom, Nigel (1981): *Frankincense and Myrrh: A Study of the Arabian Incense Trade*, London/New York: Longman.

Gutas, Dimitri (1998): *Greek Thought, Arabic Culture: The Graeco-Arabic Translation Movement in Baghdad and Early 'Abbasid society (2nd–4th/8th–10th century)*, London: Routledge.

Habib, Samar (2007): *Female Homosexuality in the Middle East: Histories and Representations*, London/New York: Routledge.

——ed. (2009): *Islam and Homosexuality*, 2 vols, Santa Barbara, CA: ABC–CLIO, LLC.

Hasselhoff, Görge (2002): 'Maimonides in the Latin Middle Ages: An Introductory Survey', *Jewish Studies Quarterly* 9, pp. 1–20.

Heine, Peter (1982): *Untersuchungen zu Anbau, Produktion und Konsom des Weins im arabisch-islamischen Mittelalter*, Wiesbaden: Harrassowitz.

Hinds, Martin, and El Said Badawi (1986): *A Dictionary of Egyptian Arabic, Arabic–English*, Beirut: Librairie du Liban.

Hinz, Walther (1970): *Islamische Masse und Gewichte umgerechnet ins metrische System*, Leiden/Cologne: Brill.

Hodgson, Michael G. S. (1977): *The Venture of Islam: Conscience and History in a World Civilization, The Classical Age of Islam*, Chicago, IL: Chicago University Press.

Holt, P. M. (1992): *The Age of the Crusades: The Near East from the Eleventh Century to 1517*, Harlow: Longman.

Hopwood, Derek (1999): *Sexual Encounters in the Middle East: The British, the French and the Arabs*, Reading: Ithaca Press.

Issa Bey, Ahmed (1930): *Dictionnaire des Noms des Plantes*, Cairo: Imprimerie Nationale.

Jacquart, Danielle (1996): 'The Influence of Arabic Medicine in the Medieval West', in R. Rashed, ed., *Encyclopedia of the History of Arabic Science*, London: Routledge, III, pp. 963–84.

Jacquart, D., and F. Micheau (1990): *La Médecine Arabe et l'Occident Médiéval*, Paris: Maisonneuve et Larose.

Jacquart, D., and C. Thomasset (1988): *Sexuality and Medicine in the Middle Ages*, Cambridge: Polity Press.

Joseph, Suad, and Afsāna Naᶜmābādī (2003): *Encyclopedia of Women and Islamic Cultures, Volume 3: Family, Body, Sexuality and Health*,

Leiden: Brill, 2003.

Kahl, Oliver (2003): *Sabur Ibn Sahl: The Small Dispensatory*, Leiden: Brill.

Kennedy, Philip F. (2007): *Abu Nuwas: A Genius of Poetry*, London: OneWorld Publications.

Kircher, Heidi Gisela (1967): *Die 'einfachen Heilmittel' aus dem 'Handbuch der Chirurgie' des Ibn al-Quff*, Bonn: Rheinischen Friedrich-Wilhelms- Universität.

Kligerman, Nicole (2007): 'Homosexuality in Islam: A Difficult Paradox', *Macalester Islam Journal* 2: 3, pp. 53–64.

Kruk, Remke (1976): 'Pseudo-Aristotle: An Arabic Version of Problemata Physica X', *Isis* 67, pp. 251–6.

Kuru, Selim Sirri (2000): *A Sixteenth-Century Scholar: Deli Birader and his Dāfi 'ü'l- ġumūm ve rafi'ü''l-humūm*, unpublished PhD dissertation, Harvard University.

de Lacy, Phillip (1992): *Galen, On Semen*, Berlin: Akademie Verlag.

Lagrange, F. (2000): 'Male Homosexuality in Modern Arabic Literature', in Mai Ghoussoub and Emma Sinclair-Webb, eds, *Imagined Masculinities: Male Identity and Culture in the Modern Middle East*, London: Saqi, pp. 169–98.

——(2008): 'The Obscenities of the Vizier', in Babayan and Najmabadi, *Islamicate Sexualities*, pp. 161–203.

Lahoucine, Ouzgane, ed. (2006): *Islamic Masculinities*, London: Zed.

Lane, W. E. (1863–74): *Arabic–English Lexicon derived from the best and the most copious Eastern sources; comprising a very large number of words and significations omitted in the Ḱámoos, with supplements to its abridged and defective explanations, ample grammatical and critical comments, and examples in prose and verse*, 5 vols, London (vols 6–8 ed. Stanley Lane Poole, London, 1877–93).

Laqueur, Thomas (1992): *Making Sex: Body and Gender from the Greeks to Freud*, Cambridge, MA: Harvard University Press.

Leclerc, Lucien (1876): *Histoire de la médecine arabe*, Paris: E. Leroux.

Leibowitz, J. Joshua Otto, and Shlomo Marcus (1974): *Moses Maimonides: On the Causes of Symptoms*, Berkeley, CA: University of California Press.

Lev, Ephraim, and Zev Amar (2008): *Practical Materia Medica of the Medieval Eastern Mediterranean according to the Cairo Genizah*, Leiden: Brill.

Levey, Martin (1966): *The Medical Formulary of Aqrābīdhīn of al-Kindī*, Madison, WI: University of Wisconsin.

Lindgren, Amy (2005): *The Wandering Womb and the Peripheral Penis: Gender and the Fertile Body in Late Medieval Infertility Treatises*, unpublished PhD dissertation, University of California.

López-Baralt, Luce (1992): *Un Kama Sutra Español*, Madrid: Ediciones Siruela.

Lowry, Joseph Edmund, and Devin J. Stewart (2009): *Essays in Arabic Literary Biography II: 1350–1850*, Wiesbaden: Otto Harrassowitz.

Mahawatte, Royce (2003): 'Loving the Asian: Race, Gay Pornography and the Essentials of Passion', in Pamela Church Gibson, ed., *More Dirty Looks: Gender, Pornography and Power*, 2nd edn, London: BFI Publishing.

Malti-Douglas, Fedwa (1991): *Woman's Body, Woman's Word: Gender and Discourse in Arabo-Islamic Writing*, Princeton, NJ: Princeton University Press.

Mande, Gabrielle (1983): *Islamische Erotik*, Fribourg: Liber.

Massad, Joseph (2002): 'Re-Orienting Desire: the Gay International and the Arab World', *Public Culture* 14, pp. 361–85.

Matar, Nabil (1994): 'Homosexuality in the Early Novels of Nageeb Mahfouz', *Journal of Homosexuality* 26: 4, pp. 77–90.

Meyerhof, M. (1940): 'Un glossaire de matière médicale, composé par Maïmonide: Šarh asmā' al-'uqqār (l'explication des noms de drogues', *Mémoires Présentés à l'Institut d'Egypte* 41, Cairo: Imprimerie de l'Institut Français d'Archéologie Orientale.

Mortel, Richard T. (1990): 'Weights and Measures in Mecca During the Late Ayyubid and Mamluk Periods', in R. B. Serjeant and R. L. Bidwell, *Arabian Studies* 8, Cambridge: Cambridge University Press, pp. 177–85.

Murray, Stephen O., and Will Roscoe, eds (1979): *Islamic Homosexualities: Culture, History, and Literature*, New York: New York University Press.

Musallam, B. F. (1983): *Sex and Society in Islam: Birth Control before the Nineteenth Century*, Cambridge: Cambridge University Press.

Muschler, Reno (1912): *A Manual Flora of Egypt*, Berlin: R. Friendländer and Son.

Najmabadi, Afsaneh (2005): *Women with Mustaches and Men without Beards: Gender and Sexual Anxieties of Iranian Modernity*, Berkeley,

CA: University of California Press.

Nasrallah, Nawal (2010): *Annals of the Caliphs' Kitchens: Ibn Sayyār Al-Warrāq's Tenth-Century Baghdadi Cookbook*, Leiden: Brill.

Nathan, B. (1994): 'Medieval Arabic Medical Views on Male Homosexuality', *Journal of Homosexuality* 26: 4, pp. 37–9.

O'Boyle, Cornelius (1998): *The Art of Medicine: Medical Teaching at the University of Paris, 1250–1400*, Leiden: Brill.

Paris, Harry S., Marie-Christine Daunay, and Jules Janick (2011): 'Occidental Diffusion of Cucumber (*Cucumis sativus*) 500–1300 CE: Two Routes to Europe', *Annals of Botany* 108: 3, pp. 471–84.

Parker, Holt N. (1992): 'Love's Body Anatomized: The Ancient Erotic Handbooks and the Rhetoric of Sexuality', in Amy Richlin, ed., *Pornography and Representation in Greece and Rome*, Oxford: Oxford University Press, pp. 90–111.

Perho, I. (1995): 'The Prophet's Medicine: A Creation of Muslim Traditionalist Scholars' (*Studia Orientalis* 74), Helsinki: Finnish Oriental Society.

Pormann, Peter E., and Emilie Savage-Smith (2007): *Medieval Islamic Medicine*, Edinburgh: Edinburgh University Press.

Rahman, Fazlur (1989): *Health and Medicine in the Islamic Tradition: Change and Identity*, New York: Crossroad.

Rasslan, W. (1934): *Mohammed und die Medizin nach den Überlieferungen*, (*Abhandlungen zur Geschichte der Medizin und der Naturwissenschaften* 1), Berlin.

Redhouse, J. W. (1880): *Redhouse's Turkish Dictionary: In Two Parts, English and Turkish, and Turkish and English*, 2 vols, London: Bernard Quaritch.

Rosenthal, Franz (1975): *The Classical Heritage in Islam*, Berkeley, CA: University of California Press.

———(1978): 'Ar-Rāzī on the Hidden Illness', *Bulletin of the History of Medicine* 52, pp. 45–60.

———(1986): *The Muqaddimah: An Introduction to History*, 3 vols, London: Routledge and Kegan Paul.

Rosner, F. (1984): *Maimonides: Medical Writings: Treatises on Poisons, Hemorrhoids, Cohabitation*, Haifa, Maimonides Research Institute.

———(1995): *Šarh Asma al-'Uqqar, Glossary of Drug Names*, Haifa: Maimonides Research Institute.

Rosner, F., and S. Muntner (1970): *The Medical Aphorisms of Moses*

Maimonides, New York: Yeshiva University Press.
Rouhi, Leyla (1999): *Mediation and Love: A Study of the Medieval Go-between in Key Romance and Near-Eastern Texts*, Leiden: Brill.
Rowson, E. K. (1991a): 'The Effeminates of Early Medina', *Journal of the American Oriental Society* 111, pp. 671–93.
——(1991b): 'The Categorization of Gender and Sexual Irregularity in Medieval Arabic Vice Lists', in J. Epstein and K. Straub, eds, *Body Guards: The Cultural Politics of Gender Ambiguity*, New York/London: Routledge, pp. 50–79.
——(1997): 'Two Homoerotic Narratives from Mamluk Literature: al-Safadi's *Law'at al-shaki* and Ibn Daniyal's *al-Mutayyam*', in J. W. Wright, Jr, and E. K. Rowson, eds, *Homoeroticism in Classical Arabic Literature*, New York: Columbia University Press, pp. 158–91
——(2003): 'Gender Irregularity as Entertainment: Institutionalized Transvestism at the Caliphal Court in Medieval Baghdad', in Sharon Farmer and Carol Braun Pasternack, eds, *Gender and Difference in the Middle Ages*, Minneapolis, MN: University of Minnesota Press, pp. 45–72
——(2004): 'Middle Eastern Literature: Arabic', *glbtq: An Encyclopedia of Gay, Lesbian, Bisexual, Transgender, and Queer Culture*, at glbtq.com.
——(2006): 'Arabic: Middle Ages to Nineteenth Century', in Gaëtan Brulotte and John Phillips, eds, *Encyclopedia of Erotic Literature* I, New York: Routledge, pp. 43–61.
——(2008): 'Homoerotic Liaisons among the Mamluk Elite in Late Medieval Egypt and Syria', in Babayan and Najmabadi, *Islamicate Sexualities*, pp. 204–38.
Rüegg, Walter and H. De Ridder-Syoens, eds (1992): *A History of the University in Europe*, Vol. 1, Cambridge: Cambridge University Press.
Sanders, Paula (1991): 'Gendering the Ungendered Body: Hermaphrodites in Medieval Islamic Law', in Beth Baron and Nikki Keddie, eds, *Women in Middle Eastern History: Shifting Boundaries in Sex and Gender*, New Haven, CT: Yale University Press, pp. 74–95.
Schild, Maarten (1988): 'The Irresistible Beauty of Boys: Middle Eastern Attitudes towards Boy-Love', *Paidika* 3, pp. 37–48.
——(1990): 'Mujun' and 'Mukhannath', in Wayne R. Dynes, ed., *Encyclopedia of Homosexuality*, New York: Garland, pp. 848–50.
Sbath, Paul (1932–33): 'Kitāb al-Azmina. Le *Livre des temps* d'Ibn

Massawaïh, médecin chrétien célèbre décédé en 857', *Bulletin de l'Institut d'Egypte* 15, pp. 235–57.
——(1938–40): *Al-Fihris. Catalogue de manuscrits arabes*, Cairo: Imprimerie Al-Chark.
Schindler, Herbert, and Helma Frank (1961): *Tiere in Pharmazie und Medizin*, Stuttgart: Hippokrates-Verlag.
Schipperges, Heinrich (1964): *Die Assimilation der arabischen Medizin durch das Lateinische Mittelalter*, Wiesbaden: F. Steiner.
——(1976): *Die arabische Medizin im lateinischen Mittelalter*, Berlin: Springer Verlag.
Schmitt, Arno (2001–2): 'Liwat im Fiqh: Männliche Homosexualität?', *Journal of Arabic and Islamic Studies* 4.
Schmitt, Arno, and Jehoeda Sofer, eds (1992): *Sexuality and Eroticism among Males in Moslem Societies*, New York/London: Haworth Press.
Schmidtke, Sabine (1999): 'Homoeroticism and Homosexuality in Islam: A Review Article', *Bulletin of the School of Oriental and African Studies* 62, pp. 260–6.
Schmucker, Werner (1969): *Die pflanzliche und mineralische Materia Medica im Firdaus al-hikma des 'Alī ibn Sahl Rabban at-Tabarī*, Bonn: Orientalischen Seminars der Universität Bonn.
Schoeler, G. (1990): *Arabische Handschriften*, Stuttgart: Franz Steiner.
Serjeant, R. B. (1965): 'Notices on the "Frankish Chancre" (Syphilis) in Yemen, Egypt, and Persia', *Journal of Semitic Studies* 10: 2, pp. 241–52.
——(1997): *The Book of Misers*, rev. Ezzedine Ibrahim, Reading: Garnet.
Sezgin, Fuat (1967–84): *Geschichte des arabischen Schrifttums*, 9 vols, Leiden: Brill.
Shalakany, Amr A. (2008): 'Islamic Legal Histories', *Berkeley Journal of Middle Eastern and Islamic Law* 1, pp. 1–82.
Sharif, M. M. (1963–66): *A History of Muslim Philosophy. With Short Accounts of Other Disciplines and the Modern Renaissance in Muslim Lands*, 2 vols, Wiesbaden: Otto Harrassowitz.
Spies, Otto (1969): 'Das erste Auftreten der Syphilis in Ägypten im Jahre 1498', *Sudhoffs Archiv Geschichte der Medizin* 52: 4, pp. 382–4.
Steckler, Paul (2007–8): 'Brotherhood of Vice: Sodomy, Islam, and the Knights Templar', *Perspectives: A Journal of Historical Inquiry* 34, pp. 13–28.
Steingass, Francis Joseph (1892): *A Comprehensive Persian–English*

Dictionary, Including the Arabic Words and Phrases To Be Met with in Persian Literature, London: Routledge and Kegan Paul.

Steinschneider, Moritz (1900): *Die Heilmittelnamen der Araber*, Frankfurt: J. Kaufmann.

——(1902): *Die arabische Literatur der Juden: ein Beitrag zur Literaturgeschichte der Araber, grossentheils aus hand- schriftlichen Quellen*, Frankfurt: J. Kaufmann.

Storey, C.A. (1972): *Persian Literature: A Bio-Biographical survey* 2: 2/E, Oxford: Royal Asiatic Society of Great Britain and Ireland.

Tziallas, Evangelos (2009): *Too Dark, Too Hairy, Too Much!': Representations of Arab Men and 'Arabness' in Contemporary Gay Male Pornography*, unpublished MFA dissertation, York University (Canada), 2009.

Ullmann, Manfred (1970): *Die Medizin im Islam*, Leiden: Brill.

——(1978): *Islamic Medicine*, Edinburgh: Edinburgh University Press.

Vajda, Georges (1953): *Index général des manuscrits arabes musulmans de la Bibliothèque Nationale de Paris*, Paris: Bibliothèque Nationale.

Walzer, R., ed. (1962): *Greek into Arabic: Essays on Islamic Philosophy*, Cambridge, MA: Harvard University Press.

Watt, W. Montgomery (1972): *The Influence of Islam on Medieval Europe*, Edinburgh: Edinburgh University Press.

Weisser, Ursula (1983): *Zeugung, Vererbung und pränatale Entwicklung in der Medizin des Arabischislamischen Mittelalters*, Erlangen: Lüling.

Wikan, Umi (1977): 'Man Becomes Woman: Transsexualism in Oman as a Key to Gender Roles', *Man* 12, pp. 304-319. Replies can be found in *Man* 13 (1978), pp. 133–4, 322–33, 473–5, 663–71; *Man* 15 (1980), pp. 541–2.

Williams, Craig A. (1999): *Roman Homosexuality*, Oxford: Oxford University Press.

Wright Jr, J. W., and E. K. Rowson, eds (1997): *Homoeroticism in Classical Arabic Literature*, New York: Columbia University Press.

Yep, Stephanie (2012): *A Hermeneutical Consideration of Islamic Jurisprudence on Same-Sex Acts*, unpublished PhD dissertation, Wake Forest University, NC.

Ze'evi, Dror (2006): *Producing Desire: Changing Sexual Discourse in the Ottoman Middle East, 1500–1900*, Berkeley, CA: University of California Press.

Index of Proper Names

Ābāqā 60
ᶜAbbās Ibn ᶜAbd al-Muṭṭalib 57
Abū Nuwās 18–19, 36
Abū Ṣāliḥ A. Ibn Ṣāliḥ al-Tadaġī 172
Abū Tammām 33
Adarrāq, ᶜAbd al-Wahhāb Muḥammad 23
Afflacius, Johannes 50
Alphanus 50
al-Anṭākī, Dā'ūd Ibn ᶜUmar 21
al-Aqfahsī, Shihāb al-Dīn 23, 164
Aretino, Pietro 55
Aristo 91
Aristotle 27–9, 31, 53, 62, 64, 91, 99, 116, 127
Avicenna, *see* Ibn Sīnā

al-Baghdādī, Abū 'Abd al-Rahmān 24, 164
al-Bājī al-Masᶜūdī 22
Bashshār Ibn Burd 18
Burton, Richard 15–18

Constantine the African 50–2, 55, 77

al-Dāmghānī, Muhammad 116
Deli Birader 36
al-Dhahabī, Shams al-Dīn 22
al-Dihmānī, Aḥmad 22–3
Dioscorides 125

al-Fārābī 62
al-Fulātī, Muḥammad

Galen of Pergamon 27–31, 50–1, 64–5, 73–4, 115–16, 125, 127, 133

Genghis Khan 59
Gerard of Cremona 51, 55, 77
al-Ghazzālī, Abū Ḥāmid 23
al-Ghazlāwī, Muḥammad Ibn ᶜUmar 164
Greaves, John 60

Hārūn al-Rashīd 27, 35, 58
al-Ḥawrānī, ᶜAbd al-Raḥīm 164
al-Ḥillī, Ṣafī al-Dīn 36
al-Ḥimṣī, al-Muẓaffar Ibn Nāṣir Ibn ᶜAlī al-Qurayshī 165
Hippocrates 27, 64, 91, 99, 116, 127
Hulagu 59–60
Ḥunayn Ibn Isḥāq 27, 50, 165

Ibn Abī Uṣaybiᶜa 33, 35
Ibn ᶜĀdī, Yaḥyā 165
Ibn al-Bayṭār, Ḍiyā' al-Dīn Abū Muḥammad 24, 147, 158
Ibn Bukhtīshūᶜ 26–7
Ibn Buṭlān 22
Ibn Falīta al-Yamanī, Aḥmad b. Muḥammad b. ᶜAlī 165
Ibn Ḥājib al-Nuᶜmān, Muḥammad Ibn ᶜAbd al-Azīz 165
Ibn Hishām, Abū Ahmad 165
Ibn Ishāq, ᶜAlī 50, 165
Ibn al-Jawzī, Abū 'l-Faraj 23, 33
Ibn al-Jazzār, Abū Jaᶜfar 24, 32, 38, 46–7, 51–2, 75, 78, 146, 153
Ibn Kannān, Muḥammad Ibn ᶜĪsā al-Khalūtī 38, 165
Ibn al-Khaṭīb 22
Ibn Lūqā, Qusṭā 22, 24, 38, 46–7, 73, 78, 141, 165–6

Ibn Mandawayh, Abū ᶜAlī 166
Ibn Marzūq, Shams al-Dīn Abu ᶜAbd Allāh 166
Ibn Māsawayh 27
Ibn Māssa, ᶜĪsa 28, 166
Ibn Maymūn, *see* Maimonides
Ibn al-Nadīm 26, 33, 35
Ibn al-Qaṭṭāᶜ 166
Ibn Qayyim al-Jawziyya 22–3
Ibn al-Quff, Abū 'l-Faraj 21, 136, 149, 157–8
Ibn Raḥmūn, Sallāma 166
Ibn Raqīqa, Maḥmūd Ibn ᶜUmar al-Shaybānī 77, 166
Ibn Sahl, Sābūr 24, 125, 153
Ibn Sīnā, Abū ᶜAlī al-Ḥusayn 21, 38, 41, 45–7, 51, 53–4, 58, 61, 69, 128, 132, 155, 157, 166
Ibn Sulaymān, Aḥmad 166
Ibn al-Takrītī, Yaḥyā Ibn Jarīr 167
Ibn Ṭayfūr, Abū Faḍl
Ibn Zuhr 52
al-Isrā'ilī, Samaw'āl Ibn Yaḥyā Ibn ᶜAbbās al-Maghribī 72, 77, 167

al-Jāḥiẓ, Abū ᶜUthmān 33–5, 37, 75, 167
al-Jildakī, Īdmar Ibn ᶜAlī ᶜIzz al-Dīn 167
John of Capua 52

al-Kātib, Abū 'l-Ḥasan ᶜAli Ibn Nasr al-Samnānī 28, 33, 36, 45, 47, 140, 167
Khān, Muḥammad al-Ṣādiq Ḥassan 167
al-Khaṭīb, Abū Naṣr 167
al-Khuwārizmī, Abū Bakr 167
al-Kindī, Yaᶜqūb Ibn Isḥāq 134, 140, 167
al-Kūhin al-ᶜAṭṭār 24

al-Ma'mūn 27
al-Maghribī, Ibrāhīm 167
al-Majūsī, ᶜAlī Ibn al-ᶜAbbās 21, 51, 78
Maimonides 38, 46, 52, 55, 77, 129, 134–5, 137, 141, 146, 153, 157, 166, 177
al-Makkī, Abū Ṭālib 23
al-Manṣūr 21, 57
al-Masīhī, ᶜIzz al-Dīn 168
al-Mawṣulī, ᶜAbd Allāh Mekka 23
al-Mufaḍḍal Ibn ᶜUmar 168
al-Mughalṭāy, al-Ḥāfiẓ 168

al-Nafzāwī, Muḥammad Ibn Muḥammad 15, 47, 168
al-Namlī, Hassān Ibn Muḥammad 47
al-Nawājī, Shams al-Dīn Muḥammad Ibn Ḥasan 36, 168
al-Niḥillī 168

Peter of Spain 52–3
Plato 91, 116

Qāzān 63, 85
al-Qusṭanṭīnī, Maḥmūd Ibn Muḥammad 21, 169

Raimondi, Marcantonio 56
al-Rāzī, Muḥammad Ibn Zakariyyā' 21–2, 35, 46–7, 51, 58, 64, 76–8, 116, 127, 146, 169
Rhazes, *see* al-Rāzī
Rufus of Ephesus 27

al-Ṣabāḥ, Ḥasan 59
al-Ṣafadī, Khalīl Aybak 36
al-Ṣaymarī, Muhammad Ibn Ishāq Abū al-'Anbas 26, 47, 169
al-Shādhilī, ᶜAbd al-Qādir Ibn Aḥmad Ibn Muḥammad al-Māliki 170
al-Shāfiᶜī, ᶜAlā 'l-Dīn 170
al-Shayzarī al-Ṭabarī, ᶜAbd al-Raḥmān Ibn Naṣr 20, 170
Soranus of Ephesus 50
al-Surramarrī 22
al-Suyūṭī, Jalāl al-Dīn 22, 35, 37–8, 46–7, 128, 170–2

al-Ṭabarī, ᶜAlī Ibn Rabbān 35, 170
al-Tamakrūtī 173
al-Tawḥīdī
Ṭayfūr, Aḥmad Ibn Abī Ṭāhir 173
al-Tīfāshī, Shihāb al-Dīn Aḥmad Ibn Yūsuf 33–4, 36, 38, 43, 45–7, 55, 135, 137, 144, 150, 157, 173, 178
al-Tījānī, Muḥammad Ibn Aḥmad 173
Trotula 54, 78
al-Ṭūsī, Abū Jaᶜfar Naṣīr 21, 36, 38–9, 46,

58–63, 67–8, 77, 79, 85, 99–100, 127, 174

Ulugh Beg 60

Vesalius, Andreas 51, 77

al-Warrāq, Ibn Sayyār 24

al-Ẓāhirī, ʿAlī Ibn Muḥammad 174
al-Ẓāhirī, Muḥammad Ibn Dāwūd 20, 47
Zarrūq, Aḥmad 174

Index of Arabic Terms

abāzīr (spices) 138
Abū zaydān (orchis root) 144
abhal, see *ardij*
ᶜ*afṣ* (gallnuts / *Quercus lusitanica*) 123, 158
afrībūn, see *ūfarbiyūn*
akhlāṭ, sg. *khilṭ* (humours) 30
alam, pl. *ālām* (pain) 22
*am*ᶜ*ā'* (intestines) 87, 134, 141
amlaj (emblic / *Phyllanthus emblica*) 149, 153
ᶜ*anbar* (amber) 143–4
anīsūn (anise / *Pimpinella anisum*) 145
ᶜ*āqir qarḥa/ā* (pellitory / *Anacyclus pyrethrum*) 147
ᶜ*ar*ᶜ*ar*, see *ardij*
ardij (juniper / *Juniperus oxycedrus*) 156
ās, see *marsīn*
ᶜ*asal naḥl* (bee honey) 130–1, 148
aṣl al-ḥasak (caltrop root) 152
aṣṭūfūlin, see *jazar*

bāh (sexual potency) 21–2, 25, 33, 166–9
balgham (phlegma) 30
balīlaj (belleric myrobalan / *Terminalia bellerica*) 149, 153
ballūṭ (acorn / *Quercus faginea*) 157–8
banafsaj (sweet violet / *Viola odorata*) 116
basbāsa (mace / *Myristica fragrans*) 148
barrī (wild) 134, 138, 140–1, 152, 156–7
barūda (coldness) 87, 96, 99, 103, 109, 111, 133
baṣl (onions / *Allium cepa*)
bawraq (borax) 148
bizr (seeds) 138
bunduq (hazelnuts / *Coryllus avellana*) 141
bustānī (cultivated) 134, 138, 140, 152, 156–7

dajāj (chickens, hens) 139
dam (blood) 30
dār fulful (long pepper / *Piper longum*) 146
dār ṣīnī (Chinese cinnamon / *Cinnamomum cassia*) 128, 133, 151
dawqū, see *jazar*
dhāt al-janab (pleurisy) 112
dhāt al-ri'a (pneumonia) 112
dhawq (taste) 89, 91, 135, 156
dīk, pl. *duyūk* (cockrel) 135
dimāgh (brain) 140
dirham 10, 93–5, 97–9, 102–10, 114–15, 117–21, 123–4, 128, 130–2, 137, 150–3, 158–9
duhn (oil) 150

farārij (pullets) 139
firākh al-Hamām (squabs) 139
fujl (radish / *Raphanus sativus*) 136
fulful (*Piper nigrum*) 131
fustuq (pistachios / *Pistacia vera*) 142

halīlaj ([chebulic] myrobalan / *Terminalia chebula* var. *citrina*) 149, 153
ḥabba sawdā' (black cumin / *Nigella sativa*) 134, 149, 159
ḥarāra (hotness) 32

ḥarāra gharīziyya (innate heat) 32
harīsa (harissa) 137
ḥasak (caltrop / *Tribulus terrestris*) 152
ḥaṣā lubān (rosemary / *Rosmarinus officinalis*) 151–2
ḥayy ʿālam (houseleek / *Sempervivum arboreum*) 158
ḥimmaṣ, see *ḥimmiṣ*
ḥimmiṣ (chickpeas / *Cicer arietinum*) 137
ḥummuṣ see *ḥimmiṣ*
ḥuqna, pl. *ḥuqan* (enema)
ḥurf see *rashād*

idhkhir (lemon-grass / *Cymbopogon citratus*) 158–9
iḥtirāq (burning [sensation]) 96, 113, 133, 155
ʿinab (grapes / *Vitis vinifera*) 139, 142–3
ʿinab al-dhi'b (black nightshade / *Solunum nigrum*) 155–6

janṭiyāna (gentian / *Gentiana lutea*) 133–4
ja/uwārish (digestive stomachic) 126
jawz (walnuts / *Juglans regia*) 69, 148–9
jawz hindī/al-hind (coconut / *Cocos nucifera*) 69, 149
jazar (carrots / *Daucus carota*) 134
jimāʿ (sexual intercourse) 25
juljulān see *simsim*
jullanār (pomegranate blossom) 156

kabāba (cubeb / *Piper cubeba*) 144
khafaqān (palpitations)
khashkhāsh (poppy / *Papaver somniferum*) 147–8
khaṭmiyat al-thaʿlab (marshmallow / *Althaea officinalis*) 147
khiṭmī see *khaṭmiyat al-thaʿlab*
khiyār (cucumber / *Cucumis satius*) 145–6
khūlinjān (galingale / *Alpinia galanga*) 147
kuḥl (kohl) 152
kundur see *lūbān*
kurrāth (leek / *Allium porrum*) 68, 140–1

lakk (lac) 144–5
lawz (almonds / *Prunus amygdalus*) 141
lift (turnip / *Brassica rapa*) 140
liḥyat tays (goatsbeard / *Tragopogon pratensis*) 147
lisān ʿuṣfūr (common ash / *Fraxinus Excelsior*) 145
lūbān (frankincense) 151–2, 158

mallūkha see *qāqullā* 129
marsīm see *marsīn*
marsīn (myrtle / *Myrtus communis*) 157
martak see *murdāsank*
maṣṭikā (mastic, *Pistacia lentiscus*) 69
misk (musk) 131
mithqāl, pl. *mathāqīl* 97, 99, 108, 122, 131, 135, 138, 151–2
mizāj, pl. *amzija* (temperament) 30–1
murdāsanj see *murdāsank*
murdāsank (litharge) 135–6
murr (myrrh / *Commiphora myrrha*) 135, 141

nafas, pl. *anfus* (breath, soul)
nārdīn see *sunbul*
narjis (narcissus / *Narcissus poeticus*) 156

qanṭāriyūn (centaury / *Centaurium*) 144
qāqulla (cardamom / *Elettaria cardamom*) 129
qāqullā (saltwort / *Salsola fruticosa*) 129
qaranful (clove / *Syzygium aromaticum*) 129
qaṭrān (tar) 147, 158
qilī see *qāqullā*
qīrāṭ 94, 97, 102, 109, 114, 117–20, 123–4, 131–2
qirfa (cinnamon bark / *Cinnamomum zeylanicum*) 128
qishr (peel) 145
qullām see *qāqullā*
qusṭ (costus / *Saussurea costus*) 146
quṭn (cotton) 153

rashād (peppergrass / *Lepidium campestre*) 136–7

rāzyānāj (fennel / *Foeniculum vulgare*) 145
rummān (pomegranate / *Punica granatum*) 143
ruṭab (fresh dates) 142, 159

sādaj (malabathrum) 68, 133
sadhāb (rue / *Ruta chalepensis*) 148
sādhaj see *sādaj*
safarjal (quince / *Cydonia oblonga*) 143
salīkha (cinnamon / *Cinnamomum aromaticum*) 128, 133
samak (fish) 139
ṣamgh ᶜarabī (gum arabic / *Acacia arabica*) 159
samn (ghee) 138–9
ṣanawbar (pine / *Pinus pinea*) 150–1
sawdāʾ (black bile) 30
shabb (alum) 159
shaḥm al-ʿasad (lion's fat) 147
shahwa (lust)
shaᶜīr (barley / *Hordeum vulgare*)
shaqāqul (parsnip / *Pastinaca sativa*) 144
sharāb (syrup, wine) 157
shibitt (dill / *Anethum graveolens*) 154–5
shīshak (one-year-old lamb) 137–8
shōnīz see *ḥabba sawdāʾ*
simsim (sesame / *Sesamum indicum*) 152
suᶜd (cyperus / Cyperus longus) 147, 149
ṣūf (wool) 155
sukkar al-qand (sugar candy) 156
sunbul (Indian spikenard / *Nardostachys jatamansi*) 132–3

tamr (dried dates / *Phoenix dactylifera*) 138, 142, 159
thuffāʾ see *rashād*
thūm (garlic / *Allium sativum*) 138, 141
tīn (figs / *Ficus carica*) 142
tuffāḥ (apples / *Malus sylvestris*) 145

ᶜūd (aloewood / *Aloexylon agallochon*) 132, 135
ᶜūd hindī (Indian aloewood / *Aquilaria agallocha*) 132
ᶜūd Salīb (peony / *Paeonia officinalis*) 150
ūfarbiyūn (resin spurge) 157
ᶜuṣfur (safflower / *Carthamus tinctorius*) 137
utrujj see *utrunj*
utrunj (lemon / *Citrus Limon*) 145

zaᶜfarān (saffron / *Crocus sativus*) 129
zabīb (raisin) 99, 139
ẓahr (back) 166
zanjabīl (ginger / *Zingiber officinale*) 93–4, 98, 101, 105–10, 120, 128, 172
zayt (olive oil) 102, 150
zurunbād (zerumbet / *Zingiber zerumbet*) 101, 148–9
zift rūmī (Greek pitch) 101, 147

Index of English Terms

acorn 121, 158
almonds 100, 116, 139, 141–2
aloewood 97, 101
  Indian - 95, 104–6, 119, 123–4, 132
alum 123–4, 150, 159
amber 101, 105–6, 117, 120, 143–4
anchomium
anise 101, 145
ants 118
apples 94, 99–100, 130, 158
armpit 97, 119, 141
ash (*common* -) 101, 103, 108, 150

back 87, 96, 99, 103, 109–10, 113, 123, 133, 146, 153, 155
bandages 87, 111
barley
billy-goat 99
black bile 30–1, 106, 109, 126, 149
black nightshade
bladder (*urinary* -) 96, 108, 113, 131, 140, 150, 153–4
blood 30–2, 66, 87, 91, 96, 102–3, 105–6, 108, 113, 118, 134–5, 139, 141–2, 155
borax 101, 148
bowels 110
breath 94, 129, 132–4, 138, 145–6, 148–9
broth 98–9, 138

caltrop 107, 117
- *root* 116
camphor 123
candy (*sugar* -) 156
cardamom 31, 95, 101–2, 106–7, 120, 124, 130–1, 137, 139, 151
carob 114, 131
carrots 101, 110
catarrh 87, 106, 108, 151, 156
centaury 101, 144
chickens 98, 100, 138
chickpeas 97–8
cinnamon 97, 133, 151
  - *bark* 93, 95, 98, 101–2, 104, 110, 120, 128, 137, 150, 153
  Chinese - 105, 107–8
clove 93–5, 101–2, 107, 119, 130–1, 135, 146, 150, 153
cockrel 135
coconut 102–3, 110, 114–15, 117, 119–20, 149–50
coitus 22, 25, 33–5, 41–2, 52, 54, 64–7, 79, 86–8, 90, 92–6, 99, 101–10, 112–16, 118–23, 126–8, 130, 132, 135–8, 140, 142, 144, 146, 151–6, 159, 163–70, 172–3
colchicum 109
cold 30–1, 92, 95–6, 118, 130, 132–3, 135–6, 139–40, 143–4, 146, 149–50, 153–4, 156–8
coldness 87, 96, 99, 103, 109, 111, 133
colic 66, 87, 110, 112–13, 138, 140–1, 147, 149, 157
costus 101
cotton 109, 111, 118, 122, 152–5
cubeb 101, 120, 144
cucumber 101, 146
cumin (*black* -) 97, 101, 103, 107, 124, 134, 149
cyperus 114–17, 121, 123–4, 127

dates 10–11, 100, 123, 138, 142

dill 110
disease 23, 45, 89, 96, 100, 144
dung (*sheep* -) 117

ejaculation 34, 42, 65, 96, 113, 133, 155
electuary 96–7, 107–8, 126, 133, 135–6, 149
emblic 101, 108, 153
enema 110, 155
ermine 111, 155

figs 32, 100, 142
fish 98, 100, 139
flatsedge (*fragrant* -) 101, 115
frankincense 106

galingale 101–2, 150
gall 67, 97, 113, 115, 136, 143
  bear – 122
  cow – 122
  wolf – 122
gallnuts 123–4, 158
garlic 98–9, 137–8, 141, 148
gentian 97, 141
ghee 99–100, 104, 139
ginger 93–4, 98, 101, 105–10, 120, 128, 131, 152–4, 172
goatsbeard 101, 103, 121, 123–4
gourd 110, 154
gout 112, 154
grapes 100, 105, 114–15, 139, 142–3, 155–6
gum arabic 124
gums 92, 150

hazelnuts 100, 141, 148
hens 140
hotness 88, 158
heat (*innate* -) 32, 64–5, 87, 89, 91, 95, 103, 106, 108, 112, 126, 132, 150–1, 153
houseleek 121
headache 87, 106
heat 61, 94, 111, 121, 137, 142, 150
hemiplegia 95
hip 87, 109–10, 153
honey 94–5, 97, 99–100, 104–5, 107–9, 119–20, 130–1, 135, 138–9, 141, 144–6, 148, 150–3
hotness 88, 158
humours 30–1, 66, 100, 133

illness 63, 66, 87, 90–1, 101, 126, 133
impotence 40, 87–8, 93, 95, 126, 136, 138, 143, 147–50, 153, 163
impotent 96, 115
incontinence 113
intercourse (*sexual* -) 16, 21, 25, 29, 33, 36, 38, 40, 44–5, 64–7, 72, 88–93, 95–6, 99, 103, 106–7, 112–13, 118, 120, 126, 128, 132–3, 144, 146, 163–5, 167–8, 170–2, 174
intestines 87, 134, 141

jaundice 87, 95, 145, 152
joints 87, 110, 112, 131, 154, 156, 158
juniper 113, 156

kernel 104, 114
kidney 90, 108, 129, 134, 140, 152–5, 158
kohl 106, 109, 118–20, 124

lac 101
lamb 98, 102, 110, 137, 155
leek
lemon 101, 104, 124, 130, 150–1, 170
lemon-grass 123
lentisk, "mastic" 134
libido 38, 65, 90, 92
lion's fat 101, 109, 147
liquorice 118
litharge 97, 135
liver 65, 90, 95, 106, 113, 129, 132–4, 136, 141–6, 150–2
lust 65, 86, 89–90, 96, 126, 133, 135, 137–8, 144, 150–1, 154

mace 101, 106–8
malabathrum 97, 101, 133
marshmallow 101
mastic 97, 119, 134
medicine 20–3, 26–9, 35, 41, 46, 50–4, 58, 61, 64, 69, 74, 78, 85–6, 125–31, 133–5, 138, 140–3, 145, 147–8, 150–1, 154, 159
moist 30–1, 92, 136, 139–40, 142, 146–7, 150–1, 154

moistness 61, 87, 93, 103, 109, 150
musk 65, 67, 94, 96–7, 101–2, 117, 119, 123, 131–2, 136, 147
myrobalan
belleric - 101, 108, 153
chebulic - 101, 108, 153
myrrh 97, 135
myrtle 121, 123, 157

narcissus 114, 155–6
nerves 130, 153, 156

obstruction 86, 125, 129, 132–3, 136, 142, 144–5, 152, 156, 158
oil 102, 110, 115–20, 148, 150, 152, 154, 156–8
- *cake* 116
sesame - 122
olive - 104, 115, 135, 138, 141, 147
ointment 116
olibanum 151
onions 97–8, 100, 102, 104, 110, 136, 148, 150

pain 22, 87, 90–1, 112–13, 154–5
palpitations 94, 112, 130–1, 134, 141, 145–6
paraplegic 63
parsnip 101, 108
pearls 101, 167
peel 94, 98, 101–2, 104, 108, 123–4, 130, 143, 145, 150–1, 159
pellitory 101, 107, 109, 114–15, 120–1
penis 33, 40–1, 65–6, 87, 91, 93, 96–7, 108, 114–22, 126, 132, 134–5, 153, 155–7, 171
peony 102, 150
pepper 101, 110, 131, 137, 139, 144, 146
long - 98, 101, 106, 108, 110
peppergrass 101
phlegma 30–1, 92, 128
pills 32, 66, 85, 88, 119–20, 129, 163
pine 147
pistachios 100–1, 116, 119–20, 134, 139
pitch (Greek -) 101
pleurisy 112
pneuma 65, 91
pneumonia 112
pomegranate 121, 124, 156
- *blossom* 116
poppy 101, 147
pot (*cooking* -) 93–4, 98, 102, 104–5, 107, 110, 118, 121–3, 155
potency 25, 66, 91, 95, 101–2, 105, 108, 140, 144, 150, 153–4
potency (*sexual* -) 65, 86, 96, 100, 103, 106, 125–7, 129, 137–8, 143, 145, 152, 173
principal organs 89–90, 103, 106, 108, 112, 150
pullets 97, 100, 103, 140
pus 113

quince 143

radish 97
rain 94
raisins 99, 114, 139
recipe 32, 66–7, 93, 95, 97–9, 102–9, 115, 117–19, 122–3, 130–2, 138, 144, 149–50, 153, 158–9, 163
remedy 47, 86, 93, 95, 103, 105, 129, 131, 136, 138–9, 147–9, 154, 156, 158
rosemary 121, 152, 158
rosewater 94–5, 131–2, 139, 157

sable tiger 111
safflower 121
saffron 93–5, 97, 99, 101, 104, 106, 129, 131–2, 139, 150–1, 154
sciatica 87, 110, 112, 140, 144, 157
seeds 94, 97, 101, 107, 109–10, 131, 134, 136, 139–40, 145, 152, 154
sesame 107–8, 122
silk 101, 104–5, 111
soul 78, 88–90, 163
sparrow 109, 140, 152
house - 98, 100, 107, 118
spices 31, 98–9, 132, 138–9, 150
spikenard (*indian* -) 65, 95, 97, 101, 105, 107, 133
squabs 100, 102, 140
squirrel 111, 155
stimulants (*sexual* -) 63, 86, 125, 128–9, 134, 136, 141, 146, 149, 154
stomach 24, 87, 90, 93–5, 97, 99–100, 106,

110, 113, 126, 130, 132–5, 139–40, 143, 145, 148–9, 151–3, 157
stomachic 106
sugar 93, 100, 105, 107–9, 113, 119–20, 128, 130, 141, 151, 156
sweet 99–100, 105, 116, 130, 132, 141, 143, 157–8
syrup 93–5, 105, 107, 121, 123, 126, 128, 130, 141, 145, 148, 151–2, 157

tar 101, 147, 158
taste 89, 91, 135, 156
temperament 30–1, 65–6, 86, 90, 92, 102–4, 111–12, 142, 150, 155
testicles 65, 90, 92, 96, 108, 110, 135, 154–5, 157
treatment 22, 31, 44, 46, 52, 63, 86, 89, 91, 93, 97, 122, 128, 130–1, 133, 136, 139–45, 152–4, 157, 159
turnip 101, 110

unguents 90, 127, 133, 138
urination 113, 155

vagina 41, 45, 66, 79, 121–2, 136, 145, 150, 157–9
veins 91–2, 96, 108, 116
vertigo 92, 128
violet (*sweet* -) 116

walnuts 101, 107, 116, 137, 142, 148
wheat 92, 110, 128, 137, 139
wine 121, 123–4, 139, 142–3, 146, 152, 156, 159, 167
womb 42, 79, 96, 121, 133, 145–6, 150
wool 111, 121–3, 155, 159

zerumbet 101

نصير الدين الطوسي

كتاب الباب الباهية والتراكيب السلطانية

كتاب الباب الباهية والتراكيب السلطانية[1]

</١[2]/١[3]/1[4]> بسم الله الرحمن الرحيم الحمد لله رب العالمين وصلى الله على سيدنا محمد خاتم النبيين وعلى اله صحبه أجمعين وبعد[5] فإن الله تعالى قد أكمل النفوس الناطقة الانسانيه بمواهب انعامه وملا معادن خواطر الحكما باعلامه لهم جواهر حكمته كما قال الله[6] {سبحانه} تعالى[7] ولقد اتينا لقمان الحكمة الايه[8] فالفضل بيده كما قال الله تعالى وان الفضل بيد الله يوتيه من يشاء

---

١. هذا كتاب الباهية في التراكيب السلطانية تأليف الشيخ العلامه والحر الفهامه ابي البركات نصير الدين الطوسي رحمه الله تعالى وجميع المسلمين. أمين. أمين. أمين. (ق)/ – (غ).

٢. ترقيم مخطوطة غلاسكو.

٣. ترقيم مخطوطة برلين.

٤. ترقيم مخطوطة القاهرة.

٥. الرحيم ... وبعد: + وبه نستعين الحمد لله الذي شهده بوده جميع الكائنات والصلاة والسّلام علي افضل الانام سيّد محمد المبعوث الأيات الواضحات وعلي اله وصحبه والتابعين لهم المكرمات (ق) / – (غ) .

٦. الله : – (ق).

٧. تعالى : – (ق) /– (غ).

٨. الايه فالفضل بيده كما قال الله تعالى: فالاحسان منه والفضل بيده كما قال سبحانه وان الفضل (ق).

والله ذو الفضل العظيم ونشرع الان فى بيان سبب[٩] تاليف هـذا الكتاب وكشف اسـرار الحكما واظهار رموزاتهم فى هذا الكتاب هو[١٠] ان خليفة الزمان سلطان قازان[١١] كان له ولد ذات جمال وبها فحصل {له} فى بدنه الريح[١٢] <2> الفالج[١٣] وابطل شقته فسال الشخ العالم ملك <٢> علماء العصر واستاد فضلآء الدهر قطب الاسلام والمسلمين ومربى الملوك والسلاطين[١٤] ابو[١٥] البركات الخواجا[١٦] ناصر الدين الطوسى رحمه الله تعالى[١٧] ان يؤ{لف} كتابا فى الطب صغير الحجم كثير الفوايد لينتفع به المسلمين[١٨] فاجابه الى سواله والف هذه الرساله وجمع فوايدها من كتب المتقدمين والمتاخرين[١٩]

٩. بيان : – (ق).
١٠. فى هذا الكتاب هو: وذلك .
١١. قازان : فازان (ق).
١٢. الريح: ريح (ق).
١٣. الفالج : + {بدانه خفيف ما اقدر الرفعة من المكان بعد رشيد الحلق} (ق).
١٤. مالك ... السلاطين: الفاضل (ق).
١٥. ابو : أبا (ق).
١٦. الخوجا: الخوجه (غ).
١٧. رحمه الله تعالى: – (غ).
١٨. المسلمين: – (ق).
١٩. وجمع ... المتاخيري : – (ق).

وجعلها حاوية الفوايد نافعة وكافية[٢٠] لحفظ صحة بدن الانسان وسبب وقوع العلة وعلاجها لا يحتاج احد بسبب مطالعتها الى معالجة طبيب ويكتفى بها فى مداوات ما يحدث من العلل والامراض وغير ذلك من الفوايد المجربه والمنافع والخواص المنتخبة[٢١] ورتبتها على ثمانية عشر بابا وسميتها[٢٢] كتاب الباب الباهيه والتراكيب السلطانيه وهذه فهرسه <٣> الكتاب واليه المرجع والماب[٢٣] الباب الاول فى بيان تدبير الانسان وبيان امزجته وغير ذلك الباب الثاني في بيان اغدية[٢٤] المفردات وبيان[٢٥] منافعها وخواصها وغير ذلك[٢٦] الباب الثالث فى بيان الادوية المفردة التى هي خلاصة الادوية خصوصا لتقوية الافعال وزيادة الباه والشهوة والمنى وغير ذلك[٢٧] الباب الرابع فى بيان الادوية المركبة لدفع الامراض وتقوية الافعال[٢٨] الجماع ودفع موانعه وزيادة

---

٢٠. وكافية: – (ق).

٢١. وسبب ... منتخبها : وسيتغني بها عن معالجة الطبيب (ق).

٢٢. سمينتها: سماها (ق).

٢٣. واليه ... الماب: – (ق) / – (غ).

٢٤. اغدية: الاغذية (ق).

٢٥. وبيان: – (ق).

٢٦. وغير ذلك: – (ق).

٢٧. الافعال ... وغير ذلك : تقوية الشهوة وزيادة المني والباه (ق).

٢٨. الافعال: افعال (ق).

المنى والشهوة وبيان <٢> الاغذية المركبات والحلاوات النافعة لمزاج الانسان والمصلح له ويزيل فلاجة المفلوج من بدن الانسان ورخاوت اعضايئه ويقوى الباه[٢٩] الباب الخامس فى بيان الاشربه التى تصلح المزاج الفاسد وتصفى الدم والبدن وتقوى افعال الجماع وتفيد فايدة <٤> عظيمة[٣٠] الباب السادس فى بيان المعاجين والجوارشات التى تفرح وتدفع الملال وتنفع المعده نفعا عظيما وتقويها وتزيل الصفرا والبلغم وتقطع السودا وتنفع الدماغ وتفتح سدد الاعضا وتفشش[٣١] الرياح الفاسده وتزيلها[٣٢] وتقوى الاعضا الريه وتدفع الصداع والنزلات ووتقى الحراره الغريزية وتقوى جميع الافعال[٣٣] الباب السابع فى بيان الاشياف التي اذا تشيفت بها تجذب الرياح[٣٤] والبرودات من الوسط والظهر والاعضا وتخرجها وتزيل الرطوبات والصفرا

---

٢٩. موانع ... الباه: وبيان الاغدية المنافعه للامزجة ورخاوة الاعضاء وغير ذلك (ق).

٣٠. وتقوى ... عظيمة: – (ق).

٣١. تفشش: تصفى (غ).

٣٢. تزيلها: يزيلها (غ).

٣٣. التي تفرح... الافعال : النافعة للمعده وازالة الصفرا والبلغم والسوداء وتنفع الدماغ وتفتح سدد الاعضاء وتفشش الرياح الفاسدة وتقوي الحرارة الغريزة (ق).

٣٤. الرياح: الارياح (غ).

والسودا من المعده والامعا وغيرها[٣٥] الباب الثامن <3> فى بيان الحقن التى تزيل وجع المفاصل وتدفع[٣٦] الرياح الفاسده وتخرجها[٣٧] من البدن وذات الريه وعرق النسا ووجع الظهر وريح القولنج وتشد الظهر <٥> والوسط[٣٨] وتقوى جميع الافعال[٣٩] الباب التاسع فى بيان الشدود التى[٤٠] يشد بها الوسط في الفصول الاربعة وما تليق من ذلك[٤١] فى كل فصل حتى لا يخالف طبيعة الانسان ولا يحصل المرض منه[٤٢] الباب العاشر فى بيان شروطه وكيفيته حتى لا يحصل منه الضرر ويقع الضعف بسبب ذلك[٤٣] الباب الحادى عشر فى ذكر الادوية التى يطلى بها على الذكر فيقويه ويطوله ويقومه[٤٤] الباب الثانى عشر فى بيان الادوية التى يطلى بها على الذكر

٣٥. والظهر... والسودا من : ما يزيل البرودات والرطوبات من الظهر والاعضاء و (ق).
٣٦. وتدفع: واخراج (ق).
٣٧. وتخرجها: – (ق).
٣٨. الظهر والوسط: الوسط والظهر (غ).
٣٩. وذات ... جميع الفعال: – (ق).
٤٠. الشدود التي : ما (ق).
٤١. من ذلك : – (ق).
٤٢. حتى لا ... منه : الاصطلاح الطبيعه (ق).
٤٣. حتى ... ذلك : ومنع ضروره (ق).
٤٤. بها .... ويقومه : به الذكر لتقويته وزياده انعاظه (ق).

فيقومه[٤٥] ويطوله كما ينبغى[٤٦] الباب الثالث عشر فى بيان الادويـة التى[٤٧] يطلى بها على[٤٨] اصابع اليدين والرجلين[٤٩] فيفيد الجماع ويقويه ولا يضعفه لكثرة الجماع[٥٠] الباب الرابع عشر فى بيان الحبوب التى تمسك في الفم عند المجامعه[٥١] فيستلذ بها الفاعل[٥٢] <٦> الباب الخامس عشر فى بيان حالة الجماع التى يحصل بها لذة عظيمة للرجل والمـراة مثل ما ذكره الحكما[٥٣] الباب السادس عشر فى الادوية التى اذا استعملها النسا تحمر بها وجوههن <٣> وخدودهن كالورد الاحمر ويحصل من مجامعتهن لذة عظيمة حتى لا يقدر احد على مجامعتهن لحرارتهن وضيقتهن[٥٤] الباب السابع عشر

٤٥. فيقومه: فيقويه (غ).
٤٦. في بيان ... ينبغى : في ذكر منافع اخر متعلق بالباه وزيادة الشهوة طلاء على الذكر (ق).
٤٧. الادويه التي : ادويه (ق).
٤٨. على : – (ق) /– (غ).
٤٩. اليدين والرجليون: الرجلين واليدين (ق) / – (غ).
٥٠. فيفيد ... الجماع : لتقوية الجماع (ق).
٥١. المجامعه: الجماع (ق).
٥٢. فيستلذ بها الفاعل: ويستلذ بها (ق).
٥٣. حالة الجماع ... الحكما : ما يحصل للرجل والمرأه من لذة الجماع وكثرتها (ق).
٥٤. إذا استعملها ... ضيقتهن : اذا استعملتها بها النساء احمرت خدودهن واستحسنت فروجهن (ق).

في بيان الادوية التى تمنع الناس من الحبل وتبقين دايما كالبنات البكر[٥٥] الباب الثامن عشر فى بيان الادوية التى اذا استعملتها المـراة لم تحبل[٥٦] بـاذن الله تعالى[٥٧] تمت فَهْرَسَتِ[٥٨] الابواب وقد قدمناها حتى تسهل على طالبها اذا احتاج منها الى شى يسهل عليه تحصيلها من غير مشقة ولا تعب وبالله استعين وهو حسبنا ونعم الوكيل <٧> اعلم ايها الطالب[٥٩] وفقنا الله واياك الى طاعته ان الله سبحانه وتعالى خلق الحيوانات واخرجهم من العدم الى الوجود وخلق لهم[٦٠] ازواجـا وجعل لهم انفسا بحيث يحتاج ويشتاق بعضهم الى بعض فى الزوجيه[٦١] <4> وفضل الانسان على الجميع وفضله[٦٢] بالعقل

---

٥٥. في بيان ...البكر: في الادوية التي تمنع الحبل وتضيق الفروج (ق).

٥٦. تحبل: + تحبل (غ).

٥٧. في بيان... تعالى : في الادوية التي للحبل وفوائدك اخر تاتي ان شاء الله تعالي (ق).

٥٨. فَهْرَسَتِ الابواب : فهرسة الكتاب والابواب (غ).

٥٩. وقد ... الوكيل: ليسهل على طالبها تحصيلها من غير مشقه وبالله المستعان وعلياه التطلا اعلم وفقنا (ق).

٦٠. وخلق لهم: خلقهم (غ).

٦١. ان الله...الزوجية : بمنه وكرمه ان الله خلق الحيوانات واخرجهم من العدم الي الوجود وخلقهم ازواجا وجعل لهم انفاسا بحيث يحتاج ويشتاق بعضهم بعضا للزواج (ق).

٦٢. على الجميع وفضله: علي جميع (ق).

وزينه وكرمه كما قال الله تعالى وهو اصدق القايلين[٦٣] ولقد كرمنا بنى ادم وحملناهم فى البر والبحر الاية وجعل غذايهم الطف الحيوانات وبسطنا الكلام فى هذا الباب لانه ما ثم شى يكون[٦٤] سببا لهلاك النفس اشد من الجماع فكل مرض يمكن مداواته الا المرض الذى يكون سَبَبُه[٦٥] كثرة الجماع فانه[٦٦] يطفى الحرارة الغريزية فلا يعود ينفع العلاج ولا المداواة ابدا نعوذ بالله من ذلك[٦٧] فان المنى اذا انصرف[٦٨] يخرج من الاعضا الرئيسه وجميع <٨> الجوارح[٦٩] كما قال على رضى الله عنه[٧٠] منيك روحك ونور عينيك ومخ راسك مع ساقيك ان شيئت فاحفظه ومتى علمت الجماع وجامعت كما ينبغى تحصل منه اربعة وعشرون فايدة منها ان[٧١] يزيل

٦٣. الله تعالى وهو أصدق القايلين: تعالى (ق).
٦٤. وجعل ... يكون: فلا شيء (ق).
٦٥. يكون سَبَبُ: يحدث من (ق).
٦٦. فانه: لكونه (ق).
٦٧. فلا يعود... ذلك: – (ق).
٦٨. اذا انصرف: – (ق).
٦٩. وجميع الجوارح: – (ق).
٧٠. كما قال على رضي الله عنه: كما قال أمير المؤمنين على كرم الله وجهه (ق).
٧١. فاحفظه ... منه ان: فاحفظ نفسك ومن يعلم بتدبير الجماع وشروط فلا يضر بل ينفعه لأنه (ق).

اسقام السوداوية ويمنع العلل الصفراوية والبلغمية[٧٢] ويحصل[٧٣] الفرح والخفة كما ذكره العلما والحكما المتقدمون والاطبا المتاخرون وعملوا ذلك بتجاربهم واستعمالاتهم واما ما ذكره بعض العلما[٧٤] ان الجماع ردى مضر لا ينبغى لاحد ان يستعمله بل يتركه فهذا كلام لا اصل له بل هذا الكلام خطا لان شرف وزينته الظاهره بوجود خمسة اشيا وهي الحواس الخمسة الظاهرة كالسمع والبصر والشم والذوق واللمس فاما الذوق الذى هو احد الخمسة عبارة غالبة عن ذوق الجماع ولذته <٩> ونتيجه لذة الجماع لحصول وجود الحيوانات وبر التوالد والتناسل فى العالم الانسانى ايضا فالقول يعدم جواز الجماع <٤> قولا باطلا والظاهر ان هذا القول ليس قولا مطلقا بل بالنسبة الى الذين يجامعون مع جهلهم باوقات المجامعة[٧٥] واحوال مباشرتها وعدم علمهم بشروطها وتدبيرها فبسبب ذلك الجماع يبتلون بتلك الامراض المذكوره ويهلكون انفسهم بخلاف من يعلم تدابير[٧٦] الجماع وشروطه فلا

---

٧٢. الصفراوية والبلغمية: البلغمية والصفراوية (غ).

٧٣. يحصب: + من (ق).

٧٤. العلما: الحكماء (غ).

٧٥. المجامعة: الجماع (غ).

٧٦. تدابير: تدبير (غ).

يضره الجماع بل ينفعه نفعا بليغا كما ذكرناه مع انه ما ثم شى فى لذات النفسانيه الذ من لذة الجماع لانها جبلية ومختلطة فى تراكيب الانسان وباقي الحيونات ومنصبه فى خلقهم ولهذا لم يمر حيوان لم تركن تلك اللذة في نفسه ولم تحصل في دماغه الا ان يكون <١٠> معلول لمزاج مرخى الاعضا ميت الشهوه فصل اعلم ان البشرة لا تضعف ولا تبلى بمرض والم الا اذا حصل للاعضا الرئيسه الم وما دام الاعضا الرئيسه تقوية بالادوية والمعالجات والاحتما عن المخالفات والاحتراز عن المضرات لها تكون الجوارح سالمة امنة من العلل والاسقام فلا يصيبها شى من الالام باذن الله تعالى الى وقت اجَله فان الاجل لا يمنعه شى لا راد لفضايه ولا مانع لحكمه[٧٧] واعلم ان الاعضا الرئيسه هو الدماغ والقلب والكبد والخصى مع اعضائه وبعض الحكما جعل الريه من الاعضا الرئيسه وبعضهم عد الكلى ايضا[٧٨] فينبغى للانسان ان يقوى هذه الاعضا ويقوى المعدة بالادوية والمعاجين والاشربة والتمريخات كما سياتى <١١> شرحهم وصفات اعمالهم وتدابيرهم ان شآء الله تعالى كما القوا ذلك الحكما المنقدمون والاطبا

٧٧. كما ذكره... حكمه: – (ق).

٧٨. وبعض الحكما ... ايضا: – (ق).

المتاخرون بتجاربهم واستعمالاتهم وبينوا ذلك فى كتبهم كافلاطون وارطاطالوس وبقراط وبلطيوس وارسطو او امثالهم[٧٩] فصل فى بيان فايدة الجماع وضرره بحسب الفصول الاربع التى هى[٨٠] الربيع والصيف والخريف والشتا[٨١] واعلم ان اولى الفصول واحسنها[٨٢] وانفعها للجماع هو فصل الربيع لانه اعدل الفصول وهواه[٨٣] اعدل الاهوية وفيها يصفوا[٨٤] الدم ويعدل[٨٥] ويزداد فى عروق الروح ويقوى الحرارة الغريزية ويزداد النشاط والذوق ويزول ضعف الذكر ويشتد فاذا كان الامر كذلك[٨٦] فلا يضره الجماع فى هذا الفصل ولا يشقل البدن ولا يجلب السقم ولا الام سواء جامع بالادوية والمعاجين <١٢> او بغير المعاجَين[٨٧] واما

---

٧٩. يقوي هذه الاعضا ... او امثالهم: يقوي هذه الاعضا بالادويه والمعاجين والاشربه والتمريخات والاحتراز عن المضرات لتكون الجوارح سالمة من العلل والاسقام (ق).

٨٠. هى: – (غ).

٨١. الصيف والخريف والشتا: الربيع والخريف والشتا والصيف (ق).

٨٢. اولى الفصول واحسنها: احسن الفصول (ق).

٨٣. لانه اعدل الفصول وهواه: لان هواه (ق) .

٨٤. يصفوا: يصف (ق).

٨٥. ويعدل: – (ق).

٨٦. فاذا كان الامر كذلك: – (ق).

٨٧. لا يشقل ... المعاجين: – (ق).

الجماع فى غير <٥> فصل الربيع فمضر[٨٨] اذا كان بالادوية فلا يضر لان الذى ينصرف من الشهوة حصل عنده بسبب قوى الادويـة[٨٩] فذلك بالحقيقة ينصرف بالادوية لا منك فحينئذ يحتاج من مجامع فى فصل الصيف والخريف والشتا الى العلاج بالادوية والمعاجين حتى يفيد ولا يضر[٩٠] الباب الاول فى تدبير ما يقتضيه <5> مزاج كل انسان وبيان العلامات التى يستدل بها على مزاج كل واحد[٩١] اعلم ان كل من كان اسمر اللون وحنطى اللون وكان لحمه قويا وليس بمرخى[٩٢] واسع العروق واسود الشعر ويكون معتدلا نظيفا اشهل العينين ويكون شعر حاجبيه كثيرا[٩٣] وخصيتيه قويا[٩٤] كان مزاجه حـارا يابسا فهذه الطايفة تكون حمسا على <١٣> الجماع لا يبالون من الجماع[٩٥] واما من يكون

---

٨٨. فمضر: + الا (غ).

٨٩. فلا يضر ... الادوية: – (غ).

٩٠. اذا كان ... ولا يضر: الا اذا كان بالادوية فلا يضر ان شاء الله تعالي (ق).

٩١. على مزاج كل واحد: على المزاج (ق).

٩٢. وحنطى... بمرخى: ولحمه قوي (ق).

٩٣. ويكون ... كثيرا: يكون معتدلا لا اشهل العينين كثير شعر الحاجبين (ق).

٩٤. قويا: قويه (ق).

٩٥. فهذه ... الجماع: فلا يضره الجماع (ق).

اصفرا اللون واحمر الوجه وابيض الجسم[٩٦] كبير البطن يكون مزاجه بارد رطب مرطوب المزاج حريص على الجماع وليكن لا يقوى عليه واذا زاد فى الجماع ضعف بسببه[٩٧] واما من كان اسود اللون ونظيف الجلد والبدن هزيلا مغيرا صغير العينين ويكون[٩٨] لحم اسنانه شديد الحمرة يدل على انه حار المزاج وهذا[٩٩] يكون حريصا على الجماع واما من كان ابيض اللون فهذا يكون على نوعين احدهما من يكون لونه صافيا وعينيه ملاحا والثانى هو الذى يكون بياضه مستويا بالصفره ويكون شعره اصفر فهو يكون حريصا على الجماع ومن كان ابيضا وبلغمى المزاج يكون مرخى الاعضا لا يكون له قوة على الجماع وان افرط فى الجماع <١٤> هلك فينبغى لهذا ان يحترز من الجماع فصل[١٠٠] اعلم ان ضعف الجوارح ورخاوة الاعضا تحصل من ضعف الدماغ وهذا يسمى ضعيف الدماغ وعلامة ذلك دوخان الراس وتغوير العينين وضعف البصر[١٠١] وضعف

٩٦. واحمر الوجه وابيض الجسم : احمر الوجه ابيض الجسم (ق).

٩٧. رطب ... بسببه: رطبا فيضره كثرية الجماع (ق).

٩٨. الجلد والبدن هزيلا صغيرا: البدن (ق).

٩٩. وهذا: فهذا (ق).

١٠٠. اما من كان... فصل: – (ق).

١٠١. ضعف الجوارح ... البصر: ضعف الجوارح الاعضاء تحصل

القوى وتغير اللون وغلبة الحيا عند رخاوة الذكر والجماع[١٠٢] من غير نشا واذا جامع لم تبق[١٠٣] له قدرة على اعادة الجماع مرة اخرى من غير توهمه ورخاوة اعضايه فينبغى لمثله[١٠٤] ان يدفع هذه العلل بتقوية الدماغ فعلاج تقوية الدماغ بشراب السكر لان هذه العلل لا تحصل الا من زيادة الرطوبات و[١٠٥]تحل[١٠٦] الفضلات ويقوى المنى ويكثر ويقوي الجماع وله منافع شتى بطول شرحها صفة عمل تركيب السكر قال[١٠٧] يوخذ زنجبيل وقرفه <١٥> لف من الاثنين خمس دراهم بالسويه[١٠٨] وقاقله درهمين وقرنفل درهمين تدق هذه الادوية كل واحد وحده ثم تجمعهم بالدق وتجعلهم فى قدره وتجعل عليهم قدرهم سبع مرات ماء عذب ويغلى نبار لينه الى

من ضعف الجماع وعلامته دوخان الراسن وضعف البصر والقواير العينين (ق).

١٠٢. رخاوت الذكر والجماع: الجماع ورخاوة الذكر (غ).

١٠٣. تبق: يبق (غ).

١٠٤. عند رخاوة ... لمثله: وقت الجماع ورخاوه الذكر وان جامع مره لم يقدر علي الاعاده ولم يكن لنشاة لرخاوه اعضائه فهذا ينبغي له (ق).

١٠٥. و: + هذا الشراب (غ).

١٠٦. تحل: يحل (غ).

١٠٧. فعلاج... قال: فعلاجه شراب السكر فإنه يحل الفضلات ويقوي الجماع ويكثر المني وله منافع شيء (ق).

١٠٨. لف... بالسوية : لف خمسة دراهم منهما (ق).

ان تخرج قوة الادوية فيه وينهرى[١٠٩] <٦> فيه الحوايج ثم يصفى الماء ويرمى التفل ثم يوخذ قوامه بوزنه اربع مرات سكر يعنى بوزن الحوايج اربع مرات سكر فيكون وزن السكر اثنين وثلاثون درهم ثم يغلى الى ان يمتزج ولا يعقد[١١٠] ثم اذا اراد ينزلها يضع فيها نصف درهم زعفران وينزله ويستعمله فى[١١١] كل يوم على <6> الريق مقدار ملعقه ويصبر عن الاكل الى الضحوه مفيد وشفا ان شا الله تعالى واما السبب الثانى فى[١١٢] ضعف الجوارح ورخاوة الاعضا التى تحصل بحدث[١١٣] <١٦> منها ضعف الجماع فهو ضعف القلب فعلامة من يكون ضعيف القلب انه اذا تحرك بحركة او مشى قوى فى طلوع عقبه او غضب على احد او اذا بشروه ببشارت او اذا راى مطلوبه او اذا اراد ان يقارن جماعة يحصل له

١٠٩. ينهرى: تنهري (غ).

١١٠. يعقد: ينعقد (غ).

١١١. وقاقله ... فى : وقرنفل وقالقله درهمين من كل منها نرقهم وتصب عليهم ماء عذبا حتي يعمهم ويغلى ذلك علي النار الي ان تخرج قوة الادوية في المء فيصفي ويرمي التفل ثم تطوح فيه اثنين وثلاثين درهما سكرا ويغلي علي النار الي أن يمتزج فيلقى عليه نصف درهم زعفران وينزل ويرفع ويستعمل منه (ق) / فى: – (غ).

١١٢. مفيد... فى: فانه في شفاء باذن الله واما (ق).

١١٣. تحصل بحدث: يحدث (غ).

فى هذه الصور كلها[١١٤] خفقان القلب وتاخذه الرعشة فى يديه وركبه ويحصل له اللهفات وضيق النفس ويتغتر لونه ويجامع بالضعف ويحصل له بعد الجماع خفقان القلب {فينبغى لمثله ان يدفع هذه العلل بتقوية الجوارح ورخاوة الاعضا بشراب التفاح لا يزيل هذه العلل} ويزيد[١١٥] فضلات المعده ويسخن المنى ويزيده وله منافع كثيره غير هذا لو ذكرناها لطال علينا كتابتها وفيه كفاية واما صفة[١١٦] تركيب شراب التفاح قال يوخذ التفاح يقشر وينقى من[١١٧] نواه ويدق ويعصر مآوه من خرقة رفيعة او[١١٨] منخل رفيع ثم <١٧> يوخذ وزن مآ التفاح مآ ورد ثم يخلطهما ثم يوخذ وزن الجميع عسل نحل مصفى منزوع الرغوه وياخذ قليلا من مآ التفاح وماء

---

١١٤. تحصل ... كلها: تحدث عند الجماع نهي من ضعف القلب وعلامة انه اذا تحرك بحركة ومشي او غضب يحصل له (ق).

١١٥. فينبغي لمثله ... يزيد: وضربات العروق فاذا سكنت العروق يحصل لها الضعف والرخاوة ومتى افرط هذه الامراض في الجماع يهلك بلا شبه فينبغى ان يعالج في وقع هذه العلل بشراب التفاح فانها يدفع هذه العلل ويقوي القلب ويزيل (غ).

١١٦. صفة: + عمل (غ).

١١٧. ويحصل... وينقي من: ويتغير لونه فهذا ايضره الجماع فينبغي ان يعالج بشراب التفاح فانه يدفع هذه العلل ويقوي القلب ويزيل فضلات المعده ويسخن المني ويزيده وله منافع شتي وصفة يؤخذ من التفاح جزء يقشر ويرمي (ق).

١١٨. او: له (غ).

الورد المخلوطان يجعل فى قدره وحده ويجعل عليه نصف درهم[١١٩] زعفران ونضف درهم فلفل ودرهم زنجبيل وقرنفل درهمين وتغليه حتى تخرج قوة الادوية فيه ثم يصفى ويرفع الى وقت الحاجة ثم ياخذ[١٢٠] وزن هذا الماء مرتين من ماء المطر وتجعل الجميع مع الما[١٢١] الذى غليته بالبزور ان فى قدره على نار لينه وانت تحركه الى ان ينعقد وترمى عليه قبل ان ينعقد قيراط مسك خالص ثم تنزله وتبرده[١٢٢] وتستعمل[١٢٣] منه كل يوم على الريق قدر ملعقه ونصف نافع واما السبب الثالث فى رخاوة الاعضا <١٨> وضعف الجوارح والجماع قال واما ضعف الكبد فعلا منه صفار الوجه مثل علة اليرقان وينشف لسانه وشفتيه وتغور عيناه <٧> ويكون هزيلا قليل الاشتها للطعام[١٢٤] واذا اكل لا ينهضم واذا وقف

١١٩. يجعل عليه نصف درهم: تجعل عليهم وزن (غ).
١٢٠. من خرقة ... ثم ياخذ: ويصفي ثم يخلط بوزنه ماء ورد وكذا وزنهما عسل نحل منزوع الرغوه ويغلي علي النار ويلقي عليه نصف زعفران ونصف درهم قاقله ودرهم زنجبيل ودرهمان قرنفل ثم يصفي ثم تاخذ (ق).
١٢١. الما: – (غ).
١٢٢. تبرده: + وترفعه (غ) .
١٢٣. وتجعل ... وتستعمل: ويغلي الجميع علي النار ثم الق عليه قيراط مسك ثم نزل وارفع ويستعمل (ق).
١٢٤. واما السبب ...للطعام: لما ذكر واما علامة ضعف الكبد تصفير الوجه وتنشف اللسان والشفتين ويكون هزيلا قليل الشهوة

يرتعد ساقيه ولا يقدرعلى القيام الا بالتكلف ويكون مرخيا لا يقدر على الجماع وان قدرعليه لا يكون له حلاوة ولا لذة ويكون منيه بارد[١٢٥] ويكون يديه ورجليه باردتان ومثل هذا الرجل اذا افرط فى الجماع يبتلى باحد هذه الامراض الثلاثة أما ان يكون مفلوجاً او مرخيا واما ان تنقطع حرارته الغر يزيه فيحدث من ذلك موت المفاجاه[١٢٦] نعوذ بالله من ذلك فينبغى ان يدفع هذه العله[١٢٧] بشراب السنبل يسخن <٧> معدته ويقوى كبده[١٢٨] ويقوى <١٩> الحرارة الغريزيه ويقوى الجماع وله ستة وعشرون منفعه ان ذكرناها يطول الكتاب واما صفة شراب السنبل قال يوخذ[١٢٩] قرفه وقاقله وعود هندى[١٣٠] من كل واحد درهم وقرنفل نصف درهم تدق

الاكل (ق) .

١٢٥. بارد: باردا (غ).

١٢٦. لا ينهضم ... المفاجاه: لا يهضم وليس له قدرة علي الجماع وان جامع لم يجد له لذة ولا شهوة ومنيه بارد وكذا اعضائه باردة فهذا ايضا يفره الجماع ويخشي عليه مرض الفالج لانقطاع الحرارة الغريزيه عنه (ق).

١٢٧. هذه العلة : + عنه (ق).

١٢٨. معدته ويقوي كبده: ويقوي الكبد (ق) / ويقوي كبده: – (غ).

١٢٩. ويقوي ... يوخذ: يزيد في الجماع وله منافع آخر يطول شرحها وصفته (ق).

١٣٠. عود هندى: + وجوز هندي (ق).

هذه الادويـة وتجعل[١٣١] عليها قدر الحوايج[١٣٢] خمس مـرات ماء ويغلى حتى ينهرى[١٣٣] الحوايج ويبقى[١٣٤] نصف المـاء ثم يصفى ويجعل قدرالماء عسل منزوع الرغوه ويغلى ساعة حتى يمتزج ثم يجعل[١٣٥] عليه نصف درهم زعفران يذاب بماء الورد ويخلط ويستعمل نافع مفيد لما ذكرناه السبب الرابع لضعف الجماع وضعف الذكر والخصيتين ورخاوتهما وهذا النوع يكون[١٣٦] على ثلاثة انواع اولها[١٣٧] ان تكون هذه[١٣٨] التى ذكرناها من رخاوة الذكر والخصيتين حبليا له صحبة[١٣٩] من بطن امه وتانيها <٢٠> يكون[١٤٠] من كثرة الجماع من[١٤١] صغره

---

١٣١. تجعل: يجعل (غ).
١٣٢. تجعل عليها قدر الحوايج: يجعل عليها بقدرها (ق).
١٣٣. ينهرى: يتهري (غ).
١٣٤. ينهرى الحوايج ويبقى : علي النار حتي يبقي (ق).
١٣٥. ويجعل ... ثـم يجعل: ويخلط بـقـدره عسلا مـنـزوع الـرغـوة ويغلي حتي يمتزج ثم يلقي (ق).
١٣٦. يذاب... النـوع يـكـون: مـذوب بمـاء ورد ويـرفـع ويستعمل منه وقت الحاجة فانه نافع لما ذكر واما رخاوة الذكر وضعفه فهو على ثلاثة انواع (ق).
١٣٧. اولها: – (غ).
١٣٨. هذه: + العلل (غ).
١٣٩. هذه التى... صحبته: خلفته (ق).
١٤٠. يكون: تكون (ق).
١٤١. من: في (ق).

وثالثها كثرة الجماع من فوق الاربعين وبعد الاربعين[١٤٢] وعلامة الاول يعنى الذى يكون رخاوته من بطن امه[١٤٣] لا يقوم ذكره ويكون مع ذلك[١٤٤] حريصا على الجماع من غير اشتهاء له ويكون مرخيا وعلاج هذا النوع معتدلا على[١٤٥] طول الزمان وعلامتها الذى حصل منها ذلك لكثرة الجماع فى زمن صغره فعلامته[١٤٦] قيام ذكره فى اوايل الليل واواخره ووقت الصبح او فى فصل الربيع فعلاج هذا النوع هين يصلح سريعا سنذكره ان شا الله فى موضعه وما حصل له من كثرة الجماع فى كبره من فوق الاربعين فعلا منه قيام ذكره فى الجملة فى الاوقات القليلة وبعض الايام و[١٤٧] جماعه بلا نشاط ينزل منيه بارد[١٤٨] او تارة <٢١> منيه بالحرقان ومثل هذا لا يكون له اولاد ولا بنين وسبب هذا النوع من البروده فى

---

١٤٢. فوق الاربعين وبعد الاربعين: فوق الاربعين من عمره (ق).

١٤٣. من بطن امه: من بطن من بطن امه (ق) ـامه: + كذلك (غ).

١٤٤. مع ذلك: – (ق).

١٤٥. معتدلا: معقد والا (غ).

١٤٦. اشتهاء... فعلامته: شهوة فلا علاج له وعلامته الثانية (ق).

١٤٧. فى اوايل... الايام و: اخر الليل فعلاجه بالادوية والمعاجين الاتية وعلامته الثالثة (ق).

١٤٨. بارد: باردا (غ).

ظهره ووسطه فان البرودة تكون <٨> غله لبة عليه[١٤٩] فينبغى ان يعالج فى مثل هـذه[١٥٠] بمعجون المسك فانه يزيل البروده والرطوبة[١٥١] التى فى الظهر وفى الوسط ينقى المثانة ويجرى المنى ويجرى[١٥٢] الدم فى العروق ويفتح السدد فينبغى ان يحمى من المآ كل المتخالفات حتى يتخلص سريعا ولا يبتلى بزيادة المرض وسنذكر احتمايه وما يفيد من الاغذية ان شا الله تعالى ولهذا المعجون ثلاثة وثلاثون فايده غير ما ذكرناه[١٥٣] وصفة تركيب[١٥٤] معجون المسك قال[١٥٥] يوخذ مسك قيراط وسليخه وسنبل وسادج <8> هند[١٥٦] مليح وجنطيانه رومى من كل واحد درهمين وزعفران[١٥٧] وكمون وبزر جزر ومصطكى من كل واحد ثلاث <٢٢> دراهم[١٥٨]

١٤٩. ينزل منيه ... لبة عليه: ومنيه بارد ينزل بحرقان بلا شهوة وسببه بروده في ظهره (ق).

١٥٠. في مثل هذه: – (ق).

١٥١. والرطوبه: – (ق).

١٥٢. يجرى: – (ق).

١٥٣. المتخالفات... تعالى: الرديه الحامضه ليتخلص من هذا المرض ولهذا المعجون ثلاث وثلاثون فايده (ق).

١٥٤. تركيب : – (ق).

١٥٥. قال: ان (ق).

١٥٦. هند: هندي (ق).

١٥٧. وزعفران: زعفران (ق).

١٥٨. ثلاث دراهم: درهم (ق).

وعود وقرنفل[١٥٩] ومر تركى من كل واحد نصف درهم يدق هذه الادوية وينخل ويوخذ قوامهم بقدر الادوية ثلاث مرات عسل نحل ويجعله[١٦٠] معجونا ويستعمل منه كل يوم مثقال نافع ان شا الله تعالى[١٦١] علاج اخر يوخذ ديوك صغار قبل ان يصيحوا ويذبحهم[١٦٢] ويجمع[١٦٣] مرارتهم مقدار[١٦٤] عشرة دراهم ثم يوخد مرداسك مقدار[١٦٥] ما يعجن به المراير المجموعه ويعجنه بها عجنا رقيقا[١٦٦] ثم يضعه فى الشمس حتى يمتزج ويخلط بعضه فى بعض واياك ان لا يجف ولا يغلظ[١٦٧] ثم يدخل الحمام وكلما خرج من الحمام[١٦٨] يطلى به ذكر وتحت ابطيه ومقعده وليكن ذلك على الريق ثم يستعمل من ذلك المعجون اى معجون المسك الذى تقدم[١٦٩] ثم

---

١٥٩. وقرنفل: – (ق).

١٦٠. يدق ... يجعله: وعسل نحل قدر الجميع ثلاث مرات ويغلي علي النار ويجعل (ق).

١٦١. تعالى: لما ذكر (ق).

١٦٢. يذبحهم: يذبحو (ق).

١٦٣. يجمع: يؤخذ (ق).

١٦٤. مقدار: بقدر (ق).

١٦٥. مقدار: بقدر (ق).

١٦٦. المجموعه ... رقيقا: – (ق).

١٦٧. ويخلط ... ولا يغلظ: – (ق).

١٦٨. وكلما خرج من الحمام: صباحا و (ق).

١٦٩. وتحت... تقدم: ومقعدته وتحت ابطيه ثم ياكل من معجون

يطبخ الادياك[١٧٠] المذبوحه التى جمعت مرايرهم بقدره مع بصل <٢٣> ويرش عليه بزر فجل وبزر رشاد اجزا سوا وياكله نافع مفيد ان شا الله تعالى[١٧١] فينبغى ان يجعل غداوه ما يناسبه ويصلح له[١٧٢] مثل الهريسة بلحم الفراريج او بلحم الغنم الشيشاع والخبز الفطير المخدوم بالعجن القوى من دقيق الجراية وماء الحمص كعادة الحكما وذلك ان ياخذ الحمص الابيض وينقع[١٧٣] ويقشر ويطبخ فى قدره الى ان ينهرى[١٧٤] وتخرج قوته الى الماء[١٧٥] ثم يصفى الماء ويرمى التفل ثم يجمع العصافير الدروريه[١٧٦] وتذبح[١٧٧] وينقوا من اوساخهم ويقطعوا كل قطعة قدرا الحمصه تجعلهم فى القدره فى ماء الحمص وتطبخهم به[١٧٨] وتسد فم القدره حتى لا يخرج

المسك بعد خروجه من الحمام (ق).

١٧٠. الادياك: الديوك (ق).

١٧١. التي جمعت ... تعالى: بقدرها بصلا ويرش عليه بزنجبيل وبزر رشاد اجزاء سواء ثم يأكلها فانه نافع المذكور (ق).

١٧٢. يناسبه ويصلح له: يناسب (ق) .

١٧٣. الشيشاع ... وينقع: وصفه اما ماء الحمص وهوان يؤخذ منه جزء ونقطع (ق).

١٧٤. ينهرى: يتهري (غ).

١٧٥. الماء: الماء المطبوخ فيه (ق).

١٧٦. يجمع العصافير الدروريه: تجمع العصافير (ق).

١٧٧. تذبح: يذبح (غ).

١٧٨. اوساخهم ... به: الاوساخ وتقطع كل قطعه مقدار الحمص

البخار وتقد عليه بنار لينه حتى لا يحترق وينهرى[١٧٩] وعلامة ذلـك ان تطلع <٢٤> رايحته مثل اللحم المشوى ثم ينزل عن النار ويجعل فيه هـذه الحوايج وهـي[١٨٠] زنجبيل خمسة دراهـم ودار فلفل درهمين ونصف وستجات جوزه وعشرة دراهم <9> قرفه يدق الجميع ويرفعوا[١٨١]<٩> وتـرش على مـا ذكرناه ويستعمل وكلما اكل مثل هذا الطعام يرش عليه من هذه الابازير وياكل وان لم يلتقى[١٨٢] العصافير ياخذ عوضهم فراخ الحمام فان ذلك يقوم مقام العصافير وكذلك ياكل تقلية الجزر بلحم الشيشك او الفراريج والديوك قبل اوان صياحها ولا يطبخ الجزر الا بعد غلسه وتتطيفه من قشره ثم يقطع صغارا ويطبخ مع ما تيسر من اللحوم التى ذكرناها ثم يرش عليه من الابازير المذكوره يوكل ويشرب عليه من الالبان الحليب البقرى مطبوخا <٢٥>

وتطبخ في ماء الحمص (ق).

١٧٩. ينهرى: تتهري (غ).

١٨٠. وتقد ... هى: فاذا ظهرت رائحته ينزل عن النار ويغلي عليه (ق).

١٨١. يرفعوا: يرفعها (غ).

١٨٢. وستجات ...لم يلتقى : وست جوزات وقرفة عشرة دراهم وتمزجهم ثم ترفعهم فاذا اكلت طعاما نفيسا فرشها عليه منه ويستعمل فانه نافع لما ذكرناه وان لم يجد (ق).

بالثمر مقداران تحليه وياكل ايضا السمك المشوى[183] بالبصل الابيض واذا اكل التسليق ياكله بالثوم نافع صفة عمل التسليق الثوم قال هو ان[184] ياخذ الثوم الشامى الجديد ويقشر فصوصا ثم[185] يوخذ دهن البقر يسلى[186] ثم يصفى ثم يوخذ من سلاه قليلا ويدق ويخلط مع الدهن ويطبخ حتى ينهرى[187] ثم يوضع فى سكروجه[188] ثم يعجن باليد عجنا قويا حتى ينماع ويكون رايق ثم يجعله على النار اللينة الى ان يشتد قليلا[189] ثم يجعل عليه الثوم المقشر ويخلط ويضرب حتى يتحدا ثم ينزله عن النار ويرمى عليه[190] من الابازير والحرارات المذكوره وقدر ما يعمل مزاجه[191] مع نصف

---

١٨٣. مطبوخا ... المشوي: المستوي (غ).

١٨٤. فان ذلك... هوان: فانها تقوم بمقامها وكذا طبيخ الجزر باللحم او الفراريج يرش عليه وصفة التسليق (ق) .

١٨٥. ويقشر فصوصا ثم: يقشر و (ق).

١٨٦. يسلى: ويسلي (ق).

١٨٧. ينهرى: يتهري (غ).

١٨٨. سكروجه: سكرجه (غ).

١٨٩. قليلا: حتى يتحد (غ).

١٩٠. يوخذ ... عليه: ويلقي عليه الثوم المقشر ثم يطبخ علي النار اللينة ويرمي عليها (ق).

١٩١. وقدر ما يعمل مزاجه: – (ق) / ما ... يعمل مزاجه: ما كيل مزاجه (غ).

درهم زعفران فى وعا قزاز[١٩٢] ويرفع ويستعمل منه فى كل يوم ثلاث مثاقيل[١٩٣] وهذا <٢٦> هو تسليق الثوم الذى ذكرناه يدفع البروده من الظهر والوسط وينقى المعده من البلاغم وينقى الصدر من البلغم والفضلات ويخرج جميع العلل من البدن باذن الله تعالى ويستعمل ايضا الورد المربا بالعسل النحل الصافى وصفنته هو ان تاخذ الورد وتجعله فى الشمس فى وعا قزاز وتجعل عليه العسل وتبسه معه وكلما خف العسل عنه تزيده عسلا الى ان ياخذ قوامه ويتربا وياكل ايضا الخبز الفطير المبسوس بالسمن البقرى الطرى ويستعمل التفاح الحلو البالغ الاحتما الذى ذكرناه فينبغى ان يحتمى من اكل الحوامض جميعها ومن الالبان ومن قديد البقرى والطرى منه ويحترز من لحم الماعز ومن الزبيب الاسود ويتناول من الاشربه الحلويه ويحترز من حامضها ومرها

<٢٧> نقل الخواجا الطوسي انه سمع روايات عن الحكيم بقراط وعن ارطاطاليس وغيرهم انه من عالج نفسه بما تقدم من الاغديه والاشربه الحامضه يامن من جميع ما ذكرناه من المضرات ومن جميع الالام

١٩٢. في وعا قزاز: – (ق).

١٩٣. كل.... مثاقيل: في كل يوم ثلاث مثاقيل فانه نافع باذن الله (ق).

والاسقام ويـزول عنه الرخاوه وتقوى جميع افعاله خصوصا على الجماع ولو جامع ما شا لا يضعف ولا يتغير وجهه من الجماع ولا يمل ابـدا ويجمل حاله وينصلح امره والسلام[١٩٤] الباب الثانى فى بيان الاغدية المفرده النافعه المقوية المصلحة لبدن الانسان وطبيعته[١٩٥] فمن ذلك الحلاوة العجمية التى يكون دقيقها من دقيق جراية معتدل الملح والنضج قال الحكيم خواجا الطوسي رحمه الله تعالى رواية عن الحكما المتقدمين انه من كل من اول عمره على <٢٨> الدوام خبزا ناشفا ولا ياكل معه اشياء اخر لا يبلى فى عمره بمرض عدا اجله لان الابتلا بالمرض لا يكون الا من زيادت الاخـلاط[١٩٦] <١٠> وزيـادت الاخـلاط لا تكون الا من اختلاف الاطعمة وايضا من الاغدية النافعة مثل لحم الغنم المشوى المهرى حتى لا تشوش المعده منه بسرعة هضمه وما اثم احسن غدا الطبيعة الانسان والطف من هذه الاثنين وبعد ذلـك[١٩٧] لحم الحمام وافراخه وافـراخ[١٩٨] الاوز

---

١٩٤. وهو تسليق ... والسلام: – (ق).

١٩٥. المصلحة ...وطبيعته: لبدن الانسان والله اعلم (ق).

١٩٦. زيادت الاخلاط: الاخلاط وزيادة (غ).

١٩٧. التي يكون دقيقها ... بعد ذلك: وهي ماخوده من الدقيق الجاريه والسمن البقري والعسل النهل وكذا اكل الخبز الناشف و (ق).

١٩٨. افراخه وافراخ: لحم (ق) / افراخ: فرخ (غ).

والدجاج والفراريج والديوك قبل اوان صياحها[199]
ولحم[200] السمك الطرى وبيض الدجاج والاوز
والبرشت وبيض غيرها يضر ويوكل بيض السمك[201]
ولحم العصافير الدرويه[202] وادمغتهم وحليب البقر
والغنم الطرى والبصل الابيض المستوى على النصف[203]
والجزر واللفت <٢٩> والحمص والكرات والسكر
والعسل والسمن البقرى[204] واللوز والبندق والفستق
والرطب والتين الاخضر والعنب والرمان الحلو
البلدى[205] والتفاح البلدى البالع[206] الحلو والسفرجل
الحلو المستوى[207] البالغ حتى لا يبْقى فيه اثر الحموضه
وهذه الاشيا التى ذكرناها جميعها مقويات للجماع
ملطفات تقوى الدماغ والاعضا وان كانت الادوية
كثيره لكن المختار منها هذا المذكور والسلام[208] الباب

١٩٩. قبل اوان صياحها: – (ق).
٢٠٠. لحم: – (ق).
٢٠١. برشت... والسمك: – (ق).
٢٠٢. الدرويه: – (ق).
٢٠٣. على النصف: – (ق).
٢٠٤. والسمن البقرى: – (ق).
٢٠٥. الحلوى البلدى: – (ق).
٢٠٦. البالغ: – (ق).
٢٠٧. المستوى: – (ق).
٢٠٨. حتى لا يبقى ... والسلام : فهذه كلها نافعه تقوي الدماغ والاعضاء (ق).

الثالث <*10*> في بيان الادوية المفرده التى هو خلاصة الادوية النافعة لجميع الامراض التى يعالج بها خصوصا لتقوية الافعال فى الجماع[٢٠٩] وزيادة المنى وقوة الباه قال اولها المسك والعنبر والزعفران والشقاقل وقنطريون وكبابه فلفل وزنجبيل وقرنفل <٣٠> وابو زيدان ولك وقرفه وعود هندي ولسان العصافير وقشر اترنج وينسون وفستق وخيار ودار فلفل وقسط وخطمية الثعلب والبض الاحمر والابيض[٢١٠] والخوالنجان وعاقرقرح[٢١١] وشحم الاسد ولحية التيس وزفت رومى وخشخاش وبزر الجزر وبزر اللفت وبزر الرشاد وجوزه وبسباسة وسنبل ومصطكى وقاقله وبورق ارضى[٢١٢] ارمنى ولؤلؤ غير مثقوب وزرنباد وسادج هندى وهليلج وبليلج واملج وحرير والحبة السودا وحوز الهندى وسعد[٢١٣] وجميع هذه الادويـة المذكوره لتقوية الجماع والباه وزيـادة المنى ودفـع الامراض وهـولاء خاصة الادويـة المستعملة المفيده ولا جل هذا ذكرناها فانتبه لها اذا ذكرت كل <٣١> واحد منها فى مقامه كما سيأتى

٢٠٩. الافعال فى الجماع : افعال الجماع (غ).

٢١٠. البض الاحمر والابيض: الهنا الابيض والاحمر (غ).

٢١١. عاقرقرح: عاقرقرحا (غ).

٢١٢. ارضى: – (غ).

٢١٣. سعد: السعد (غ).

ذلك عند الاحتاج الى ذكرها الباب الرابع[٢١٤] فى بيان الادويـة والاغدية المركبة[٢١٥] والحلويات التي تصلح مزاج[٢١٦] الانسان وتزيل علة[٢١٧] الفالج ورخاوة الاعضا وتقوى افعال الجماع والباه قال[٢١٨] يوخذ من[٢١٩] البصل الابيض و[٢٢٠] يقشر ويقطع ويطبخ بقليل زيت وماء حتى ينـهرى[٢٢١] ثـم يطبخ افـراخ الحـمـام <١١> بالملح الاندرانى[٢٢٢] فاذا استوى وتهرى[٢٢٣] يصب عليه البصل الذي طبخته بالزيت وتقلية معه حتى يختلطا جيدا ثم يوخذ وزن درهم قرفه ودرهم خولنجان ودرهم عود صليب تسحق هـذه الادويـة وترش على البصل[٢٢٤] المطبوخ ويوكل بالخبز الفطير ويشرب مرقته نافع

---

٢١٤. في بان الادوية المفرده... الباب الرابع: – (ق).
٢١٥. المركبة: – (ق).
٢١٦. مزاج: – (ق).
٢١٧. علة: – (ق).
٢١٨. قال: فمن ذلك (ق).
٢١٩. من: – (ق).
٢٢٠. و: – (ق).
٢٢١. ينهرى: يتهري (غ).
٢٢٢. بالملح الاندرانى: (ق).
٢٢٣. وتهرى: – (ق).
٢٢٤. الـذي طبخته... البصل: ويغلي حتي تختلط بـه ثـم يؤخذ قرفة وخولنجان وعود صليب من كل واحد درهم يدق ويرش علي ذلك المطبوخ (ق).

مفيد[٢٢٥] يصلح المزاج الفاسد وينور الوجه ويصفى اللون والدم ويقوى <٣٢> الجماع وله سبعة عشر فايده غير ما ذكرناه ولو عددناها لطال الكلام وتظهر تلك الفوايد عند استعمالها ان شا الله تعالى غيره قال[٢٢٦] يوخذ لحم الخروف يكون لا سمينا ولا هزيلا معتدلا بين الشيئين وتدق كبيبان ويطبخ بقدره[٢٢٧] بصل ابيض حتى ينهرى[٢٢٨] ثم يوخذ قليل[٢٢٩] من دهن الجوز ويجعل عليه قاقلا ودرهم قرفه ونصف درهم قرنفل[٢٣٠] وقيراط مسك ويسحق هذه الادوية[٢٣١] وتخلط[٢٣٢] بدهن الجوز وتصب[٢٣٣] على اللحم في القدر وتحرك حتى تتخطا جميعا ويغلى شويه فينزل وهو مسدود الغطا[٢٣٤] حتى لا يخرج بخاره ويترك ساعة حتى يبرد ويعتدل يوكل منه

٢٢٥. يشرب مرقته نافع مفيد: يشرب عليه المسرفه فانه نافع (ق).
٢٢٦. وله سبعة .... قال: نوع آخر (ق).
٢٢٧. الخروف... بقدره: الضاءن الصغير ويدق ويعمل الكباب ويطبخ ويرمي عليه (ق).
٢٢٨. ينهرى: يتهرى (غ).
٢٢٩. ثم يوخذ قليل: ويؤخذ (ق).
٢٣٠. ويجعل ... قرنفل: حزء وقاقله وقرفه وقرنفل من كل واحد درهم (ق).
٢٣١. ويسحق هذه الادوية: – (ق).
٢٣٢. تخلط: يخلط – (ق).
٢٣٣. تصب: يصب (ق).
٢٣٤. الغطا: الفم (غ).

وقت الغدا فانه يصلح المزاج الفاسد ويزيل الرخاوه ويشد الباه ويزيد المنى ويقوى الجماع كما ينبغى وله منافع كثيره هذا تظهر <٣٣> عند استعمالها والسلام غيره قال[٢٣٥] يوخذ الفراريج وتذبح وتنشف وتغسل ثم تشرح شرحات وترش على ناحية منها[٢٣٦] ملح اندرانى وتشوى على جمر وتقلب ظهرا وبطنا حتى تستوى معتدلا فيوخذ قدر خمسة دراهم حبة السودا وثلاثة دراهم[٢٣٧] من لحية التيس واربعة دراهم لسان عصفور ونصف درهم جوز الهند[٢٣٨] الجميع ويرش منهم على اللحم ثم يتعشى به من بحين فانه يقوى الاعضا الرئيسه ويزيد فى الحرارة الغريزية ويزيل البرودات من الظهر والوسط ويخرج الرطوبات والفضلات من البدن ويحمر الوجه ويصفى الدم ويقوى الجماع ولو جامع ثلاثة ايام متواليه لا يبالى ولا يضعف ومع ذلك يرضى كل ليلة عشر من الجوار ومن النساء <٣٤> الاحرار من غير تشويش وانزعاج كذا ذكروه الحكما والاطبا المتقدمون وقالوا ان هذه الاسرار لا ينبغى {لاحد}

---

٢٣٥. تحرك حتى ... قال: يحرك حتي يمنزج بها وينزل ويشرب فانه نافع لما ذكر ان شاء الله وغيره (ق).

٢٣٦. منها: منهم (غ).

٢٣٧. دراهم: – (غ).

٢٣٨. الهند: الهندي + يسحق (غ).

كشفها الا على اهلها واذا استعملها الانسان ودوام عليها يظهر له زوايد ومنافع فى اسرع وقت والسلام فصل فى بيان الحلاوات اذا استعملها الانسان يصلح[٢٣٩] مزاجه وتصلح المفلوج وتزيل الرخاوة وتقوى الاعضا الرئيسه وتزيد الحرارة الغريزية وتقوى الجماع وتزيد المنى وذلك ان ياخذ وزن[٢٤٠] ماية درهم عسل نحل الابيض منزوح الرغوه مع وزنه بصل ابيض يقشر ويقطع صغارا <١٢> ويطبخ مع العسل ويجعل عليه[٢٤١] <*11*> قليل ماء[٢٤٢] حتى ينهرى[٢٤٣] البصل ثم يجعل عليه قليل زيت وينقل ويجعل فى قدره ويوقد[٢٤٤] علي نار لينه الى ان ينعقد نصف انعقاد ثم يصفى <٣٥> ويصبر قليلا حتى يبرد ثم يرش علي[٢٤٥] هذا السحوق وهو من القرفه

---

٢٣٩. يصلح: تصلح (غ).

٢٤٠. وتذبج وتنشف.... وزن: وتطبخ ويرمي عليها خمسة دراهم لسان عصفور ودرهم جوز هندي ودرهم قرفة وقرنفل ويحرره حتي يمتزج بها وينزل ويتعشا به فانه عاية لما ذكر واما الحلويات في اصلح المزاج وتقوي الاعضاء الرئيسة وتزيل الرخاوه وتزيد الحرارة الغريزيه ومنها يؤخذ (ق).

٢٤١. الابيض... عليه: ومثله بصل ابيض يقطع ويرمي العسل المنزوع الرغوه ويصب عليه (ق).

٢٤٢. ماء: الماء (غ).

٢٤٣. ينهرى: تتهري (غ).

٢٤٤. يوقد: يغلي (غ).

٢٤٥. علي: عليه (غ).

خمسة دراهم ومن قشر الاترنج[٢٤٦] خمسة دراهم وعود هندى درهمين ونصف درهم زعفران يدقوا ناعما[٢٤٧] وينخلوا من خرقة حرير ويضافوا الى العسل والبصل ويضربوا بالملعقة وترفعهم فى اناء قزاز وتستعمل منه كل ليلة عند النوم ترى[٢٤٨] العجب نوع اخر قال يوخذ حمص اصفر ينقع فى الماء ثم يقشر و[٢٤٩]يغلى فى سمن بقرى الى ان يحمر واياك ان يسود ويحترق ثم يدق ناعما ويجعل عليه وزنه لب صنوبر[٢٥٠] شامى مدقوق ويخلط في عسل نحل ابيض منزوع الرغوه ويرش عليه هذه الادوية مسحوقه وهي نصف درهم زعفران وخمسة دراهم قشر اترنج ودرهم قرفه لف ونصف درهم عود هندى وعشرة <٣٦> دراهم عود صيني يسحقوا ناعما وترش على الادوية ويحركوا ثم

٢٤٦. ثم يجعل ... الاترنج : ويأخذ العسل في الانعقاد فيرش عليه وقرفه وقشر الاترنج من كل (ق).

٢٤٧. ناعما: + ويسحقوا (غ).

٢٤٨. ونصف... يرى: مدقوق ودرهم زعفران وينزل ويرفع في اناء زجاج ويستعمل منه عند النوم كل ليلة يرا (ق) / كل ليلة عند النوم ترى: عند النوم في كل ليلة (غ).

٢٤٩. اصفر... و: مقشر بعد نقعه في ماء ثم (ق).

٢٥٠. واياك ... صنوبر: ثم يدق ناعما ويضاف وزنه لب شونيز (ق) / صنوبر: شونيز (غ).

ترفعوا[٢٥١] ويستعملوا عند النوم كل يوم ترى العجب ولو كان لك عشر جوار ترضيهن فى ليلة من غير انزعاج ولا تغير مزاج مجرب والسلام[٢٥٢] الباب الخامس فى بيان الاشربه التى تصلح المزاج الفاسد وتصفى الدم وتقوى جميع الافعال للجماع والباه اعلم ان الشراب اذا كان حلوا واحمر اللون يقال له الشراب للعلى فهو مفيد واما الشراب الذي يميل الى الصفر يقال له الشراب اليزدى ويكون حلوا[٢٥٣] بيض مفيد واما الشراب الذى يعتصر من العنب الابيض المستوى البالغ يقال له الشراب الريحاني وهو ايضا مفيد ولكن احسنهم ان يكون ممزوجا مطبوخا لان الشراب[٢٥٤] يضر بل ينبغى ان يكون مثلثا <٣٧> كعادة الحكما مطبوخا بالادوية حتى يناسب الطبيعة ويحصل[٢٥٥] الفوايد كما علموا ذلك بالتجارب صفة الشراب المثلث قال هو على عادة الحكما هو يوخذ من اى نوع اردت من الاشربة

---

٢٥١. ترفعوا: يرفعوا (غ).

٢٥٢. مدقوق ويخلط... والسلام: ويصب عليه بقدره عسل نحل منزوع الرغوه حتي يمتزج به ثم يرش عليه قشر اترنج خمس دراهم وزعفران نصف درهم ويحرك وينزل ويستعمل منه كل يوم عند النوم مثقال تر العجب العجيب لما ذكر (ق).

٢٥٣. حلوا: + فهو (غ).

٢٥٤. الشراب: + الصرف (غ).

٢٥٥. يحصل: تحصل (غ).

المذكورة وتجعل عليه قدره ثلاث مرات ماء عذب صافى يغلى حتى يذهب ثلثى الماء ويبقى الثلث فيوخذ من هذا المطبوخ وزن ثلاثماية درهم ووزن خمسين درهم من عسل النحل الابيض[٢٥٦] او سكر ابيض ويغلى الي ان يوخذ رغوته ثم يوخذ[٢٥٧] زنجبيل ودار صينى من كل واحد درهمين وعود هندى وعنبر وسنبل من كل واحد درهم يدق الجميع ناعما كالغبار وينخلوا من خرقة حرير ثم يضعهم[٢٥٨] على الشراب ثم يغلى ثانيا بنار لينه ساعة لطيفه حتى يمتزج <١٣> بعضها[٢٥٩] <٣٨> ببعض ثم ينزل وتصبر عليه حتى يبرد ثم يرفع فى اناء زجاج واذا اراد الاستعمال منه ياخذ منه وزن اربعين درهما وتمزج بوزنهم ماء وتشربهم نافع ان شاء الله تعالى يقوى المعده ويسخن الكبد وينور الوجة ويصفى الدم ويقوى الحرارة الغريزية والجماع ولو جامع عشر جوار لأرضاهن من غير تعب ولا ضعف ولا ازعاج بل يزداد

---

٢٥٦. جميع الافعال... الابيض: الجماع ويسمي بالشراب المثلث يؤخذ من ماء العنب جزء ويجعل عليه ماء عذب قدره بثلاث مرات ويغلي حتي يبقي الثلث فيوخذ منه وزن ثلاث مائة درهم ومن العسل النحل خمسين درهما (ق).

٢٥٧. الى ان ... يوخذ: ثم يضاف له (ق).

٢٥٨. يضعهم: تضعهم (غ).

٢٥٩. يمتزج بعضها: تمتزج بعضهم (غ).

نشاطا ولكن يصبر بعد[٢٦٠] ساعتين ثم يجامع ولا ياكل شيءٌ الابعد الجماع يرى عجبا ان شا الله تعالى[٢٦١] الباب السادس <12> فى بيان المعاجين والجوارشات[٢٦٢] المفرحه الدافعة للملال[٢٦٣] التى تقوى المعده وتدفع[٢٦٤] البلغم والسودا وتدفع سدد الدماغ والاعضا[٢٦٥] وتصفى الدم وتحلل الرياح الفاسده وتقوى <٣٩> الاعضا الرئيسه وتزيل الصداع ووجع الراس والنزلات و[٢٦٦]الحرارة الغريزية[٢٦٧] وتقوى الجماع قوة عظيمة حتى لو جامع عشرين امراة لم يحصل له كلل ولا ملل ولا ارتخاء عضو بسبب هذا المعجون وفوايده لا تعد ولا تحصى خصوصا فايدته عند الجماع والاستعمال صفة جوارش القاقله قال مولفه عفى الله عنه[٢٦٨] يوخذ حصا

---

٢٦٠. بعد: + شربه (غ).

٢٦١. يدق الجميع... تعالى: حتي يمنزج وينزل ثم يرفع في اناء زجاج فاذا اراد استعمال يؤخذ منه وزن اربعين درهما ويمزج بوزنه ماء عدب ويشرب فانه نافع لما ذكر ان شاء الله (ق).

٢٦٢. والجوارشات: – (ق).

٢٦٣. الدافعة للملال: – (ق).

٢٦٤. وتدفع: + الصفراء و (غ).

٢٦٥. البلغم ... الاعضاء: الصفرا والبلغم والسوداء وتفتح السدد في المعدة (ق).

٢٦٦. و: + تقوي (غ).

٢٦٧. ووجع... الغريزية: – (ق).

٢٦٨. حتى لو... الله عنه: صفة جوارش القاقلة (ق).

لبان[٢٦٩] وقاقلة وبسباسه من كل واحد اربعة دراهم ودار فلفل فزنجبيل[٢٧٠] من كل واحد ثمانية دراهم وعنبر وعود هندى من كل واحد درهم ومن الزعفران عشرة دراهم[٢٧١] تدق[٢٧٢] الادوية وتنخل ناعما كالكحل ويوخذ قوامه[٢٧٣] عسل نحل منزوع الرغوه ويكون على نصف قوامه ثم يضاف اليه الادوية ويرفع ويستعمل عند الحاجة اليه ترى عجبا والسلام[٢٧٤] <٤٠> صفة معجون السنبل قال يوخذ سنبل وبسباسه وحوز وقرنفل وحبة السودا[٢٧٥] وقاقلة ودار صينى من كل واحد نصف[٢٧٦] درهم وسمسم ابيض[٢٧٧] مقشر ستين درهما تدق الادوية وحدهم والسمسم وحده ناعما كالغبار ثم يخلطا[٢٧٨] ويعجن بعسل منزوع الرغوه على نصف قوامه

---

٢٦٩. حصا لبان: + ذكر (ق).

٢٧٠. فزنجبيل: وزنجبيل (ق) / (غ).

٢٧١. وعنبر ... عشرة دراهم: وعوده درهم وعنبر درهم وزعفران ثلث دراهم (ق).

٢٧٢. تدق: يدق (غ).

٢٧٣. وتنخل... قوامه: وترمي في (ق).

٢٧٤. ويكون... والسلام حتي ينعقد ويرفع ويستعمل منه وزن مثقال بعد العشاء تر العجب (ق).

٢٧٥. السوداء: سوداء (ق).

٢٧٦. نصف: – (ق).

٢٧٧. ابيض: – (ق).

٢٧٨. تدق... ويخلطا: – (ق).

ويستعمل منه عند الحاجه اليه وزن ثلاث دراهم ترى عجبا خصوصا عند الجماع صفة معجون ذوى الحسك قال يوخذ[٢٧٩] شوك الحسك ما اردت يقطع صغار ويوضع في قدره ويغلى عليه بالمآ حتى يخرج قوة الحسك[٢٨٠] فى الماء ثم يصفى المآ المنتخب فى الحسك الذى يبقى قشره ويوخذ قشره وورقه ويسقى المآ الذى صفيته في الشمس الحاره ايام الصيف وكلما جف ونشف تسقيه وحركه <٤١> الى ان يشرب المآ الذى صفيته ويبقى ليناً مستويا[٢٨١] فيوخذ منه درهم وعاقرقرح درهم وزنجيل نصف درهم وعشرة دراهم من ادمغة العصافير <١٤> الدرورية ثم تسحق[٢٨٢] الادوية سحقا بليغا وتخلط مع الادمغة خلطا جيدا ويضاف اليهم قوامهم من السكر او من العسل النحل المنزوع الرغوه

٢٧٩. يعجن ... يوخذ: بعد الدق بالعسل النحل حتي ينعقد ويستعمل منه عند الحاجة ثلاث دراهم تر العجب معجون الحسك يؤخذ من (ق).

٢٨٠. ما اردت... الحسك: جزء يقطع ويغمر بالماء ويغلي علي النار حتي تخرج قوته (ق).

٢٨١. ثم يصفى... مستويا: فيصفي ويتبقي من قشره ومرقه ثم يوضع في الشمس الحاره فكلما نشف اسقه من ذلك الماء حتي يلين (ق).

٢٨٢. تسحق: يسحق (غ).

ويعقد معجونا[٢٨٣] ويجعل فى آنا زجاج ويستعمل منه عند الحاجة اليه واذا[٢٨٤] اراد الجماع يشرب عليه قد حين ثلاثه من الشراب المثلث الذى تقدم وصفه يرى عجبا حتى لو جامع عشر[٢٨٥] من النسا فى ليلة لارضاهن والسلام[٢٨٦] <*13*> صفة الاطريفل وله منافع عظيمة وفوايد لا تعد ولا تحصى منها انه يزيد فى العقل[٢٨٧] وينقى[٢٨٨] الدماغ من جميع العلل والنزلا[٢٨٩] ويحد البصر ويزيد <٤٢> نوره ويفتح سدد الراس والعين[٢٩٠] ويقوي سمع الاذان[٢٩١] ويصفى الدم وسمن ويقوي الاعضا الرئيسه والحرارة الغريزية ويقوى الباه ويشد الاعصاب[٢٩٢] وعروق الذكر والخصيتين ويسخن الكلا

---

٢٨٣. درهم وزنجبيل ... معجونا: وزنجبيل من كل درهم وادمغة العصافير عشرة دراهم ويسحقهم سحقا جيدا ثم يعقد بالعسل النحل (ق).

٢٨٤. واذا: فاذا (ق).

٢٨٥. عشر: عشرة (غ).

٢٨٦. يشرب ... والسلام: تشرب عليه قد حين الشراب المثلث المتقدم ذكره فانه غايه والله اعلم (ق).

٢٨٧. ولو ... العقل: – (ق).

٢٨٨. ينقى: ينفع (ق).

٢٨٩. النزلا: النزلات (غ).

٢٩٠. نوره ويفتح سدد الراس والعين: العقل (ق).

٢٩١. الاذن: – (ق).

٢٩٢. الرئيسه ...الاعصاب: – (غ).

والمثانه والمنى ويقوى الجماع تقوية عظيمه بحيث لو جامع ما شا لا يمل ولا يضعف ولا يرتخي ولا يضره وصفته يوخذ قشره وهليله صفرا وبليله واملج[٢٩٣] ودار فلفل من كل واحد ثلاثة دراهم وبسباسه وزنجبيل من كل واحد اربعة دراهم وشقاقل[٢٩٤] درهم ولسان عصفور[٢٩٥] خمسة دراهم ودار صينى سبعة دراهم وسمسم ابيض مقشور عشرون[٢٩٦] درهما يدق هذه الادوية ناعما وينخل من خرقة رفيعة[٢٩٧] ويضاف اليهم نصف قوامهم[٢٩٨] سكر ابيض <٤٣> او عسل نحل منزوع الرغوه ويعجن الحوايج به ويرفع فى آنا قزاز[٢٩٩] ويسد راسه ويدفن فى الشعير اربعين يوما ثم يستعمل منه عند الحاجة اليه ثلاث مثاقيل ويشرب بالماء نافع ان شا الله تعالى مجرب[٣٠٠] الباب السابع فى بيان الشفايات

٢٩٣. يقوي الباه... واملج: يشد العصب والذكر ويسخن الكلا والمثانه ومني ويقوي الجماع قوة عطيمة وصفة اهليلج واملج وبليلج (ق).

٢٩٤. وبسباسه ... وشقاقل: بسباسه وشقاقل (ق).

٢٩٥. عصفور: العصافير (ق) / (غ).

٢٩٦. عشرون: عشرين (ق).

٢٩٧. هذه الادوية... رفيع: الادويه وتنخل (ق).

٢٩٨. اليهم نصف قوامهم: اليها (ق).

٢٩٩. الرغوة... قزاز: ويرفع في اناء زجاج (ق).

٣٠٠. نافع ... مجرب: فانه نافع لما ذكر ان شاء الله (ق).

التى تدفع الرطوبات من الاعضا ويزيل[٣٠١] البرودات من الظهر والوسط[٣٠٢] وتجذب البلغم والصفرا والسودا ويقوى الجماع بالغا وصفته قال[٣٠٣] يوخذ سكر ابيض خمسة[٣٠٤] دراهم وزنجبيل درهمين[٣٠٥] وعاقرقرح[٣٠٦] قيراط يسحق الجميع ناعما كالكحل[٣٠٧] ويعجن بعسل نحل منزوع الرغوه ماخود القوام ويجعلوا اشيافا ويشتف[٣٠٨] منه عند النوم نافع ان شاء الله تعالى نوع اخر قال[٣٠٩] المفيد[٣١٠] يوخذ ادمغة ثلاث عصافير وقيراط عاقرقرح[٣١١] اجزا <٤٤> سواء يدقوا ناعما وينخلوا ويعجنوا بالعسل النحل ويجعلوا اشيافا ويشف منها عند

---

٣٠١. يزيل: تزيل (غ).

٣٠٢. تدفع .... والوسط: – (ق).

٣٠٣. بالغا وصفته قال: جدا ويهيج الشهوة يهيجا عظيما وصفة (ق).

٣٠٤. خمسة: خمس (ق).

٣٠٥. درهمين: درهمان (ق).

٣٠٦. عاقرقرح: عاقرقرحا (غ).

٣٠٧. يسحق الجميع ناعما كالكحل: ويدق (ق).

٣٠٨. ماخود القوام ويجعلوا اشيافا ويشتف: ويستعمل (ق) / يشتف: يشيف (غ).

٣٠٩. ان شاء الله تعالى نوع اخر قال المفيد: لما ذكر نوع اخر (ق).

٣١٠. المفيد: – (غ).

٣١١. عاقرقرح: عاقرقرحا (غ).

النوم يحصل المقصود[٣١٢] نافع نوع اخر قال يوخذ[٣١٣] لب القطن وسورنجان من كل واحد ثلاث[٣١٤] دراهم يدق ناعما ويعجن <14> بشحم الاسد ويجعلا الشيافا[٣١٥] ويتشف به[٣١٦] عند النوم <١٥> بالقطن يرى عجبا خصوصا فى قوة الجماع يحصل المقصود نافع ان شا الله تعالى[٣١٧] الباب الثامن فى بيان الحقن التى تمنع وجع المفاصل وذات عرق النساء ووجع الظهر والوسط ويدفع الارياح الفاسده والقولنج ويشد الظهر ويقوى افعال الجماع قال يوخذ خصي[٣١٨] الخرفان يدق دقا

---

٣١٢. اجزا... المقصود : يدق ناعما وينخل من خرقة رفيعة ويخلط مع الادوية ويوضعهم فوامهم عسل نحل ويجعل شافا ويستعمل عند النوم ويكن بعد الاحتماء والتسقية من المغلظات (غ).

٣١٣. اجزا... يوخذ: وقرفة وقرنفل وزنجبيل من كل درهم ويجق ويخلط مع العسل ويستعمل عند النوم نافع لم ذكر جدا ونوع يؤخذ لب القطن وعاقرقرحا وزنجبيل يدق ويعجن بالعسل ويستعمل عند النوم يحصل المقصود نوع آخر (ق).

٣١٤. ثلاث: ثلاثة (ق).

٣١٥. والسورنجان ... الشيافا: وعاقرقرحا اجزا سواء ويدقوا ناعما وينخلوا ويعجنوه بالعسل النحل ويجعلوا مشيافا (غ).

٣١٦. به: بها (غ).

٣١٧. ناعما... تعالى: ويعجن بشحم الاسد مع السل ويستعمل عند النوم يري العجب معجب (ق).

٣١٨. التي تمنع... خصي: لوجع المفاصل وعرق النساء والقولنج وتدفع الارياح الفاسده وتقوي الجمع وتنفع وجع الظهر وصفة يؤخذ خصا (ق).

جريشا ويوخذ قدره قمح احمر[٣١٩] وقبضة بزر لفت ويجعل فى قدر برام[٣٢٠] ويصب فوقه غمره ماء[٣٢١] <٤٥> ويسد راس القدر بغطا ويوضع[٣٢٢] فى الفرن ليلة حتى يتهرى فاذا اصبح يخرجه وياخذ من مائية وزن ثلاثين درهما يوضع عليه وزن درهمين من دهن الجوز الهندى[٣٢٣] ويحتقن به وقت الصبح[٣٢٤] بعد الاحتما ويكون خالى البطن[٣٢٥] وبجعل تحت وسطه مخده لا عاليه حتى راسه الى اسفل ورجليه الى فوق[٣٢٦] بحيث يصل الماء الى بطنه وتجرى فى مصارنيه يرى[٣٢٧] عجبا ولو احتقن به فى كل سنة مرتين مر فى فصل الربيع ومره فى فصْل الخريف يامن من جميع الامراض والاسقام باذن الله تعالى نوع اخر قال[٣٢٨] يوخذ بزر الجزر وبزر القرع

---

٣١٩. دقا جريشا ويوخذ قدره قمح احمر: وقدره قمح (ق).
٣٢٠. ويجعل فى قدر برام: ويوضع في قدر (ق).
٣٢١. غمره ماء: ماء حتي يغمره (ق).
٣٢٢. راس...فرن: راسها ويرفع (ق).
٣٢٣. الجوز الهندى: جوز الهند (غ).
٣٢٤. يتهرى ... الصبح: يتهرا فيؤمن ماية صباحا وزن ثلاثين درهما ويوضع عليه درهمان من دهن جوز الهند ومحتقون به صباحا (ق).
٣٢٥. ويكون خالى البطن: – (ق).
٣٢٦. فوق: + ويحقن (غ).
٣٢٧. يرى: ترى (غ).
٣٢٨. لا عاليه ... قال: بحيث يصل الدواء الي بطنه ويجري في

وشبت[٣٢٩] وبزر بصل وكراث وقرفه وزنجبيل وفلفل[٣٣٠] ودار فلفل من كل واحد ثلاثة دراهم وكبشة حمص مقشر وكبشة قمح مدقوق <٤٦> وقطعة ليّنه وقليل من دهن الخـروف الضأن وخصى الخـروف ويجعل هذا المجموع[٣٣١] فى قدره ويسد راسها بغطا وتوضع فى تنور حامى او فرن حامى ليلة حتى يتهرى ثم يوخذ ويحتقن به وهى {التى} يسمونها[٣٣٢] الحقنه الملينه ولها سبعة وعشرون فايدة اذا[٣٣٣] احتفن بها فى فصل الربيع مرة يامن فى سنة الى الربيع الاخر من[٣٣٤] جميع الامراض والاسقام باذن الله تعالى الباب التاسع فى بيان الشدود والثياب التى تناسب طبيعة الانسان <*15*> اذا اشتد بها فى وسطه فى كل فصل من الفصول الاربعة فان الشدود اذا خالف طبيعة الانسان بحسب الفصول ربما يبتلى

مصاريه فانه نافع لجميع الامراض فيفعل في فصل الريع مره وفي فصل الصيف وعجبا نوع اخر (ق).

٣٢٩. وشبت: – (ق).

٣٣٠. وكراث وقرفه وزنجبيل وفلفل: بزر كراث وبزر شبت وقرفه وقرنفل وزنجبيل (ق) فلفل: قرنفل (غ).

٣٣١. المجموع: الجميع (غ).

٣٣٢. وقطعة لينة ... يسمونها: وقليل دهن ضان وقطعه لينه خروف ويوضع في قدر ويغمر با لمء ويسد راسها ويوضع في الفرن ليله حتي يتهي ويحتقن به وتسمي بالمليه (ق).

٣٣٣. اذا: فاذا (ق).

٣٣٤. الى الربيع الاخر من: – (ق).

بمرض من الامراض فينبغى ان يكون الشدود والثياب منسابا للاوقات التي <٤٧> ينبغى فيها لبس ذلك حتى تشد اعضاوه وتقويها ولا يفسد مزاجه فطهرات المناسب من الشدود ومن ذلك اللباس والملابس فى فصل الربيع الذى هو اعدل الفصول الذى يستوى فيه الحر والبرد ان يكون من القطن لانه معتدل الحرارة والبرود لا يخرج الاعضا من الاعتدال ولا يفسد المراج واما الفصل الثانى <١٦> الذى هو فصل الصيف الذى يقوى فيه الحر فينبغى ان تكون الدكك والشدود فى هذا الفصل كلها ملمعه منسوجه من الحرير والكتان او الكتان وحده ولا تكون من الحرير وحده واما فصل الخريف فينبغى ان تكون الشدود والملابس في هذا الفصل من الصوف والمنسوج من التنكيك[٣٣٥] واما الفرا فينبغى ان تكون من <٤٨> السمور والقاقم والسنجاب او فرا الخرفان الابيض منه والاسود منه ويكون شده من صوف الجمال ومن جلد السمور الذى يصفونه على هيئية شد يقال له بالتركى كمر قشاق فاذا دبر على هذا التدبير مشى على هذا المنوال يحصل له الامن من ارتخاء[٣٣٦] الاعضا الرئيسه ضعفا ويامن من

٣٣٥. من التنكيك: والتفكيك (غ).

٣٣٦. الارتخاء: + وضعف الجراح والمنى بسبب اختلاف الادوية

وجاع المفاصل والضربان والقولنج ومن الامراض المختلفة[٣٣٧] .بمشيئة الله تعالى الباب العاشر فى بيان شروط الجماع وكيف يبغى ان يجمع حتى لا يصل اليه ضعف ولا ضرر ولا سرعة الشيب والشيخوخه قال اعلم ان الجماع[٣٣٨] قايما يضر الانسان غاية الضرر[٣٣٩] ويورث له الخفقان وذات الجنب وعرق النساء وذات[٣٤٠] الريه والنقرس والصداع نعوذ بالله من ذلك كله فانها امراض مهلكة <٤٩> صعبة المداواة يحدث غالبها من الجماع واقفا وبعض الناس لا يعتمد على هذا الكلام ويقول انا جامعت هكذا ولا حصل لى من هذا الامراض شى فنقول ان هذه الامراض التى تحصل من الجماع قايما تارة تحدث على الفرور وتارة على التراخي الى اخر عمره عند ضعف الحرارة الغريزية بحسب قوة المزاج وضعفه

ولا يكون (غ).

٣٣٧. فان الشدود...القولنج ومن: وكذا لبس الثياب المناسب للاوقات لاشتداد الاعضاء وتقويتها فمما يناسب في فصل الربيع لبس القطن فانه لايخرج الاعضاء من الاعتدال ولا يفسد المزاج ومما يناسب لبسه في فصل الصيف لبس الكتان وحده وفي فصل الخريف لبس الصوف المنسوج واما لبس الفر فالسمون والقاقم والسنجاب والغنم الابيض والاسود فينفع من ارتخاء الاعضاء ومنعو المزاج و (ق).

٣٣٨. وكيف... اعلم ان: وكيفيته فالجماع (ق).

٣٣٩. غاية الضرر: – (ق).

٣٤٠. ذات: – (ق).

من اين علم هذا القايل بانه سلم من الحوق شى من هذه الامراض ربما يعرض له ذلك على التراخى على انا قلنا هذا القول اذا اكثر من الجماع قايما اما اذا لم يكثر بل فعله مرة او مرتين فى عمره فلا لان الذى يفعل هذا الشى ما يفعله الامر كثرة الشغف والمحبة فى حال الشبوبية فربما دافع الم ذلك <٥٠> وضرره كثرة حرارته الغريزية وقوة اعضايه الرئيسه وبعض هذه الابدان يوثر فيه ضرر ذلك الانه لم يميز حاله لجهله باحوال نفسه وقواه هذا القدر يكفى للعاقل والسلام واما الجماع وهو قايم على ضلعه فهو مضر غاية الضرر[٣٤١] يحدث منه[٣٤٢] وجع الفواد {والقلب} والكبد ويبتلى عرض[٣٤٣] القولنج وسلس البول نعوذ بالله من ذلك كله خصوصا اذا جامع على شقه الايمن فانه اضروا نحس من اليسر وكذلك الجماع <١٧> قايما على قفاه والمراة من فوقه[٣٤٤] يورث وجع المثانه وانعقاد البول والتنقيط واحتراق البول ويبتلى بوجع المرء وهو سيلان الدم والقيح مع البول اذا بال او وحده بلا بول نعوذ باالله من ذلك فينبغى <٥١>

---

٣٤١. نعوذ بالله ...الضرر: نايما (ق).
٣٤٢. منه: – (ق).
٣٤٣. يبتلى عرض: – (ق).
٣٤٤. نعوذ بالله... فوق: والجماع علي الايمن اضر من الايسر وقائم علي القفاء وهو علي المرأة عليه (ق) .

للعاقل ان يحترز من الجماع على الهيئات المذكوره المضره حينئذ حتى لا يبتلى بما ذكرناه من الامراض اما علاج هذه الامراض هو ان يوخذ[٣٤٥] من عنب الديب المستوى البالغ ويعصره ثم ياخذ الاردج البالغ المستوى ويستخرج ما وه بالطبخ ثم يجعل عليه من سكر القند قوامه ثم يخلط المايز ماءين ماء عنب الديب ومآ الاردج وياخذ قوامها على النار اللينه ثم يستعمل منه قدر ملعقه على الريق وملعقه عند النوم نافع ان شا الله تعالى فصل واعلم ان احسن الهيئات واولى الاشكال من الجماع ان تستلقى المراه على قفاها استلقاء مستويا وتضع تحت وسطها مخده رقيقه وترفع المراه فخذيها بنفسها ولا يرفعها الرجل فان ذلك مشقة على <٥٢> الرجل عند المجامعه تضره وان يقوم الرجل على يدية واصابع رجليه الى ان يقرب انزال المنى فاذا اخذ فى الانزال يضع الرجل ركبتيه على الارض ويلقى نفسه على المراه تعانقه بيديها ورجليها وتلم الرجل على صدرها لماً قوياً الى ان يتم انزال المنى وينقطع انزاله فى الرحم مستقيما مستويا ولا ينتصب منحرفا ولا يضيع المنى فيحصل من اضاعته عدم حصول التولد والتناسل ويحصل الضرر للرجل واذا وقع الجماع على الوجه والشروط الذي ذكرناه يحصل له

٣٤٥. يوخذ: يأخذ (غ).

الفوايد التى ويامن العلل التى قدمناها الباب الحادى عشر فى بيان الادوية التى اذا طلابها على الذكر تغلظه وتشده وتجعله قايمًا من غير رخاوة خصوصا اذا كان الرجل <٥٣> لا يقدر على اكل الادوية الحاره يعالج بالادوية التى تطلى على الذكر وذلك ان تاخذ بصل النرجس[٣٤٦] وعاقر قرح[٣٤٧] وزبيب احمر منزوع النوى اجزا سواء وتدق الادوية مع ربعها جوز الهند[٣٤٨] <*16*> وتسحق الجميع ناعما ثم تغسل ذكره قبل الجماع بساعة بالماء الحار ويدلكه دلكا قويا حالة الغسل ثم يطلى ذكره بالادوية مقابل حرارة النار يحصل له ما ذكرناه من الغلظ والقوة واحكامه كما ينبغى نوع اخر قال يوخذ لب بزر القطن نصف درهم وسعد درهمين ونصف ولد نوى الخروب <١٨> الشامى نصف درهم وقيراط

---

٣٤٦. انعقاد البول ... النرجس: احتراق البول والنقطه وسيلان الدم فينبغي للعاقل ان يحترز من الجماع علي الهيأت المذكورة فينبغي هذا ان تستلقي المراه علي قفاه وتضع تحتها وسطها يجده وترفع مخدتها ويقوم الرجل علي اصابع رجليه الى ان يقرب انزال المني يلقي نفسه علي المرأة وتعانقه بيديها الي الن يتم انزال المني فيحصل له الفايدة ويامن العلل المتقدمه ان شاء الله تعالي الباب الحادي عشر في بيان الادوية لتقويته وتغليظه يؤخذ بصل نرجس (ق).

٣٤٧. عاقر قرح: عاقرقرحا (غ).

٣٤٨. تدق الادوية مع ربعها جوز الهند: يدق مع ربعه جوز الهندي (ق).

جوز الهند يدق الجميع ناعما[٣٤٩] ويجعل عليه ماء العنب او الزبيب الرازقى ويغلى على النار الليلنه الى ان يمتزجا ويشد الما ثم ينزل ويرفع ويطلى به <٥٤> الذكر عند الحاجة اليه[٣٥٠] نوع اخر قال هذا العمل لمن به رخاوة فى اعضاءيه وذكره وليس له قوة على الجماع وهذا لا يخلوا ما ان يعرض له بعد او من عدم استعماله الجماع وعلى اى تقدير يركان فعلاجه ان[٣٥١] يوخذ مرارة تيس[٣٥٢] وعاقرقرح[٣٥٣] عشرة دراهم يسحق ناعما ثم يخلط مع دهن[٣٥٤] السعد الريحانى[٣٥٥] وتوضع فى الشمس ثلاثة ايام حتى يمتزجوا فى بعضهم بعضا ثم تاخذ من جوز الهند[٣٥٦] درهم ونصف يدق ويخلط معهم خلطا جيدا ويرفع فاذا اراد الجماع يطلى به ذكره[٣٥٧] قبل الجماع بثلاثة ايام كل يوم مرارا فانه ينصلح امره ويقوى رخاوته

٣٤٩. ناعما: – (غ).
٣٥٠. اليه: – (غ).
٣٥١. وتسحق ...فعلاجه ان: يدق ناعما ويرمي في ماء العنب والزيت ويغلي علي النار الي ان ينزل ويطلى به الذكرنوع آخر (ق).
٣٥٢. تيس: التيس (ق).
٣٥٣. عاقرقرح: عاقرقرحا (غ).
٣٥٤. ثم يخلط مع دهن: ويخلط بدهن (ق).
٣٥٥. السعد الريحانى: سعد (ق).
٣٥٦. توضع... الهند: يوضع في الشمس ثلاث ايام ثم يوضع عليه جوز هندي (ق).
٣٥٧. يدق ... : ويخلط ويطلى الذكر (ق).

وذكر جالينوس انه من عالج نفسه بهذا العلاج[٣٥٨] يصلح حاله ويشتد رخاوته عضوه ويلقى قوة الشباب فى حالة الشيخوخة فكيف <٥٤> اذا كان شباب لا ينبغى فيه رخاوة ابدا ولو كان من عشرين سنه لزالت وانصلح امره فصل فى بيان عمل دهن الريحان وهو دهن السعد وساير الادهان قال اذا اردت[٣٥٩] عمل دهن من الادهان فحذ من ايهما شيئت مثلا فيوخذ من الريحان فيقطع او من السعد فيدق فيوضع[٣٦٠] فى قنينيه ويوضع عليه قدره مرتين زيت طيب[٣٦١] ويسدد راسها سدا محكما[٣٦٢] بالشمع حتى لا يداخل هو او يعلق[٣٦٣] فى الشمس الحاره فى ايام الصيف اربعين يوما فى موضع لا تنقطع الشمس عنه من طلوعها الى غروبها فاذا تم الاربعين يوما تم الدهن ثم يصفى من منخل رفيع او خرقة رفيعه ويرفع واعلم ان هذا دهن الريحان والسعد والبنفسج يخرج

٣٥٨. العلاج: + عشرة ايام (غ).

٣٥٩. بثلاثة ايام ... اذا اردت: ثلثة ايام ير العجب فصل في الادهان فاردت (ق).

٣٦٠. من الادهان... فيوضع: السعد فيؤخذ جزء من السعد ويوضع (ق).

٣٦١. قدره مرتين زيت طيب: زيت طيب قدره مرتين (ق).

٣٦٢. سدا محكما: – (ق).

٣٦٣. حتى لا يداخل هو او يعلق: ويعلق (ق).

على هذا المنوال وعلى هذه الطريقة[٣٦٤] واما دهن القلوب مثل <٥٦> دهن[٣٦٥] الفستق ودهن اللوز والبندق وقلب حب القطن وقلب الجوز وساير القلوب ودهن الجلنار وامثاله على غير هذه الطريقة بل يخرج على هذا الوجْه[٣٦٦] هو ان تاخذ ما شيئت من القلوب فيدق دقا ناعما حتى يبقى مثل الكسب الناعم ثم تاخذ[٣٦٧] صينيه نحاس مبيضه وتجعل على النار[٣٦٨] رماد سخن وتبل يدك بالماء الفاتر وتعرك القلب المدقوق على الصينيه وتلفه وتدحرجه على الصينيه تفعل به ذلك حتى يخرج جميع دهنه وكذا تفعل بساير القلوب والسلام[٣٦٩] الباب الثانى عشر فى بيان الادوية التى تطلى على الذكر <١٩> فتطوله تقويه كما تريد وتشهى واعلم ان الذكر كله[٣٧٠] مركب من جميع العروق

٣٦٤. في ايام الصيف ... الطريقة: في الصيف اربعين يوما ثم يصفي من منخل رفيع ويرفع (ق).

٣٦٥. مثل دهن: كدهن (ق).

٣٦٦. وقلب حب القطن ... الوجه: القطن والجوز والجلنار (ق).

٣٦٧. يدق دقا ... تاخذ: تدق ناعم حتي يبقي كالكحل ثم تضع في (ق).

٣٦٨. مبيضه وتجعل على النار: (ق).

٣٦٩. تعرك ... السلام: تعجن القلب المذكور حتي تخرج دهنه وكذا تفعل سائر القلوب (ق) / والسلام: (غ).

٣٧٠. فتطوله... كله: لتنعيظه وتقويته وتطويله اعلم ان الذكر (ق).

وهو[٣٧١] يطول بالجماع وبالدلك ولكن لا يكون ذلك مثل الطلى فان الطلى يكون <٥٧> اقوى بسبب الادوية كما ذكره افلاطون وارطاطاليس وبقراط وجالينوس الحكيم وقالوا بوقوعه ومما عملوا به وجربوه وروى محمد الدامغانى والامام الرازى رحمه الله تعالى[٣٧٢] عن افلاطون هذا العمل طويل الذكر قال[٣٧٣] يوخذ اصل الحسك الذى نبت اكثر من سنه وتغسله نظيفا وتجففه وتسحقه ناعما وتنخله من منخل رفيع وتدخل الحمام وتدلك به ذكرك بالماء السخن وتغسله حتى يحمر وتدر عليه من اصل الحسك المسحوق بعد دلكه ثم يدهن بدهن السعد المسحوق معه وزن نصف درهم جوز الهند وان كنت عملت هذه النسخه عندك ودهنت به منها فى الحمام ثلاث مرات الى ان يخرج من الحمام فانه يطول الى ان تتعجب منه لكن حكمه من ذلك <٥٨> اليوم الى عشرة ايام فقط ويريد ان تجدده والسلام نوع غريب وهو من اسرار الحكما يطول الذكر ويجعله قدر نفسه مرتين قال <*17*> يوخذ بعر الغنم الطرى المرق والعنبر اليابس مقدار ما تطلى به الذكر[٣٧٤]

٣٧١. هو: قد (ق).

٣٧٢. رحمه الله تعالى: – (غ).

٣٧٣. بالدلك ... قال: الدلك (ق).

٣٧٤. الذى نبت اكثر ...الذكر: فيغسل ويجفف ويسحق وينخل

وقيراط مسك يسحق ويوخذ من جوز الهند درهمين ويدق ناعما فى غاية النعومة ويخلط الجميع فى بعضهم بعضا خلطا قوياً ثم تدخل الحمام وتدلك ذكرك[٣٧٥] بدهن السعد دلكا قويا الى ان يحمر ثم يطْلا بالحوايج الذى خلطت بالبعر مثل ما تطلى الخاتم ثم يلف بخرقة من الصبح الى المغرب ثم تحله وتغسله ترى عجبا لانه يطول الذكر قدر ما كان مرتين ولكن حكمه الى عشرين يوما ثم تجدد العمل والسلام[٣٧٦] الباب الثالث عشر فى بيان الادوية التى يطلى بها بين اصابع اليدين <٥٩> والرجلين[٣٧٧] فيقوى الجماع ويشد الذكر[٣٧٨] ومهما جامع لم يضعف و لم يمل و لم يرتخى ابدا قال يوخذ فراخ العصافير الدوريه قبل ان ينبت عليهم الريش وتربط بخيط وتعلق على باب بيت النحل ثم يهوش على النحل

ويدلك به الذكر في الحمام بعد غسل بالماء الساخره ثم يدهن بدهن السعد مع نصف درهم بفعل ذلك ثلاث مرات او اكثر فانه غاية في تطويله نوع يؤخذ عنبر يابس جزء (ق).

٣٧٥. ويسحق ... ذكرك: وبعر غنم طري جزء ودرهمان جوز هند يدق ناعما الي ان يختلطوا فيدخل الحمام ويدلك الذكر (ق).

٣٧٦. ثم يطلا ... الخام: فيطلي بالادويه ثم يلف بخرقه من الصبح الي الغروب ثم يغسله ير العجب من تطويله ولكن حكمه الي عشرين يوما لم يجدد العمل والله اعلم (ق).

٣٧٧. اليدين والرجلين: الرجلين واليدين (غ).

٣٧٨. بين اصابع اليدين والرجلين فيقوى الجماع ويشد الذكر: علي اصابع الرجلين واليدين لتقوية الجما وشد الذكر (ق).

حتى تلذع الفراخ فاذا الذغوها مرار توخذ بالعجله وتذبح ولا يدع دماهم يقطر ابدا بل وعاء وتضعهم فى قدره وتغمرهم من دهن الريحان المذكور وتسد فم القدره وترفع على النار الى ان ينهرى[٣٧٩] الافراخ ثم يخرجوا ويصفوا من خرقة حتى تخرج قوتهم فى الدهن ثم يسحق قيراط افريبون ناعما مثل الكحل ويخلط مع الدهن خلطا جيدا ثم يجعل الدهن فى قنينيه ويسد فمها وتوضع فى الشمس الحاره ثلاثة ايام فاذا كان وقت الحاجة <٢٠> يوخذ منه بقطنه ويدهن <٦٠> بها بين اصابع اليدين والرجلين يرى عجبا ولو جامع ما شا لا يضعف ولا يرتخى ولا يمل ابدا ولا ينام ذكره ولا يزال منتصبا حتى يغسله بالماءالبارد مرارا كثيرة والسلام نوع اخر قال[٣٨٠] يوخذماية نملة من النمل الاسود الكبار والصغار يجعلوا[٣٨١] فى قنينيه ويسكب عليهم خمسة دراهم من دهن السوس الازرق ويسد فم القنينيه[٣٨٢] وتعلق فى الشمس الحاره عشرين يوما وبعد ذلك يسحق الجميع سحقا قويا حتى يتخمر وافاذا كان وقت الحاجة

٣٧٩. ينهرى: تتهري (غ).

٣٨٠. ومهما جامع ... قال: – (ق).

٣٨١. يجعلوا: تجعلها (ق) .

٣٨٢. يسكب ... القنينه: يسكب عليها من دهن السوسن الازرق وشد فمها (ق).

يوخذ قيراط عود هندى يدق[٣٨٣] ناعما ويجعل فى ماء حار وزن عشرة دراهم ثم يغسل ذكره من هذا الماء ويغسل يديه ورجليه وتحت ابطيه ثم ياخذ من ذلك الدهن الذى فى القنينية دهن النحل نقطه <٦١> اوشى قليل صرفا بلا مآ ويدهن به اصابع يديه ورجليه وابطيه ومرافقه ثم يلبث ساعة ثم يجامع فلو جامع عشرة من النسا فى ليلة لم يعجز ولم يرتخى[٣٨٤] الباب الرابع عشر فى بيان الحبوب التى اذا امسكها الانسان تلذذ الرجل بالجماع لذة عظيمة قال[٣٨٥] يوخذ درهم مصطكى وقيراط ونصف مسك ونصف درهم قرنقل وخمس دراهم سكر ونصف درهم جوزة هند ويسحق الجميع ناعما كالكحل ثم تضعهم فى قنينية وتغمرهم بدهن وتعلق فى الشمس ثلاثة ايام حتى تمزج بالدهن ثم يوخذ له قوامه عسل نحل ابيض منزوع الرغوه ويعقد الحوايج ويحبب كل حبة وزن درهم وقت الحاجه <٦٢>

---

٣٨٣. بعد ذلك ... يدق: ثم يسحقها قويا ثم قيراط عود هند يسحق (ق).

٣٨٤. وزن عشرة ...يرتخى: ويغسل ذكر بهذا الماء وكذا يديه ورجليه وابطيه ثم يدلك الدهن اصابع اليدين والرجلين والابطين والمرفقين ير العجب (ق).

٣٨٥. اذا امسكها ... قال: تمسك في الفم تلذذ الجماع جدا (ق).

للجماع يجعل فى حبة يرى عجبا والسلام[٣٨٦] نوع اخر قال[٣٨٧] يوخذ فستق بقشر ويوخذ قلبه ويستوى على النار ويحترز من حرقه فاذا انقلا وجف يسحق منه قدر[٣٨٨] درهم ويضاف اليه وزن درهم قرنفل <*18*> وقيراط مسك ودرهم عنبر ويسحق ناعما كالكحل ويدروا على دهن الفستق الذى قلاه حتى يبقى كالعجين ثم يوضع فى الشمس ثلاثة ايام ثم يحبب بالسكر او بالعسل النحل المنزوع الرغوه ويعقد كالعادة كل حبة وزن درهم ويرفع فاذا اردت ذلك ضع[٣٨٩] فى فمك حبة وجامع[٣٩٠] ترى عجبا[٣٩١] الباب الخامس عشر فى بيان حالة الجماع التى يحصل منها لذة عظيمة للرجل والمراه

٣٨٦. ونصف مسك... السلام: مسك وقرنفل نصف درهم وسكر خمسة دراهيم وجوزهند درهم يسحق ناعما ويوضع في قنينه ويغمر بدهن زنبق وتعلقها في الشمس ثلاث ايام ثم يؤخذ عسل نحل ويعقد بها ويحبب كل حبه وزن درهم ويجعل في فمه حبه وزن درهم ويجعل في فمه حبه وقت الجماع ير العجب (ق).

٣٨٧. قال: – (ق).

٣٨٨. قدر: وزن (غ).

٣٨٩. ضع: يضع (غ).

٣٩٠. جامع: يجامع + فانه (غ).

٣٩١. فستق ... عجبا: قلب فستق ويحط في طاسيه علي النار ويسحق منه درهم حتي يظهر دهنه فيؤخذ قرنفل درهم ودرهم عنبر وقيراط مسك ويدرهن الفستق ويمزج ويجعل في الشمس ثلاث ايام ثم يحلب بالسكر والعسل ويحبب كل حبه درهم ويؤخذ في الفم حبه وقت الجماع فانه ير العجب (ق) / عجبا: + والسلام (غ).

مثل ما ذكره الحكما المتقدمون والاطبا المتاخرون <٦٣> وعلموا ذلك بتجاريبهم قال يوخذ وزن درهم قرفه لف ونصف درهم <٢١> عاقرقرح[٣٩٢] وقيراط قاقله يسحق الجميع كالغبار ثم يخلطوا[٣٩٣] بماء عنب رازقى ويطلى به على جميع ذكره ويصبر[٣٩٤] ساعة ثم يغسله بماء سخن ثم ياخذ {فى فمه نضف درهم دار صينى ويمضغه ثم ياخذ} ريقه ويطلى به ذكره ويجامع يرى الرجل والمراة عجبا من اللذة ولا يتشوش منهما واحد والسلام[٣٩٥] نوع اخر قال[٣٩٦] يوخذ كبابه وعاقرقرح[٣٩٧] ودار صينى وزنجبيل[٣٩٨] وجوز هندى من كل واحد قيراط ويسحق الجميع ويعجنوا بالعسل النحل المعقود ثم ياخذ منه فى فمه ويطلى من ريقه على ذكره ويجامع يرى عجبا من اللذة للرجل والمراة ما لم يوصف

٣٩٢. عاقرقرح: عاقرقرحا (غ).

٣٩٣. حالة الجماع... يخلط: ما يحصل للرجل والمرأة من لذة النكاح يؤخذ قرفة درهم وعاقر قرحا نصف درهم وقاقله قيراط يخلط (ق).

٣٩٤. على جميع ذكره ويصبر: الذكر (ق).

٣٩٥. يمصغه ... السلام: ويطلي الذكر بريقه ويجامع فانهما يجد ان لذة عظيمة (ق).

٣٩٦. قال: – (ق).

٣٩٧. عاقرقرح: عاقرقرحا (غ).

٣٩٨. كبابه ... وزنجبيل: كبا ودار صيني وزنجبيل وعاقر قرحا (ق).

والسلام[٣٩٩] الباب السادس عشر فى بيان الادوية التى اذا تحملت بها المراة تصير فى ضيق رحمها وحرارتها ولذتها وذلك <٦٤> ان تاخذ[٤٠٠] عاقرقرح[٤٠١] وزن[٤٠٢] درهمين ولحية تيس خمسة دراهم وشراب صرف ستة عشر درهما وتمر مرسين يدقو ناعما ويجعلوا فى قدره ويغمروا بالماء ثم يغلوا على النار الى ان ينقص ثلاث الماء وبعض الشراب فاذا بقيت القدره على هذه الحاله تقف المراه على بخارها[٤٠٣] سبع مرات ثم تنزل القدرة وترفع فاذا احتاجت المراة اليها[٤٠٤] تبل صوفه وتتحمل بها فانها تصير اقوى من البكر في الصيف والحراره[٤٠٥] *<19>* نوع اخر يوخذ من ثمرة[٤٠٦] المرسين وقشر رمان وعاقرقرحا اجزا سوا ويدقوا ناعما ويغلوا[٤٠٧] شراب

---

٣٩٩. الجميع ... السلام: ويعقد بعسل ثم يأخذ منه في فمه ويطلي ذكره بريقه ويجامع يري من اللذة شيء عجيب (ق).

٤٠٠. اذا تحملت ...تاخذ: تضيق الرحم وتسخنه يؤخذ (ق).

٤٠١. عاقرقرح: عاقرقرحا (غ).

٤٠٢. عاقرقرح وزن : عاقرقرحا (ق).

٤٠٣. يدقو ... بخارها: يدق ناعما ويغمر في قدر بالماء ويغلي الان ينقص الثلث من الم‍ء فتتلقى المرأة بخاره (ق) .

٤٠٤. تنزل ... اليها: ثم ترفع القدره عندها فاذا احتجاجت (ق) / اليها: بها (غ).

٤٠٥. الحراره: + والسلام (غ).

٤٠٦. ثمرة: تمر (ق).

٤٠٧. ويدقوا ناعما ويغلوا: تدق ناعما وتغلي (ق).

عتيق صرف ثم تبل صوفه وتتحل بها[٤٠٨] ساعه فانها تصير كالبكر فى الضيق والحـراره[٤٠٩] نوع اخر يوخذ بلوط وبزرعصفر[٤١٠] وسعد وكليل[٤١١] وحي علم اجزا سوا يخلطوا فى بعضهم <٦٥> بعضا بالدق الجريش ويغلوا ويصفوا ويصفى عليهم وزن خمسة دراهم عاقرقرحا ثم[٤١٢] يغلى على النار غليا قويا ثم ينزل فاذا احتاجت المراه اليه تستنجى منه مرتين او ثلاثة فانها تصير كالبنت البكر فى الضيق والحـراره والسلام[٤١٣] الباب السابع عشر فى بيان الادوية التى اذا تحملت بها المراه ما تحبل ما دامت تستعملها وتصير كالبنات ضيقا وحـرارة قال يوخذ مـرارت دب تخلط مع مآ العنب الرازقى خلطا قويا ثم تتحمل منها المراة بقليل دقيق لم تحبل تبقى[٤١٤] كالبكر نوع اخر قال يوخذ من مرارة البقر

---

٤٠٨. بها: + المرأة (غ).

٤٠٩. ثم تبل ... الحراره: − (ق).

٤١٠. وبزرعصفر: ونور عصفور (ق).

٤١١. كليل: اكليل (ق).

٤١٢. يخلطو ... ثم: تدق وتغلي وتصفي ثم يضاف اليها عاقرقرحا خمسة دراهم و(ق).

٤١٣. ثم ينزل... السلام: وينزل وتستجي به المأه مرتين او ثلاث فانه تصير كالبنت في الضقيق والحراره واللذة والله اعلم (ق).

٤١٤. الادوية التي... تبقى: ما يمنع الحمل ويسخن الحم يؤخذ مرارة دب تخلط في ماء العنب الراز في بكف دقيق وتعمل صوفه وتتحمل بها لم تحبل مده وتسخن الرحم وتضيقه (ق).

وزن مثقال ومثله من مـرارت الذيب يجعلا بقدر ما يغمرها شيرج ثم تتحمل منه المراه بقطنه او صوفه فانها تصير كالبكر ولا تحبل ابدا[415] نوع اخر قال من اخذ[416] قطران زجاجى وطلى به وقت <٦٦> الجماع ذكره تلذذ به غاية اللذه ولا تعود المراه تحبل ابدا الا اذا كان بالعلاج[417] الباب الثامن عشر فى بيان الادوية التى اذا تحملت بها المراه تحبل باذن الله تعالى قال[418] يوخذ عود هندى[419] وورق مرسين اخضر من كل واحد نصف درهـم ومـن[420] المسك قـيراط يـدق الجميع[421] ناعما

---

٤١٥. قـال يـوخـذ ... ابـدا: يـؤخـذ مـرارة بقر مثقال وكـذا مـرارة ذئب ويعمر بشريج وتحمل المراه بصوفه منه فانها تصير و لم محبل (ق) / ابدا: + والسلام (غ).

٤١٦. قال من اخذ: يؤخذ (ق).

٤١٧. طلى بـه ...بالعلاج: يطلي بـه الـذكـر وقـت الجـمـاع يمنع الحبل منه ويلذ نوع آخر اقاقيا وجنت البلوط من كل واحد عشرة دراهيم وعفص وباذنجان يابس من كل واحد خمسة عشرة درهما تدق ناعما وتنخل ثم تسحق في هاون سحقا بليغا وتتحمل المرأه منها بقطعه مبلولة بالماء في ثلاث ايام فانها تر العجب في الضيق والحراره (ق).

٤١٨. اذا تحملت ...قال: تحبل بها المأة (ق).

٤١٩. هندي: هند (ق).

٤٢٠. من: – (ق).

٤٢١. الجميع: – (ق).

ويصرو[٤٢٢] <٢٢> فى[٤٢٣] خرقة رفيعه ويجعل[٤٢٤] فى قدره ويصب عليه قليل شراب عتيق ويغلى على نار[٤٢٥] لينه حتى تخرج قوة الادوية فيه ثم يصفى بالماء ويجعل فى قنينيه فاذا احتاجت المـراه اليه تتحمل منه بصوفه تكون كالبكر وتحبل بـاذن[٤٢٦] الله تعالى نوع اخر قال يوخذ[٤٢٧] عفص <*20*> اخضر وادخـر مكى من كل واحد درهمين وبلح اخضر درهم يسحقوا[٤٢٨] ناعما حتى تخرج قوة الادوية فى الشراب ثم يرفعوا[٤٢٩] عند الحاجة تتحمل منه المراه[٤٣٠] بصوفه[٤٣١] تحبل باذن <٦٧> الله تعالى نوع اخر قال يوخذ[٤٣٢] قشر كافور خام[٤٣٣]

---

٤٢٢. يصرو: تصر (ق) ناعما/ ويصرو: دقا ناعما ويصير (غ).
٤٢٣. فى: – (غ).
٤٢٤. رفيعه ويجعل: من شاش وتوضع (ق).
٤٢٥. على نار: بنار (ق).
٤٢٦. حتى تخرج ...باذن: وصفي المـاء ويحبل في قنينه وتحبل منها بصوفه قبل الجماع فانها تحبل ان شاء (ق).
٤٢٧. قال يوخذ: – (ق).
٤٢٨. يسحقوا: يسحق (غ).
٤٢٩. ناعما حتى تخرج قوة الادويـة فى الشراب ثـم: بقليل شراب ويرفع (ق).
٤٣٠. منه المراه: المرءه منه (ق).
٤٣١. بصوفه: + قبل الجماع (ق) / بصوفه: بصوف (غ).
٤٣٢. يوخذ: (ق).
٤٣٣. خام: + مدقوق (غ).

اربعة دراهم وشب احمر درهمين و[٤٣٤]سعد درهم وعفص اخضر مدقوق[٤٣٥] اربعة دراهم ونصف وتراب مكه نصف قيراط يسحق الجميع غير العفص فانه يدق جريشا لا ناعما ويغلى بشراب كالعادة ويصفى ويوخذ ماوه ويرفع وعند الحاجة اليه تبل المراه منه بصوفه[٤٣٦] وتتحمل بها وهى مستلقيه على قفاها قبل الجماع بساعة[٤٣٧] فانها تصير كالبكر وتحبل باذن الله تعالى نوع اخر قال[٤٣٨] يوخذ لحية التيس تدق وتسحق[٤٣٩] ويستخرج ماءوها ثم يوخذ عفص اخضر وقشر[٤٤٠] رمان وعود هندى[٤٤١] وقشر اترنج من كل واحد نصف درهم وشب احمر اربعة دراهم وسعد درهم يسحق[٤٤٢] الجميع ويغلى[٤٤٣] بشراب عتيق حتى تخرج قوة الادوية فى الشراب ثم <٦٨> تتحمل منها المراه فانها تصير

٤٣٤. و: – (ق).

٤٣٥. مدقوق: + جريش (غ).

٤٣٦. بصوفه: صوفه (غ).

٤٣٧. اربعة دراهم ... بساعة: يغلي بالشراب ويصفي ماءه ويرفع وتتحمل منه المرءه بصوفي وهي مستلقيه قبل الجماع (ق).

٤٣٨. قال: – (ق).

٤٣٩. تدق وتسحق: يدق (ق) / تدق وتسحق: يدق ويسحق (غ).

٤٤٠. قشر: قشور (ق).

٤٤١. هندى: هند (ق).

٤٤٢. يسحق: تسحق (ق).

٤٤٣. يغلى: تغلي (ق).

كالبكر[٤٤٤] وتحبل باذن الله تعالى نوع اخر قال[٤٤٥] يوخذ قاقله نصف درهم وصمغ عربى وحبة سوده[٤٤٦] من كل واحد قيراط وكحل اصبهانى نضف دراهم وقشر اترنج نصف درهم يسحق الجميع ويغلى بشراب عتيق حتى تخرج قوة الادوية فى الشراب ثم تتحمل منه المراه بصوفه عند الحاجه فانها تصير كالبكر الذى لم يصبها رجل وتحبل باذن الله تعالى ثم ذلك تحمد الله وعونه وحسن توفيقه والحمد لله على كل حال[٤٤٧] وصلى الله على سيدنا محمد وعلى اله وصحبه وسلم تسليما كثيرا الى يوم الدين يا رب العالمين بسم الله الرحمن الرحيم.[٤٤٨] [١٢٠٨]

٤٤٤. حتى تخرج ... كالبكر: وتتحمل المرأة منه بصوفه (ق).
٤٤٥. قال: – (ق).
٤٤٦. سوده: سوداء (ق) / السوداء (غ).
٤٤٧. ثم ذلك... حال: – (غ).
٤٤٨. اترنج ... الرحيم: نارنج درهم تسحق وتغلي بشراب عتيق وتتحمل منه بصوفه قبل الجماع فانها تصير بكر وتحبل بحول الله تم الكتاب بعون الملك الوهاب ثمانية عشر ايام من شهر ربيع الاول ليلة الربوع ١٢٢٩ (ق) / تسليما ... الرحيم: ولا حول ولا قوة الا بالله العلى العظيم تم وكمل لحمدالله وعون وحسن بالله (غ).

فهرس الأعلام

أرسطو ١٣
أرطاطالوس ١٣
أرطاطاليس ٢٨، ٥٦
أفلاطون ١٣، ٥٦

بقراط ١٣، ٢٨
بلطيوس ١٣

جالينوس ٥٤، ٥٦

الدامغاني ٥٦

الرازي ٥٦

الطوسي، ناصر الدين ٤

علي (ابن ابي طالب) ١٠

فهرس المصطلحات

الأدوية ٥، ٧–٩، ١٢، ١٣، ١٦، ١٧، ٢١، ٣٠–٣٢، ٣٦، ٤٠، ٤١، ٥٢، ٦٢، ٦٤–٦٧
الأدوية المركبة ٥
الأدوية المفردة ٣١
الأدوية النافعة ٣١
الأشربة ٦، ١٢، ٢٨، ٣٧
الأشربة الحامضة ٢٨
الأشياف ٦
الأطريقل ٤٢
الأعضا الريه ٦
أغذية المفردات ٥، ٢٩
الأغذية المركبات ٦، ٣٢

الباه ٥، ٦، ٣١، ٣٤، ٣٧
بدن الإنسان ٥، ٦، ٢٨، ٢٩، ٣٣
البرودة ٦، ٢٣، ٢٨، ٣٣، ٤٤
بزر البصل ٤٧
بزر جزر ٢٣، ٣١، ٤٦
بزر رشاد ٢٥، ٣١
بزر عصفر ٦٣
بزر فجل ٢٥
بزر القرع ٤٦
بزر القطن ٥٢
بزر اللفت ٣١، ٤٦
بسباسة ٤٠
البصر ١١
البصل الأبيض ٢٧، ٣٠، ٣٢، ٣٣، ٣٥
بصل النرجس ٥٢
البض ٣١
بلح أخضر ٦٥
البلغم ٦، ٢٨، ٣٩، ٤٤
بلوط ٦٣
بليلج ٣١
البندق ٣٠
بورق أرضي ٣١
البول ٥٠
بيض السمك ٣٠

التفاح الحلو ٢٨، ٣٠
تمر مرسين ٦٢
التمريخات ١٢
التناسل ١١، ٥١
التوالد ١١، ٥١
التين الأخضر ٣٠

الثوم ٢٧، ٢٨

الجزر ٣٠
الجماع ٥، ٦، ٨، ١٠، ١١–٢٢، ٢٩–٣١، ٣٣، ٣٥، ٣٧، ٣٩، ٤١–٤٣، ٤٥، ٤٩–٥١، ٥٣، ٥٦، ٥٧، ٦٠، ٦٤، ٦٦
جنطيانه رومي ٢٣
الجوارشات ٦، ٣٩
الجوزة ٢٦
جوز الهند ٣٣، ٤٦، ٥٢، ٥٣، ٥٦، ٥٧، ٥٩، ٦١

الحبة السوداء ٣١، ٣٣، ٤٠، ٦٧
الحبل ٩
الحبوب ٨
الحرارة الغريزية ٦، ٣٩، ٤٢، ٤٩
الحسك ٥٦

الحقن ٧
الحلاوات ٦
الحلاوة العجمية ٢٩
الحلويات ٣٢
الحليب البقري ٢٦، ٣٠
الحمص ٢٥، ٣٠، ٣٦، ٤٧
حوز ٤٠
الحوق ٥٠
الخبز الفطير ٢٨، ٣٢

الخصى ١٢
خطمية الثعلب ٣١
خولنجان ٣٢
الخيار ٣١

دارصيني ٤٠، ٤٣، ٦١
الدجاج ٣٠
الدم ٦، ٢٣، ٣٣، ٣٨، ٤٢، ٥٠
الدماغ ٦، ١٢، ١٥، ٣٠، ٤٢
دهن البندق ٥٥
دهن الريحان ٥٤، ٥٨
دهن السوس الأزرق ٥٨
دهن الفستق ٥٥، ٦٠
دهن اللوز ٥٥
دهن النحل ٥٩

الذكر ٧، ١٣، ١٦، ٢١، ٢٢، ٢٤، ٤٢، ٥٢
الذوق ١١

الرطب ٣٠
الرطوبة ٢٣
الرمان الحلو ٣٠، ٦٢
الرياح الفاسدة ٦، ٧، ٤٥
الريه ٧، ١٢، ٤٩
الريح ٤
ريح القولنج ٧

الزبيب الأحمر ٥٢
الزبيب الأسود ٢٨
الزبيب الرازقي ٥٣
زرنباد ٣١
زعفران ١٧، ١٩، ٢١، ٢٣، ٢٨، ٣١، ٣٦، ٤٠
زنجبيل ١٦، ١٩، ٢٦، ٣١، ٣٨، ٤٠، ٤١، ٤٤، ٤٧، ٦١

سادج هندي ٢٣، ٣١
سعد ٦٣، ٦٦
السفرجل ٣٠
السقم ١٣
السكر ١٦، ١٧، ٣٠، ٣٨، ٤١، ٤٣، ٦٠
سلطان قازان ٤
السمع ١١
السمسم ٤٠
السمك ٢٧
السمن البقري ٢٨، ٣٠، ٣٦
سنبل ٢٣، ٣١، ٣٨، ٤٠
السودا ٦، ٧، ٣٩، ٤٤
سورنجان ٤٥

شب أحمر ٦٦
الشدود ٧
شراب التفاح ١٨
شراب السنبل ٢٠
الشعير ٤٣
الشقاقل ٣١
الشم ١١
شوك الحسك ٤١
الشهوة ٥، ٦، ١٢، ١٤
الشيخوخة ٥٤

الصداع ٦، ٣٩، ٤٩
الصفرا ٦، ١٥، ٤٤
صمغ عربي ٦٧
الصنوبر ٣٦

عاقر قرح ٤١، ٤٤، ٥٢، ٥٣، ٦١، ٦٢
عرق النسا ٧، ٤٥، ٤٩
العروق ٢٣
عسل النحل ١٨، ٢٤، ٢٨، ٣٠، ٣٥، ٣٨، ٤٠، ٤١، ٤٤، ٦٠
العصافير الدروية ٣٠
عفص أخضر ٦٥، ٦٦
العلل البلغمية ١١
العلل الصفراوية ١١
العنب ٣٠، ٣٧، ٥١، ٥٣، ٦١
العنبر ٣١، ٣٨، ٤٠، ٥٦، ٦٠
عود صليب ٣٢
العود الصيني ٣٦
عود هندي ٢٠، ٢٤، ٣١، ٣٦، ٤٠، ٥٩، ٦٤، ٦٦

الفالج ٤
الفراريج ٣٠
الفستق ٣٠، ٣١
الفضلات ٢٨، ٣٣
فلاجة المفلوج ٦
فلفل ١٩، ٢٦، ٣١، ٤٠، ٤٣، ٤٧

قاقلة ٢٠، ٣١، ٣٣، ٣٩، ٤٠، ٦١، ٦٧
قرفة ١٦، ٢٠، ٢٦، ٣٢، ٣٥، ٤٧، ٦١
قرنفل ١٦، ١٩، ٢٤، ٣٣، ٤٠، ٥٩
قشر الأترنج ٣١، ٣٦، ٦٧
قطران زجاجي ٦٤
القطن ٤٥، ٤٨
القلب ١٢
القمح ٤٧
قنطريون ٣١
القولنج ٤٥، ٤٩

كافور ٦٥
كبابه ٣١، ٦١
الكبد ١٢، ١٩، ٣٨، ٥٠
الكرات ٣٠، ٤٧
كليل ٦٣
كمون ٢٣

لسان عصافير ٣٤
اللفت ٣٠
اللمس ١١
اللوز ٣٠

ماء الورد ٢١
المثانة ٢٣، ٤٣، ٥٠
مرارت الذيب ٦٤
مرداسك ٢٤
المسك ٣١، ٣٣، ٥٧، ٦٠
مصطكي ٢٣، ٣١، ٥٩
المعاجين ٦، ٣١، ٣٩
معجون المسك ٢٣، ٢٤
المعدة ٦، ٧، ٣٨
المفاصل ٧
الملال ٦
ملح اندراني ٣٤
المنى ٥، ٦، ١٠، ١٦، ١٨، ٢٣، ٣١، ٣٣، ٣٥، ٤٣، ٥١
موت المفاجأة ٢٠

النزلات ٦، ٣٩
النقرس ٤٩
النمل الأسود ٥٨

هليلج ٣١

الورد المربا ٢٨
ورق مرسين ٦٤

ينسون ٣١
اليرقان ١٩